FAT DISTRIBUTION DURING GROWTH AND LATER HEALTH OUTCOMES

A Symposium Held at Manoir St-Castin, Lac Beauport, Québec, June 9–11, 1987

Editors

Claude Bouchard
Physical Activity Sciences Laboratory
Laval University
Ste-Foy, Québec

Francis E. Johnston
Department of Anthropology
University of Pennsylvania
Philadelphia, Pennsylvania

Alan R. Liss, Inc., New York

Address all Inquiries to the Publisher
Alan R. Liss, Inc., 41 East 11th Street, New York, NY 10003

Copyright © 1988 Alan R. Liss, Inc.

Printed in the United States of America

Library of Congress Cataloging-in-Publication Data

Fat distribution during growth and later health outcomes: a symposium
  held at Manoir St-Castin, Lac Beauport, Quebec, June 9–11, 1987 /
  editors, Claude Bouchard and Francis E. Johnston.
    p. cm.—(Current topics in nutrition and disease ; v. 17)
  Includes index.
  ISBN 0-8451-1616-9
  1. Age factors in disease—Congresses. 2. Adipose tissues—
—Congresses. 3. Body composition—Congresses. 4. Lipids—
—Metabolism—Disorders—Age factors—Congresses. 5. Human growth—
—Congresses. 6. Man—Constitution—Congresses. I. Bouchard,
Claude. II. Johnston, Francis E., 1931-   . III. Series.
  [DNLM: 1. Adipose Tissue—anatomy & histology—congresses.
2. Body Composition—congresses. 3. Growth—congresses.   W1 CU82R
v. 17 / QS 532.5.A3 F252 1987]
RB210.F38 1988
612'.397—dc 19
DNLM/DLC
for Library of Congress   87-32504
                                                      CIP

Contents

Contributors

Annie Barré, University Clinic of Endocrinology, 13008 Marseille, France **[9]**

Richard N. Baumgartner, Department of Pediatrics, Division of Human Biology, Wright State University School of Medicine, Yellow Springs, OH 45387-1695 **[147,243]**

Per Björntorp, Department of Medicine I, Sahlgren's Hospital, S-413 45 Göteborg, Sweden **[175]**

Claude Bouchard, Physical Activity Sciences Laboratory, Laval University, Ste-Foy, Québec G1K 7P4, Canada **[ix,1,63,103,221,297]**

George A. Bray, Department of Medicine, University of Southern California, Los Angeles, CA 90033 **[333]**

Jean-Pierre Després, Physical Activity Sciences Laboratory, Laval University, Ste-Foy, Québec G1K 7P4, Canada **[221,297]**

David J. Evans, Clinical Research Center, Medical College of Wisconsin, Milwaukee, WI 53226 **[203]**

Frank L. Greenway, Department of Medicine, University of California at Los Angeles, CA 90291 **[333]**

M.R.C. Greenwood, Department of Biology, Vassar College, Poughkeepsie, NY 12601 **[285]**

John H. Himes, Department of Health and Nutrition Sciences, Brooklyn College, City University of New York, Brooklyn, NY 11210 **[313]**

Francis E. Johnston, Department of Anthropology, University of Pennsylvania, Philadelphia, PA 19104-6398 **[ix,85]**

Jacques Jubelin, University Clinic of Endocrinology, 13008 Marseille, France **[9]**

Solomon H. Katz, Krogman Growth Center, University of Pennsylvania, Department of Psychiatry, Einstein Northern Hospital, Philadelphia, PA 19103 **[263]**

Ruth Kava, Department of Biology, Vassar College, Poughkeepsie, NY 12601 **[285]**

Ahmed H. Kissebah, Clinical Research Center, Medical College of Wisconsin, Milwaukee, WI 53226 **[203]**

The numbers in brackets are the opening page numbers of the contributors' articles.

Bo Larsson, Department of Medicine I, University of Göteborg, S-413 45 Göteborg, Sweden **[193]**

Robert M. Malina, Department of Anthropology, University of Texas, Austin, TX 78712 **[63]**

William H. Mueller, School of Public Health, University of Texas, Health Science Center, Houston, TX 77225 **[127]**

Alan Peiris, Clinical Research Center, Medical College of Wisconsin, Milwaukee, WI 53226 **[203]**

Marielle Rebuffé-Scrive, Department of Medicine I, Sahlgren's Hospital, S-413 45 Göteborg, Sweden **[163]**

Alex F. Roche, Department of Pediatrics, Division of Human Biology, Wright State University School of Medicine, Yellow Springs, OH 45387-1695 **[147]**

Roland Savard, Department of Physical Education, University of Montreal, Montreal, Québec H3C 3J7, Canada **[285]**

R.M. Siervogel, Division of Human Biology, Department of Pediatrics, Wright State University School of Medicine, Yellow Springs, OH 45387-1695 **[243]**

Lars Sjöström, Department of Medicine I, Sahlgren's Hospital, S-413 45 Göteborg, Sweden **[43]**

Angelo Tremblay, Physical Activity Sciences Laboratory, Laval University, Ste-Foy, Québec G1K 7P4, Canada **[221,297]**

Jean Vague, University Clinic of Endocrinology, 13008 Marseille, France **[9]**

Philippe Vague, University Clinic of Endocrinology, 13008 Marseille, France **[9]**

David B. West, Department of Physiology, Hampton Veterans Administration Center, Hampton, VA 23667; present address: Eastern Virginia Medical School, Norfolk, VA **[285]**

Preface

These proceedings are from a two-day international meeting held in June 1987 at Lac Beauport, near Québec City, Canada. The theme of the symposium was fat distribution during the growing years, with implications for health outcomes later in life. Topics covered included various aspects of fat distribution, including patterns during growth and development in both sexes, tracking of the indicators of fat distribution, defining the metabolic correlates of variation in fat distribution, as well as its possible role as a risk factor for morbidity and mortality later in life. Intervention strategies that could be helpful in altering fat distribution characteristics were also discussed.

Invited participants came from France, Sweden, the United States, and Canada. The work of these investigators represents the convergence of a number of lines of scientific inquiry, yet all are focused upon a single characteristic now known to be of great importance: variation in the distribution of fat on the human body. The first line is human-biological and stems from the study of fat patterns in individuals and groups. Included in this set of concerns are the delineation and characterization of patterns of distribution. The papers dealing with this topic show clearly that there are systematic differences by virtue of sex, age, and ethnicity. Furthermore, the patterns that characterize adults are shown to have their roots in the early years of childhood as well as in the changing endocrine relationships of adolescence, and to reflect the interaction of the genotype with the environment.

The second line of inquiry is epidemiological and focuses on the relationship between fat distribution and disease risk, particularly in the adult years. The results summarized in this book are striking and indicate that the distribution of fat on the body's surface, as well as the deep and superficial deposits, is a significant predictor of morbidity and mortality, independent of the amount of fat.

The third line of inquiry seeks to provide mechanisms that could account for differences in the deposition and mobilization of fat in the body, as well as for the accompanying risk. Several possible mechanisms are explored, ranging from broad ones to those that are specific for individual anatomical regions.

The papers published here cover the great majority of topics relevant to the issue of fat distribution and health, and they provide up-to-date summaries of current thinking. Discussions, which are not included in this text, resulted in a stimulating set of ideas and hypotheses that will surely be seen in the research literature of the next several years. Differences in the distribution of fat, long known to be a characteristic of humans, has been shown irrevocably to be of significant health concern. It is hoped that this volume will move us closer to an understanding of the biological, epidemiological, and clinical relationships that exist.

It is a pleasure to acknowledge the financial support provided by Fonds pour la recherche en santé du Québec, Ministère de la santé et des services sociaux du Québec, Medical Research Council of Canada, Health and Welfare Canada, National Institute of Nutrition of Canada, Fisher Scientific, Hoffmann-LaRoche of the USA, Servier Amérique, Merck Frosst, Mandel Scientific, Parke Davis and Hoffmann-LaRoche of Canada. We are also grateful for the contribution extended to us by the Department of Anthropology of the University of Pennsylvania and by the Department of Physical Education, the Faculty of Medicine, and other entities of Université Laval, Sainte-Foy, Québec. Our thanks also to Drs. Paul Lupien, André Nadeau, and Sital Moorjani from the Centre Hospitalier de l'Université Laval, and Dr. Errol Marliss of McGill University, who served as chairpersons for some of our sessions. The efficient collaboration of the Alan R. Liss staff in the preparation of this volume is gratefully acknowledged.

Claude Bouchard
Francis E. Johnston

Fat Distribution During Growth and Later Health Outcomes
pages 1–8 © 1988 Alan R. Liss, Inc.

INTRODUCTORY NOTES ON THE TOPIC OF FAT DISTRIBUTION

Claude Bouchard

Physical Activity Sciences Laboratory
Laval University
Ste-Foy Quebec G1K 7P4
Canada

This symposium deals with fat distribution during growth and its metabolic and health implications. It is commonly recognized that excess body fat or obesity is a risk factor associated with increased susceptibility to a variety of disorders and a higher mortality rate (Simopoulos and Van Itallie, 1984; Andres, 1985). This is particularly evident when the individuals have been maintaining an obese state for a decade and more as if it took a good number of years for obesity to exert its negative influences.

On the other hand, a growing body of data suggest that fat distribution, more specifically the male (or android) type of fat distribution, is by itself a risk factor and one that seems to be at least partly independent of obesity. Two recent symposia held in Marseilles and in London have dealt with some aspects of this issue (Vague et al, 1985; Norgan, 1985). They have provided us with a variety of data demonstrating that excess truncal or abdominal fat is accompanied by a higher incidence of blood lipid disorders, diabetes and hypertension, and increased mortality rate.

In this context, the problem of fat distribution during growth has not been considered to any extent. Little has been reported about tracking of fat distribution characteristics over the years and from childhood to adolescence and adulthood. In addition, the implications of fat distribution characteristics during growth for later metabolic complications and health outcomes have never been delineated. With these considerations in mind, the objectives of the present symposium were: a) to review the data concerning fat distribution and obesity in health and disease; b) to describe the fat distribution characteristics and their determinants during growth; and c) to assess the health implications of variation in fat distribution during growth and identify some of the issues that should be addressed in the future.

For the purpose of the symposium, three concepts need to be defined. <u>Total body fat</u> represents the absolute amount of fat or adipose tissue in the body. Total body fat can also be considered in terms of its relative contribution to total body mass, i.e. precent of the body as fat. <u>Fat distribution</u> represents the amount of fat in various compartments or regions of the body. It can be described in absolute or in relative terms. <u>Fat patterning</u> is the notion used when describing the relative anatomical location of subcutaneous fat. Table 1 identifies the main purposes for using these concepts in various contexts and some of the techniques for their assessment.

The concept of main interest here is that of fat distribution as opposed to those of total body fat and subcutaneous fat pattern. Several dimensions of the fat distribution concepts are important and should be clarified. For instance, the characteristics of fat distribution can be considered in terms of upper body versus lower body, trunk versus extremities, trunk versus lower extremities, upper trunk versus lower trunk, upper extremities versus lower extremities, subcutaneous fat versus total fat mass, subcutaneous fat versus internal fat, subcutaneous abdominal fat versus internal abdominal fat, and each of these indicators can be approched from a relative and an absolute size point of view. There are good reasons to justify an emphasis on the trunk, particularly lower trunk or abdominal fat in the study of the metabolic consequences of variation in fat distribution.

Among the studies that have reported a clear

Table 1:   Interests and techniques for the
assessment of fat characteristics

Characteristic	Main purpose	Technique
Total body fat		
	- Study of human variation	Underwater weighing
	- Economy and industry	Potassium 40
	- Clinical applications	TOBEC
	- Fitness and performance	Isotope dilution, etc.
Regional fat distribution		
	- Study of human variation	CT scan
	- Ergonomy and industry	Skinfolds
	- Clinical applications	Circumferences, etc.
	- Physical fitness	
Subcutaneous fat pattern		
	- Study of human variation	Skinfolds
		Ultrasound
		X-ray

relationship between the male pattern of fat distribution and mortality or morbidity data, the size of the lower trunk (abdominal) compartment by itself or in relation to the upper leg and buttock compartment seemed to be the most predictive. Some of the other associations described, particularly those pertaining to the upper arm fat (biceps or triceps) or the upper trunk (subcapular), were perhaps the result of the rather high correlation that exists among the various subcutaneous fat measurements (generally about 0.6 to 0.7). Moreover, all the studies that have considered the biological mechanisms involved in the fat distribution issue have done so in the context of lower trunk fat or lower trunk in relation to hip size.

Only a few papers have dealt with the potential mechanisms linking fat distribution characteristics or male obesity and insulin, glucose and lipid metabolism, hyperlipidemia or hypertension (Vague et al, 1984; Björntorp, 1984; Kissebah et al, 1982, 1985; Landsberg, 1986) . Some of these mechanisms are reviewed, and others are proposed, in the various papers of this symposium. Table 2 identifies some of the biochemical or physiological events previously described by several authors and that could be helpful in an attempt to delineate the mechanisms involved in the disturbances associated with a male type of fat topography. Of course, the greatest difficulty lies in the establishment of the cause and effect relationships and the specification of the various interactions among these events. In addition, one has to recognize that unknown genetic factors are also operating not only in determining some of the fat distribution characteristics but also in creating differences in the susceptibility to abnormal fat topography (Bouchard, 1985, 1987).

We will also be concerned with the fat distribution characteristics that may be apparent during growth and their immediate and delayed clinical implications. In this context, genetically determined variation, and gender and ethnic differences have to be taken into account. Strategies to alter the course of growth in fat mass as well as in fat distribution become particularly critical given the health outcomes of persisting excess body fat and excessive fat diposition in the lower trunk

Table 2: A partial list of biochemical or physiological phenomenon involved in the relationship between abdominal obesity and metabolic disturbances[a]

A) Positive energy balance
B) Increased fat deposition (total fat mass)
C) Preferential fat deposition in lower trunk
D) Enlarged abdominal fat cells
E) Increased sympathetic activity
F) Increased metabolic rates
G) Increased abdominal fat cell lipolysis
H) Increased FFA flux in hepatic circulation
I) Decreased hepatic glucose uptake
J) Decreased skeletal muscle glucose uptake
K) Maintenance of hepatic glucose production
L) Decrease of insulin antilipolytic effect
M) Increased secretion of pancreatic insulin
N) Decreased hepatic insulin extraction
O) Decreased SHGB and increased free testosterone
P) Increased insulin resistance
Q) Increased hepatic synthesis of VLDL, TG and ApoB
R) Increased hepatic TG lipase
S) Blood hypertriglyriceridemia
T) Increased transfer of cholesterol ester to adipose tissue
U) Decreased blood level of HDL
V) Increased vasoconstriction of blood vessels
W) Increased cardiac output
X) Increased renal Na reabsorption
Y) Increased blood pressure
Z) Increased aromatization of steroids

---

[a] Cause and effect relationships and interactions are not defined

area. These issues are of prime interest if successful primary and secondary prevention strategies are to be developed for the growing children and adolescents.

It should be obvious to the reader of the proceedings of this symposium that several major conclusions can be reached at this time but also that several problems remain. First, if one accepts the findings of several prospective epidemiological studies, the relative risk of death or of experiencing a coronary event associated with abdominal obesity is generally higher than the risk of obesity per se, namely relative risks of about 2.0 versus 1.5. Second, from the epidemological studies, the relative risk of abdominal obesity is about as high as that for smoking, hypercholesterolemia and hypertension. Third, the male pattern of fat distribution is established around puberty and the androgens are apparently involved in generating this android characteristic although the exact mechanisms remain to be defined. Fourth, alterations in fat distribution are difficult if not impossible to induce unless they are secondary to total fat mass changes given the present state of knowledge and technology. Fifth, several causal mechanisms have been suggested for the initiation of the events leading to metabolic disturbances secondary to abdominal obesity. Among them, the most obvious are the following: habitual positive energy balance, increased sympathetic activity secondary to positive energy balance or chronic stress, increased androgenic activity, increased FFA flux in hepatic circulation, reduced glucose uptake in skeletal muscle, inherited predisposition to store fat in the abdominal area, and others as well (see table 2 for a list of potential primary and secondary mechanisms).

Finally, one must recognize that several problems remain in this field. They are of the utmost importance as they have the potential to influence the quality of the experimental and clinical research carried in the field as well as to hinder communication among the scientists involved. One of these problems is that of the terminology of fat distribution. Secondly, the issues of measurement and quantitative standards are still very much with us. More direct methods are now available to assess the importance of the various fat compartments including the abdominal compartments while indirect techniques remain more commonly used. Conflicting results could perhaps be accounted for by these methodological differences. Thirdly, the problem of tracking of fat distribution pattern from chilhood to adolescence, to adulthood and later years is not satisfactorily resolved at this time. Studies are urgently needed in this area incorporating both total fat mass and fat distribution indicators. Fourth, in prospective studies and clinical investigations it will be very important to monitor both variations in total fat mass and fat distribution as they appear to carry possibly independent and cumulative risks.

LITERATURE CITED

Andres, R. Mortality and obesity: the rationale for age-specific height-weight tables. In: R. Andres, E.L. Bierman and W.R. Hazzard (eds), Principles of geriatric medicine. New-York: McGraw-Hill, 1985, pp.311-318.

Björntorp, P. Hazards in subgroups of human obesity. European Journal of Clinical Investigation, 14: 239-241, 1984.

Bouchard, C., and A. Tremblay. Genetics of body composition and fat distribution. In: N. G. Norgan (ed.), Human body composition and fat distribution. EuroNut report 8, 1985, pp 175-188.

Bouchard, C. Genetics of body fat, energy expenditure and adipose tissue metabolism. In: E.M. Berry, S.H. Blondheim, H.E. Eliahou, and E. Shafrir (eds), Recent advances in obesity research: V. John Libbey: London, 1986, pp 16-25.

Kissebah, A. H., N. Vydelingum, R. Murray, D.J. Evans, A.J. Hartz, R.K. Kalkhoff, and P.W. Adams. Relation of body fat distribution to metabolic complications of obesity. Journal of Clinical Endocrinology and Metabolism, 54: 254-260, 1982.

Kissebah, A.H., D.J. Evans, A. Peiris, and C.R. Wilson. Endocrine characteristics in regional obesities: role of sex steroids. In: J. Vague et al. (eds), Metabolic complications of human obesities. Elsevier: Amsterdam, 1985, pp 115-130.

Landsberg, L. Diet, obesity and hypertension: an hypothesis involving insulin, the sympathetic nervous system, and adaptive thermogenesis. Quaterly Journal of Medicine, 61; 1081-1090, 1986.

Norgan, N.G. (ed.) Human body composition and fat distribution. Euro-Nut, report 8, 1985.

Simopoulos, A.P., and T.B. Van Itallie. Body weight, health and longevity. Annals of Internal Medicine, 100: 285-295, 1984.

Vague, J., J.M. Meignen, J.F. Negrin, M. Thomas, M. Tarmoni et J. Jubelin. Androgènes, oestrogènes et cortisol dans la physiopathologie du tissu adipeux. (Première partie). Sem. Hôp. Paris, 60:1389-1393, 1984.

Vague, J., P. Björntorp, B. Guy-Grand, M. Rebuffé-Scrive and P. Vague (eds). Metabolic complications of human obesities. Elsevier: Amsterdam, 1985.

Fat Distribution During Growth and Later Health Outcomes
pages 9–41 © 1988 Alan R. Liss, Inc.

FAT DISTRIBUTION, OBESITIES AND HEALTH : EVOLUTION OF
CONCEPTS.

Jean Vague, Philippe Vague, Jacques Jubelin et
Annie Barré
University Clinic of Endocrinology
Prado Parc 6 - 411, avenue du Prado
F. 13008 Marseille

First of all, I wish to express my congratulations to
Prof. Bouchard, Prof. Johnston and their co-wokers for
initiating this international symposium titled " Fat distribution and metabolic risk factors during growth and
later health outcomes ". The fundamental work of Laval U-
niversity's group about the genetics of fat distribution
justified this meeting in Quebec.

I am very grateful to Prof. Bouchard and his colleagues-
gues for entrusting me with the honour to pronounce the
opening address. The choice of the other participants enables us to foresee that all the aspects of the topic will
be approached with pertinence.

Morgagni (1717) was probably the first to describe android obesity on the corpse of a woman, in latin, "virili
aspectu et valde obesa ", whose fat filled abdomen and
thorax and in whom he also found hyperostosis frontalis
interna.

106 years later, a french magistrate, gastronome and
musician, neither physician nor physiologist, Brillat-
Savarin (1825), in his excellent, from a literary point
of view, "Physiology of taste ", writes : "There is a type of obesity which is limited to the belly. I have never
observed it in women (which by the way was an error of
observation) .. I name this variety gastrophorie and gas-
trophores those who have caught it. I am myself among
them. But, although a bearer of a rather prominent belly,
I still have the bottom of my leg lean and the nerve sa-

lient as an arab horse's ". That last detail completes
the discription of android obesity in which the relative
thinness of the lower limb is characteristic.

Still a little more than a century, a group of clinicians, in France, Italy, U.S.A. investigates human bioty-
pes by measurements and photographs. Sigaud (1914), Pende
(1939), Sheldon (1940) describe hypertonic and hypotonic,
plethoric and anemic obesities. Marañón (1927, 1932, 1940),
Bauer (1935) give a good description of the characters of
hypercortical obesity pointing out its predominance on the
upper body, which Sicard and Reilly (1913) had already a-
nalyzed without discerning its origin. The masterly description of pituitary basophilism by Cushing (1932) enga-
ges the attention on the importance of adipose tissue topography in physiology and in clinic. Yet, the word facio-
truncular obesity, commonly used later on overlooks the
fat of nape, neck and shoulders.

Multiplying the measurements of adipose tissue thickness in various areas of the body in both sexes, from
birth to old age, in controls and in the abnormalities of
weight regulation, we have concluded to the determining
role of adipose tissue's sexual differentiation in the e-
volution of obesities (J. Vague 1947 a-b, 1949, 1953).

The sexual differences of adipose tissue are present
in many animals, as we shall see to morrow, but usually
discrete, even in Apes, the nearest to man. About 2 million years ago our ancestor stood up for the first time
and used only his lower limbs to walk, run, jump, dance.
Probably at the same time, the uniform layer of subcutaneous fat in Primates of both sexes got differentiated in
man and woman, realizing a specific human character.

Obviously in relation with upright posture, the mecha-
nical conditions of pregnancy and the necessity of important reserves for the fetus and the newborn, fat in women
developed in the lower part of the body, in the pelvis
area where it produced less discomfort.

In man, fat, less useful, was reduced by half and pre-
dominated on the upper body, where it did not oppose to
mobility and struggle capabilities which were favoured by
the broadening of the shoulders and the narrowing of the

pelvis, both effects of testosterone. Natural selection probably increased this differentiation, which brought a-bout the sexual attraction that we find in the symbolism of fecondity and prosperity in the paleolithic times 20 thousand years ago.

Nevertheless, in a minority of men and women other-wise normal, adipose tissue exhibits the sexual differen-tiation of the opposite sex.

BIPOLAR OPPOSITION OF OBESITIES

From many measurements we had held (J. Vague 1947, 1949, 1953, 1956, 1958):on the trunk, the thickness of fat in the nape of the neck (the only area where, every-thing being equal, fat is thicker in man than in woman) and behind the third sacral piece - on the limbs, the brachio-femoral adipo-muscular ratio (BFAMR) calculated by the thickness of fat in the 4 cardinal points of limb emergence and the perimeter of the limb at this level. That interference of musculature's parameter was justified by the fact, that every thing being equal, the development of fat is more or less inversely proportional to that of muscle.

In spite of the possibility of mathematic correcting, the use of the nape-sacrum fat ratio is unpractical in obe-sity and leanness. Other things being equal in both sexes, it increases in leanness and decreases in overweight, be-cause retro-sacral fat is more sensible than nape fat to weight variations.

Having ascertained that, with a steady weight, nape-sacrum ratio is proportional to brachio-femoral adipo-muscular ratio, we have neglected the former owing to its variation, though regular and computable, with weight. We had the proof that masculine and feminine direction of fat was the same in the trunk and in the limbs.

We have observed that the sexual differentiation of human white adipose tissue appears as early as the age of 5. From then on the adipose mass of females will become twice that of males. The subcutaneous area is differentia-ted by its local development. After puberty, fat still predominates in females, as it does in girls and boys, in the lower half of the body. In men, it predominates in the upper half (Fig. 1, 2)

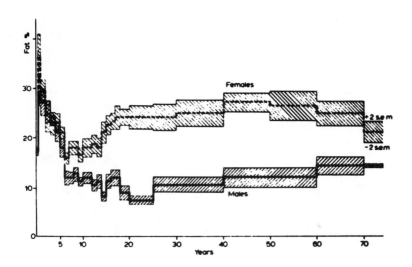

Figure 1. Body fat percentage in males and females.

Now, it was well known that :
1/ Fat reserve is necessary to preserve the glucose amount required by the brain during fasting
2/ Fat excess is dangerous by its metabolic complications.
3/ A woman has normally twice a man's fat mass, the mass of an obese man. As often obese as man is and fatter, she dies later and less often from obesity metabolic complications.

Why ? The answer : an obese woman is protected when she keeps her gynoid fat mass, an evidence of her child bearing nature. When her fat is android she dies like a man.

Our initial description of android and gynoid obesity was founded on the sexual topography of fat. In android o-

besity of both sexes fat shows virile characteristics and
predominates in the upper half of the body, nape of the
neck, shoulders, supra-umbilical abdomen. Musculature is
usually strong and adipo-muscular ratio relatively little
raised. Later on, the group of Björntorp (1985) will demonstrate the masculine histo-chemical type of muscle fibers. The course towards diabetes, hyperlipemia, hyperuricemia, hypertension, atherosclerosis is very frequent. In
contrast, in gynoid obesity of both sexes, the fat shows
feminine characteristics and predominates in the lower
half, hips, buttocks, thighs, sub-umbilical abdomen ; musculature is usually less developed and adipo-muscular ratio high. Metabolic complications are rare and weak(Fig.3).

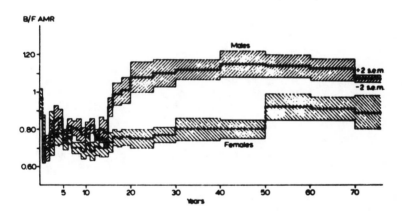

Figure 2, BFAMR in males and females.

    In our first statistics 40 years ago, according as
intermediate cases were put on one side or the other, the
diabetic and arterial risk of android obesity was multiplied by 6 or 20.

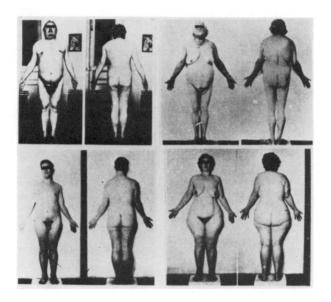

Figure 3. (Above) Android obesity in a male and female. Almost constant progression towards diabetes, hyperlipo-proteinaemia, hyperuricaemia and atherosclerosis. (Below) Gynoid obesity in a male and female. Exceptional progres-sion towards metabolic complications.

As for us, in 1956, at the latest, our opinion is ma-de. Metabolic and vascular complications of obesity are not linked to the degree of fat excess but to the predomi-nance of fat on the upper body, as well for the fat of the trunk as for the fat of the limbs. Many parameters and the mechanism of the phenomenon remain to be analyzed. But the anatomo-clinic reality of the role of sexual differentia-tion of adipose tissue in the evolution of obesity seems to us demonstrated.

A long period of hesitation follows. Langeron (1952) is the first to entirely admit our view. But several works, essentially founded on the thickness of subscapular and tri-ceps skinfolds, draw the attention more on the "centripe-tal ", yet " a masculine character " according to Feldman et al (1969) and its relations with metabolic complications.

The notion of upper and lower body is unfortunately forgotten, and the sexual differentiation of adipose tissue too in metabology, in spite of anthropometric data from Edwards (1951), from Skerlj, Brozek and Hunt (1953) and of Craig and Bayer (1967) who perfectly describe android woman, but neglect the metabolic complications of her obesity. The spider like obesity of Skamenova and Parizkova (1963) who acknowledge the relation with diabetes, completes the opposition between centripetal or central obesity and peripheral obesity.

Öker (1969), however, speaks, noting its relation with diabetes, of the chicken leg obesity, expressing what Brillat-Savarin had already observed (1825), what we had explicitly described (1947 a-b) and what de Gennes will confirm (1974), the weak development of lower limb fat in android obesity.

Meanwhile, Lister and Tanner (1955) revert to the relation of endomorphy, after all hereditary, with diabetes.

Later on, adipocytometry, after Hirsch's et al (1960) initial technics,has induced Björntorp and his group (1966, 1971) to the well founded opposition between hypertrophic and hyperplasic obesities, the former much more threatened by metabolic complications, with the necessary complement that bad prognosis hypertrophic obesity is on the upper body (J. Vague et al 1974).

The easy, quick and useful waist-hip ratio (Kissebah et al, 1980 - Krotkiewski et al, 1983 - Hartz et al, 1983 - Szathmary and Holt, 1983 - Larsson et al, 1984 - Lapidus et al, 1984) induces the opposition between abdominal and gluteal femoral obesity, or between apple and pear obesity (Krotkiewski and Björntorp, 1985), the latter also named by Björntorp and Sjöström (1985) lower body obesity, metabolic and vascular complications being peculiar to the former.

A new parameter, for a long time known by pathologists (Morgagni, 1719) and by surgeons, but which had escaped usual measurements, was revealed by computed tomography, the importance of visceral, peritoneal, omental fat in diabetogenic and atherogenic obesity opposed to subcutaneous obesity (Borkan et al, 1982 - Dixon, 1983 - Tokunaga et al, 1983 - Sjöström et al, 1983,1985 - Ashwell et

al, 1985 - Sparrow et al, 1986 - Fujioka et al, 1987).
This justified opposition is yet somewhat simplified and,
as regards to upper limb,erroneous.

However, many authors keep on using the words upper
body and lower body obesities, frequently associated with
the words android and gynoid obesities,central and peripheral obesities, with their respective metabolic and vascular prognosis (Kissebah et al, 1979,1980,1982,1985 -
Kalkhoff, 1983 - Hartz et al, 1983 - Evans, 1984 -
Björntorp et al, 1984 - Joos et al, 1984 - Lapidus et al,
1984 - Larsson et al, 1984 - Mueller et al, 1986 -
Basdevant et al, 1987 - Haffner, 1987).

Our experience induces us to think that each of those oppositions brings a parameter to be kept.

Diabetogenic and atherogenic obesity is more central
or centripetal than peripheral. But we must add that
the periphery of lower limb is specially concerned.

It is more abdominal than gluteo-femoral. Of course. But we must add that it is question, as we have said
from 1947, of the supra-umbilical abdomen, "in howitzer",
contrarily to gynoid obesity which affects the abdomen
below the navel. We must still add that diabetogenic and
atherogenic obesity is more perivisceral than subcutaneous,
eventhough the phenomenon depends on the degree of weight
excess (Björntorp and Sjöström, 1985).

Finally, we must add that nape, cheeks, neck, shoulders, thorax bear an important part of fat in all android
obesity.

The horizontal line which divides masculine fat and
feminine fat (the latter defined by the fact that testosterone strongly lessens the number of its adipocytes and that
estrogens increase their volume) crosses the navel, as we
demonstrated 40 years ago,and the L4-L5 disk, as computer
tomography in the hands of Sjöström and Göteborg's group
around Björntorp has recently confirmed (1983, 1985). In
surface as well as in depth, adrenergic innervation of those two territories originates respectively above and below
the 10th-11th dorsal spinal nerves (Fig. 4).

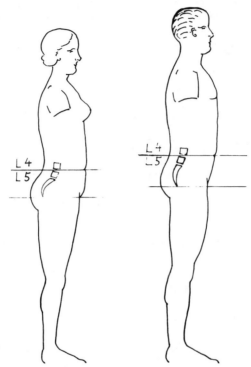

Figure 4 . The horizontal line between feminine and masculine fat.

The effects of steroid hormones on human adipose tissue are not the same as in animals, whence the difficulty in utilizing experimental data. We have demonstrated (J. Vague et al, 1973, 1974 a-b, 1976, 1979, 1984 a-b) that : a/ androgens decrease the number of adipocytes in the lower body, b/ cortisol increases the volume of adipocytes in the upper body, c/ estrogens increase the volume of adipocytes in the lower body.

Those two areas still differ by their sensibility to catecholamines. β lipolytic adrenergic activity predominates in the upper body (Lafontan, 1979,1985 - Kissebah 1979, 1985 - Ostman et al, 1979 - Rebuffé-Scrive 1985,1986 a-b - Garçon et al, 1983 - Ardissone et al, 1985), including o-mentum (Carlson et al, 1969 - Goldrich et al, 1970), anti-lipolytic α-adrenergic activity in the lower body.

M. Rebuffé-Scrive (1985, 1986 a-b), in the group of
Björntorp, demonstrated that lipoprotein lipase activity
in the gluteo-femoral region is higher than in the abdominal region (at the level of the umbilicus), in women before the menopause, except during lactation.

The different secretions of sexual steroids in man
and woman are obviously the cause of the differences in
the topographic distribution of adipose tissue, differences which proceed along with the evolution of those steroid secretions. However, from reasons which result at once from the secretion of hormones and still more from the
sensibility of adipose tissue to their action, we already
saw that, in a minority of men and women, adipose tissue's
sexual differentiation is more or less that of the opposite
sex.

The comparative use of the various methods of measurement of adipose tissue topography demonstrates that each
of the terms of the bipolar opposition of obesities is justified to distinguish pathogenic from not pathogenic obesities. But each of them is restrictive to one sector and
exclusive of others.
   a/ Those various manners of approaching distribution
lead to the same result as to metabolic complications of
its excess.
   b/ The relationships are very important between those
various morphologic parameters(Fig. 5). Besides our already ancient own findings, the concordance between waist-dia-
meter / thigh diameter ratio, waist circumference / thigh
circumference ratio, waist-hip ratio demonstrates once more
that trunk fat and limbs fat evolve in the same direction
towards the upper or the lower body(Ashwell et al, 1978,
1982, 1985 - Seidell et al, 1985 - Haffner et al, 1987).
One exception only. Triceps skinfold, although its situation and its innervation by the second dorsal root, belongs
to feminine fat.
   c/ Masculine differentiation and ageing determine the
predominance of fat in the upper body, trunk, deep and upper areas of the abdomen. This evolution which starts with
puberty in man, when he has achieved his growth, from menopause in woman, when she has achieved her reproductive activity, is obviously related to the production and action
of sexual hormones.

Fig. 5 - 113 OBESE MEN, 327 OBESE WOMEN 41 — 50 Y. OLD

RELATIONSHIP BETWEEN BRACHIO-FEMORAL ADIPOMUSCULAR RATIO (BFAMR)

AND

		ON THE LIMBS		ON THE TRUNK	
		DELTO/TROCHANTER FAT RATIO	ARM/THIGH EMERGENCE CIRCUMFERENCE RATIO	EPIGAST./HYPOGAST. FAT RATIO	WAIST /HIP CIRCUMFERENCE RATIO
MEN	n	113	113	113	96
	r	0.799	0.383	0.569	0.479
	p	< 0.001	< 0.001	< 0.001	< 0.001
WOMEN	n	327	327	327	209
	r	0.808	0.599	0.781	0.775
	p	< 0.001	< 0.001	< 0.001	< 0.001

Fig. 6   BIPOLAR OPPOSITION OF OBESITIES

CENTRAL CENTRIPETAL TRUNKAL SPIDER TYPE	PERIPHERAL
ABDOMINAL APPLE-SHAPED	GLUTEAL FEMORAL PEAR-SHAPED
INTRA-ABDOMINAL VISCERAL	EXTRA-ABDOMINAL SUBCUTANEOUS
UPPER BODY WITH CHICKEN LEG	LOWER BODY

ALL TOGETHER = ANDROID OBESITY   ALL TOGETHER = GYNOID OBESITY

= EXCESS OF FAT IN THE AREAS

WHERE ADIPOCYTES ARE NOT DECREASED BY ANDROGENS AND NOT INCREASED BY ESTROGENS	WHERE ADIPOCYTES ARE DECREASED BY ANDROGENS AND INCREASED BY ESTROGENS

In both sexes, the obesity predominating on the upper body, nape, cheeks, neck, shoulders, upper half of trunk and abdomen, peritoneum, mesentery, omentum, areas whose adrenergic innervation proceeds from above the 11th dorsal spinal root and where adipocytes are not partially destroyed by androgens nor swollen by estrogens, is consequently android obesity. The number and the volume of its adipocytes are increased in the upper body (J. Vague et al,1973, 1974 a-b, 1976, 1979,1984a-b).The obesity which exhibits the opposite characters is gynoid obesity. That is why the terms android, gynoid, intermediate obesities, identified and measured by the various equivalent means at our disposal, seem to day the most qualified to express reality and promote the success of our researches. Each of the others draws attention on one sector only of fat distribution and is unaware of the hormonal mechanism of that distribution (Fig. 6).

METABOLIC AND VASCULAR COMPLICATIONS OF OBESITIES

We have just seen that 30 years ago the statistical relationship between metabolic and vascular complications of obesities and their android topography of fat was already demonstrated. That relationship was confirmed by many works (Langeron, 1952 - Skamenova and Parizkova, 1963 - Oker, 1969 - Feldman et al, 1969 - de Gennes, 1974), particularly in the last years (Kissebah et al, 1978, 1982, 1985 - Bonnet and Lefebvre, 1979 - Kalkhoff et al, 1983 - Hartz et al, 1983, 1984 - Evans et al, 1983 - Björntorp et al, 1984, 1985 - Blair et al, 1984 - Mueller et al,1985- Joos et al, 1984 - Lapidus et al, 1984 - Larsson et al,1984 Ohlson et al, 1985 - Ducimetiere et al, 1985 - Despres et al, 1985 - Raison et al, 1985 - Sims et al, 1985 - Seidell et al, 1985 - Sparrow et al, 1986 - Mouroux and Nicolino, 1986 - Basdevant et al, 1987 - Haffner et al, 1987).

As for us we have carried on our researches. Diabetogenic obesity led us to distinguish 5 stages : D0, with normal glucose tolerance - D1, with glucose intolerance, usually contemporaneous with maximum weight - D2, overt diabetes, after the usual loss of 2-3 kgs - D3, overt still non insulin dependent diabetes, in spite of the progression of weight loss - D4, insulin dependent diabetes, after spontaneous, important but too late weight loss, observed in 15% of diabetogenic obesity.(J. VAGUE et al. 1979).

Spontaneous loss of weight, as weak it may be expresses the progressive failure of insulin secretion, initially much increased, an evidence of insulin resistance. However, almost until the end of stage D3,weight loss, non spontaneous but intentional, is able to stop the evolution of diabetes and to go back more or less to the previous stages.

A statistical study of 3012 cases of obesity observed for 10 years, 1974 women, 1038 men, clearly established in 1978 relationship between the product of maximum fat mass by the brachio-femoral adipo-muscular ratio raised to the power of 2, realizing a maximum pathogenic fat mass, and overt diabetes D2 in both sexes. The lesser relationship with stages D3 and D4 suggests the interference of other factors at the origin of the last stages (Fig. 7)

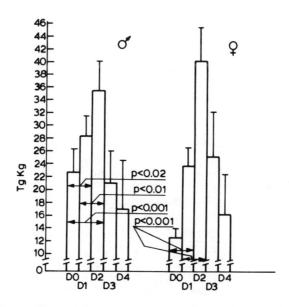

Maximum diabetogenic fat mass excess. Means ± 2 S.E.M.

Figure 7

The same methodology was employed to study 240 obese patients aged 40 to 50 years (158 women, 82 men) with or without diabetes, in whom unequivocal signs of atherosclerosis were sought in coronary, cerebral, aortic or lower limb arteries. Carbohydrate metabolism was explored concomi-

tantly. No correlation was found between fat mass and atherosclerosis hereas signs of atherosclerosis correlated well
with both the brachio-femoral adipo-muscular ratio and maximum pathogenic fat mass (Fig. 8, 9) (J. Vague et al.1979)

*Atherosclerosis vs brachiofemoral adipomuscular ratio (BF AMR) and
maximum fat mass excess in 82 obese males aged 40–50*

M ± 2 SEM	Atherosclerosis, clinical symptoms: 0				Atherosclerosis, clinical symptoms: +		
N	44				38		
Diabetes	20 D0	12 D1	12 D2		4 D0	17 D1	17 D2
Age	42	(.8)			45	(1.5)	
Maximum weight index	1.48	(.08)			1.59	(.11)	
BF AMR / Normal BF AMR	1.09	(.08)		$p < 0.001$	1.43	(.14)	
Fat mass index	2.25	(.3)			2.82	(.5)	
Maximum diabetogenic fat mass excess	18.90	(4.76)		$p < 0.001$	55.50	(15.08)	

Figure 8

*Atherosclerosis vs brachiofemoral adipomuscular ratio (BF AMR) and
maximum fat mass excess in 158 females aged 40–50*

M ± 2 SEM	Atherosclerosis, clinical symptoms: 0				Atherosclerosis clinical symptoms: +		
N	112				46		
Diabetes	46 D0	44 D1	22 D2		4 D0	23 D1	19 D2
Age	44	(.6)			45	(1.3)	
Maximum weight index	1.48	(.04)			1.50	(.10)	
BF AMR / Normal BF AMR	1.20	(.06)		$p < 0.001$	1.64	(.16)	
Fat mass index	1.60	(.06)			1.53	(.12)	
Maximum diabetogenic fat mass excess	17.15	(2.98)		$p < 0.001$	48.16	(9.02)	

Figure 9

Our last retrospective study of 327 obese women and 113 obese men, aged 41 to 50 years, different from the preceding ones, but seen by the same practitioner, confirms those correlations. (Fig. 10, 11, 12) (J. Vague et al.1987)

113 OBESE MEN, 327 OBESE WOMEN 41 — 50 Y. OLD

RELATIONSHIP BETWEEN BRACHIO—FEMORAL ADIPO—MUSCULAR RATIO (BFAMR) AND

FASTING PLASMA LEVEL OF

		GLUCOSE	CHOLESTEROL	TRIGLYCERIDES	URIC ACID	SYST. B.P.	DIAST. B.P.
	n	113	113	66	113	113	113
MEN	r	0.288	0.318	0.377	0.252	0.337	0.294
	p	< 0.005	< 0.001	< 0.005	< 0.01	< 0.001	< 0.005
	n	327	327	171	327	327	327
WOMEN	r	0.394	0.283	0.601	0.424	0.319	0.364
	p	< 0.001	< 0.001	< 0.001	< 0.001	< 0.001	< 0.001

Figure 10

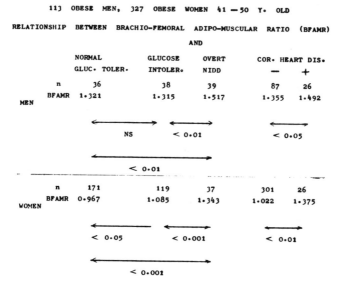

113 OBESE MEN, 327 OBESE WOMEN 41 — 50 Y. OLD

RELATIONSHIP BETWEEN BRACHIO—FEMORAL ADIPO—MUSCULAR RATIO (BFAMR)

AND

		NORMAL GLUC. TOLER.	GLUCOSE INTOLER.	OVERT NIDD	COR. HEART DIS. —	COR. HEART DIS. +
MEN	n	36	38	39	87	26
	BFAMR	1.321	1.315	1.517	1.355	1.492

NS   < 0.01   < 0.05

< 0.01

WOMEN	n	171	119	37	301	26
	BFAMR	0.967	1.085	1.343	1.022	1.375

< 0.05   < 0.001   < 0.01

< 0.001

Figure 11

Fig. 12 113 OBESE MEN, 327 OBESE WOMEN 41 — 50 Y. OLD

RELATIONSHIP BETWEEN BRACHIO-FEMORAL ADIPO-MUSCULAR RATIO (BFAMR)

AND

	GOUT		URIC LITHIASIS		STRIAE GRAVIDARUM		
	−	+	−	+	0	WHITE	PURPLE
MEN n	108	5	98	15			
MEN BFAMR	1·385	1·390	1·385	1·394			
	NS		NS				
WOMEN n	322	5	319	8	61	64	110
WOMEN BFAMR	1·046	1·370	1·045	1·275	0·994	0·895	1·204
	< 0·02		< 0·05			< 0·001	
						< 0·001	

At the same time, our group had been carrying on, since 1950, a prospective study. We have followed up the course of a homogeneous group of obese women (weight index ⩾ 1.30) aged 25 to 30 between 1950 and 1953, the period of our first investigation, until 1983. In 74 cases the course was followed from stage D0 and D1, ascertained in 1950-53 up to 1983.

The figure 13 shows : a/ the course of BFAMR in normal weight men and women from 25-30 to 60 years of age - b/ the mean of the obese women who did not lose weight and evolved towards diabetes had an initial BFAMR above 1.1.- c/ The mean of the obese women who also had an initial high BFAMR and voluntarily got normal weight did not develop diabetes. They would probably have develop diabetes, if they had kept their overweight. - d/ In contrast, the groups who had low initial BFAMR, did not develop diabetes, whether they had lost weight or not. The patients of former group would probably have never developed diabetes had they kept their overweight. (J. Vague et al. 1985)

Unquestionable symptoms of atherosclerosis were searched for on the various territories in the same series. They were absent in 1950-53. 30 years later we observe the following data : (Fig. 14)(J. Vague et al. 1987)

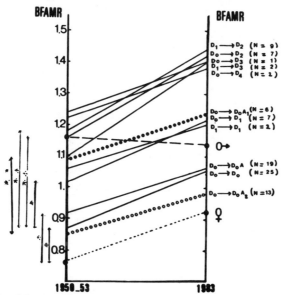

74 OBESE WOMEN (WEIGHT INDEX ≥ 1.30)
25 – 30 Y. OLD BETWEEN 1950 AND 1953
PROGRESS TOWARDS DIABETES FROM 1950–53 TO 1983

Figure 13. DO. 1. 2. 3. 4. see text. DOA : sustained intentional weight loss. DOA1 in the group DOA, 6 patients whose initial BFAMR was ≥ 1. DOA2 in the group DOA, 13 patients
whose initial BFAMR was < 1. Broken lines : male and female normal weight controls.

a/ Atherosclerosis is constant in diabetics. It is present
in some diabetics. b/ Voluntarily loss of weight with the
maintenance of an almost normal weight have prevented diabetes in spite of the predominance of fat in the upper body
and of the familial history of diabetes. They did not cons-
tantly prevent atherosclerosis. In 19 cases, 7 of them with
familial history ·of atherosclerosis, 6 display symptoms of
moderate atherosclerosis. c/ Excluding the 5 obese women
who lost weight by the evolution of their diabetes (D3 and
D4) 50 obese women did not lose weight. 16 of them have pro-
gressed towards diabetes and atherosclerosis. They significantly differ from the other 34 by their high BFAMR and the
frequency of familial history of diabetes and atherosclerosis. d/ Among the remaining 34 obese women, 15 display symptoms of atherosclerosis, without significant difference between

the 9 cases of glucose intolerance and the 25 cases of normal glucose tolerance, with borderline significant effect
of pathologic familial history. Yet we observe that in spite of 5 cases of familial history of diabetes and atherosclerosis, 15 obese women with an initial BFAMR very lower than
1 display neither glucose intolerance nor atherosclerosis
after 30 years evolution of untreated obesity.

The relation between android obesity and atherosclerosis is then the same as between android obesity and diabetes. But atherosclerosis is more frequent than diabetes
and its prevention a little less accessible to weight loss.

Fig. 14   AMONG 74 OBESE ♀ (WEIGHT INDEX ≥1.30)
25-30 Y. OLD BETWEEN 1950-53, 50 WHO DID
NOT LOSE WEIGHT. PROGRESS TOWARDS DIAB.
AND ATHEROSCLEROSIS FROM 1950-53 TO 1983

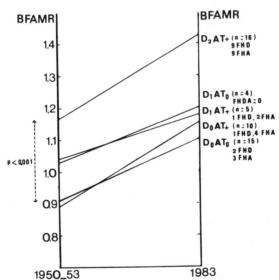

BFAMR = BRACHIO-FEMORAL ADIPO-MUSCULAR RATIO
D_0 = NORMAL GLUCOSE TOLERANCE_D_1 = GLUC. INTOLER.
D_2 = OVERT DIABETES _ AT = ATHEROSCLEROSIS
FHD = FAM. HIST. OF DIAB._FHA = FAM. HIST. OF ATHEROS.

The hormonal abnormalities observed in obesities related to adipose tissue's sexual differentiation will be extensively discussed during this symposium by those who have
best investigated the topic. Allow me to try and classify

the available data :

1/ What seems unquestionable and important :
a/ Increased insulin secretion, an evidence of insulin resistance which , as we demonstrated long time ago, is not proportional to fat excess, but to the predominance of fat in upper body, as long as B cells have not started their failing (Ph. Vague, 1966 - Ph. Vague et al,1969, 1979, 1985 - J. Vague et al, 1979, 1985) (Fig.15)- b/ Minor but long standing hypercorticism of obesity, revealed for instance by purple gravidae striae (Fig.12) and the increased response of adrenals to ACTH (Fig. 16), is too not related to fat excess, but to its predominance in upper body, such predominance being either cause or consequence, probably a shuttle phenomenon (J. Vague et al, 1960 - Krotkiewski et al. 1966 - J. Vague et al, 1971, 1979, 1985 - Schteingart and Conn, 1969) - c/ Lipolytic adrenergic activity is predominant in upper body adipocytes.
2/ What seems less important :
Hyperandrogenism of android obese women cannot entirely explain the intensity of adipose tissue's masculine differentiation. After all, except the rare cases of ovarian polykystosis with hyperandrogenism, insulin resistance and consecutive hyperinsulinemia, the other symptoms of hyperandrogenism are weak in obese android women, who, for most of them, have normal genital functions, incompatible with major hyperandrogenism. Besides the real but discrete hypercorticism we must have recourse for the explanation of woman's android constitution to increased sensitivity of adipocytes to androgens and perhaps cortisol, sensitivity which is transmitted by dominant autosomy, as demonstrated by numerous genealogic tables.

Speaking here about heredity of obesities and their topographic aspects would be rather presumptuous. Let us only recall before the better information of this afternoon :
1/ The predisposition to obesity is obviously hereditary in the majority of cases (Withers, 1964 - Seltzer, 1969 - Brook et al, 1975 - Fabsitz et al, 1980 - Annest et al,1983- Bouchard, 1984 - VAGUE (1984) - Stunkard et al, 1986). 2/ It is the same for the predisposition to the type of fat distribution (J. Vague 1953) (Fig. 17) (Bouchard 1985) and the predisposition to metabolic and arterial disturbances observed in obesity, but, with less frequency and gravity, in normal weight too (Fig. 14, 18, 19). 3/ Overtly from the association of all those genetic factors, before the effects of

environment, obesity, its morphologic type and its metabolic complications appear or not.

Finally, perhaps will you allow me to approach only the question of the mechanisms of the complications of obesity in function of fat distribution, mechanisms which will be discussed extensively to morrow. We note 3 groups of data : 1/ Insulin resistance, related : to fat acids, particularly in the portal circulation - to adipocytes hypertrophy in the upper body - to increased metabolic activity of upper body adipocytes linked in either direction to hyperphagia usually more important in android obesity than in gynoid obesity - to hypercortisolism. 2/ Hyperinsulinism reactional to insulin resistance, with its evil consequences on arterial wall and the secondary exhaustion of B cells - later effects of hyperglycemia on the other metabolisms, arterial endothelium and media. 3/ Direct effect of sexual hormones on carbohydrate, lipid and uric metabolisms, probably the less important.

All that is exciting hypothesis, the most attractive of them being increased metabolic activity of upper body adipose tissue and hyperphagia whose it seems at once cause and consequence.

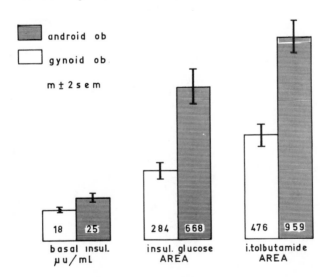

Fig. 15. Plasma insulin after glucose and tolbutamide in 76 obese females with glucose intolerance.

		t -5'.0	30'	60'	90'	120'
CORTISOL	FAT MASS %	r = 0.13 NS	r = 0.15 NS	r = 0.18 NS	r = 0.20 NS	r = 0.17 NS
	BFAMR	r = 0.20 NS	r = 0.35 $p < 0.01$	r = 0.38 $p < 0.01$	r = 0.40 $p < 0.01$	r = 0.33 $p < 0.02$
ANDROSTENEDIONE	FAT MASS %	r = 0.17 NS	r = 0.20 NS	r = 0.25 NS	r = 0.22 NS	r = 0.17 NS
	BFAMR	r = 0.23 NS	r = 0.35 $p < 0.02$	r = 0.44 $p < 0.01$	r = 0.42 $p < 0.01$	r = 0.39 $p < 0.02$
TESTOSTERONE	FAT MASS %	r = 0.15 NS	r = 0.15 NS	r = 0.18 NS	r = 0.23 NS	r = 0.21 NS
	BFAMR	r = 0.23 NS	r = 0.25 NS	r = 0.40 $p < 0.01$	r = 0.42 $p < 0.01$	r = 0.37 $p < 0.02$

34 OBESE WOMEN. 30-40 Y. WI 1.50 ± 0.12. NORMAL GLUCOSE TOLERANCE.
TETRACOSACTID 2.5 MCG/KG INFUSION FOR 60'. CORRELATION COEFFICIENT
BETWEEN PLASMA LEVELS OF CORTISOL, ANDROSTENEDIONE, TESTOSTERONE.
FAT MASS % AND BFAMR.

Figure 16

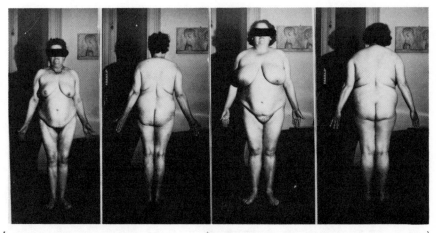

F.P. 3122. 1951. 62 Y.
W.I. 1.36. MAX. W.I. 1.68
BFAMR 1.26. 2 LARGE BABIES
NID DIABETES SINCE 1930
DEATH 1966

F.P. 3140. DAUGHTER OF FP 3122
1951. 37 Y. W.I. 1.58 (MAX)
BFAMR 1.26. NORMAL GLUC. TOLER.
1 LARGE BABY. 1966 NID DIABETES
1975 CORON. STENOSIS. W.I.1.55

Figure 17

Fig. 18

OBESE WOMEN WHO WERE <u>NOT DIABETIC</u> AT THE AGE
OF 25-30 AND THEIR GLUCOSE METABOLISM 30 YEARS
LATER IN RELATION TO :
- B/F AMR
- FAM. HISTORY OF DIAB.

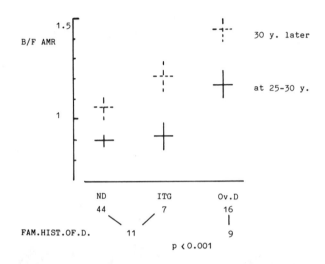

Fig. 19

ASSOCIATIONS TESTED BY χ^2 TEST

	113 OB. MEN 41 - 50 Y. OLD		327 OB. WOMEN 41 - 50 Y. OLD	
	FAM. HISTORY NIDD		FAM. HISTORY NIDD	
	+	−	+	−
NORMAL GLUC. TOLER.	7	28	37	133
GLUCOSE INTOLER.	13	26	47	73
OVERT NIDD	31	8	33	4
	χ^2 28.57		χ^2 60.66	
	$p < 0.001$		$p < 0.001$	

COR. HEART DISEASE	FAM. HISTORY COR. HEART DIS.		FAM. HISTORY COR. HEART DIS.	
	+	−	+	−
−	38	49	131	170
+	22	4	23	3
	χ^2 13.49		χ^2 19.42	
	$p < 0.001$		$p < 0.001$	

CONCLUSION

The conclusions of this opening address, the validity of which is submitted to the talks and discussions of to day and tomorrow, could be the following:
1) The predominance of fat in the upper body: nape, neck, cheeks, shoulders, supra-umbilical abdomen, including peritoneal fat, realizing android obesity, whose degree can be easily measured by various but concordant methods, is the clinical reflexion of the factors which induce the evolution towards metabolic complications: diabetes, carbohydrate sensitive hyperlipoproteinemia, high blood pressure, atheromatosis, hyperuricemia in women, gout, uric lithiasis.
2) Insulin resistance, insulin, cortisol and androgens secretions are not related to fat mass excess but to the predominance of fat in upper body, in areas whose adipocytes are neither partially destroyed by androgens nor swollen by estrogens.
3) Increased secretion of androgens and cortisol, real, but weak, does not fully account for android topography of fat in woman. Apparently genetic increased sensibility of adipocytes to those hormones must be considered.
4) Genetic independant factors determine obesity, predominance of fat in the masculine areas and the biochemical mechanisms of metabolic and vascular complications. Their association seems to be the main cause of those complications.
5) The mechanisms by which android obesity evolves towards metabolic and vascular complications require further research. Increased metabolic activity of masculine fat seems to play an important role.
6) Pathogenic predominance of fat on upper body can be detected in woman, obese or not obese, before the age of 30, whereas biological investigation is entirely normal, except hyperinsulinemia, if the woman is already obese. With the notion of metabolic and/or vascular disturbances in the familial history, that information enables us to evaluate the degree of voluntary weight loss, necessary and sufficient to an efficacious prophylaxis.

But it is now high time for the thorough study of the topic which is the reason of our presence around Claude Bouchard, Frank Johnston and their co-workers.

REFERENCES

ANNEST, J.L., SING, C.F., BIRON, P., MONGEAU, J.G. (1983). Family aggregation of blood pressure and weight in adoptive families. Am. J. Epidem. 117, 492-506.

ARDISSONE, J.P., GARCON, D., MEIGNEN, J.M., CALAF, R., BARLATIER, A., JUHAN, C., VAGUE, J. (1985). Comparative study of lipolysis in epigastric and hypogastric human adipose...J. VAGUE ET al. eds. Marseille 1985 (abstract).

ASHWELL, S., CHINN, S., STALLEY, S., GARROW, J.S. (1978). Female fat distribution - a photographic and cellularity study. Internat. J. of Obesity 2, 289-302.

ASHWELL, M., CHINN, S., STALLEY, S., GARROW, J.S. (1982). Female fat distribution - a simple classification based on two circumference measurements. Internat. J. of obesity, 6, 143-152.

ASHWELL, M., COLE, T.J., DIXON, A.K. (1985). Obesity: new insight into the anthropometric classification of fat distribution shown by computed tomography. British Med. J. 290, 1692-1694.

BASDEVANT, A., RAISON, J., GUY-GRAND, D. (1987). Influence de la distribution de la masse grasse sur le risque vasculaire. Presse Méd., 16, 167-170.

BAUER, J. (1935). Der Einfluss der Nebennieren und Hypophyse auf die Blutdruckregulation und Umstimmung der Geschlechtscharaktere beim Menschen. Klin. Woch., 14, 361-367.

BJORNTORP, P., HOOD, B., MARTINSSON, A., PERSSON, B. (1966) The composition of human subcutaneous adipose tissue in obesity. Acta Med. Scand., 180, 117-127.

BJORNTORP, P., SJOSTROM, L. (1971). Number and size of adipose tissue fat cells in relation to metabolism in human obesity. Metabolism, 20, 703-713.

BJORNTORP, P. (1984a). Morphological classifications of obesity: what they tell us, what they don't, Internat. J. of Obesity, 8, 525-533.

BJORNTORP, P., KROTKIEWSKI, M., REBUFFE-SCRIVE, M., SJOSTROM, L., SMITH, U., STROMBLAD, G. (1984b). Obésité et tissus adipeux - Journées Diabétol. Hôtel-Dieu, Paris Flammarion ed. Paris, p. 45-49.

BJORNTORP, P., SJOSTROM, L. (1985). Adipose tissue dysfunction and its consequences in New Perspective in Adipose Tissue - A. CRYER and R.L.V. VAN eds. Butterworths London, p. 447-458.

BLAIR, D., HABICHT, J., SIMS, E.A.H., SYLVESTER, D., ABRA-
HAM, S. (1984). Evidence for an increase risk for hyper-
tension with centrally located body fat and the effect of
race and sex on the risk. Am.J.Epidemiol., 119, 526-540.
BONNET, F., LEFEBVRE, F. (1979). Cellularity evolution and
prognosis of human obesities in Diabetes and Obesity - J.
VAGUE and Ph. VAGUE eds. Excerpta Med. Amsterdan p. 12-
40.
BORKAN, G.A., GERZOF, S.G., ROBBINS, A.H., HULTS, D.E.,
SILBERT, C.K., SILBERT, J.E. (1982). Assessment of
abdominal fat content by computed tomography. Am. J.
Clin. Nut., 36, 172-177.
BOUCHARD, C.,(1985). Inheritance of fat distribution and
adipose tissue metabolism in Metabolic complications of
human obesities - J. VAGUE, P. BJORNTORP, B. GUY-GRAND,
M. REBUFFE-SCRIVE, P. VAGUE eds. Excerpta Med. Amsterdam
p. 87-96.
BRILLAT-SAVARIN, J.A. (1825). Physiologie du goût - de
Bonnot Paris 1968.
BROOK, C.G.D., HUNTLEY, R.M.C., SLACK, J. (1975).
Influence of heredity and environment in determination of
skinfold thickness in children, Br. Med. J., 2, 719-721.
CARLSON, L.A., HALLBERG, D., MICHELI, H. (1969). Quantitative studies on the lipolytic response of human subcutaneous and omental adipose tissue to noradrenaline and
theophylline, Acta. Med. Scand., 185, 465-469.
CRAIG, L.S., BAYER, L.M. (1967). Androgynic phenotypes
in obese women. Am. J. Phys. Anthrop., 26, 23-34.
CUSHING, H. (1932). The basophil adenomas of the pituitary body and their clinical manifestations (pituitary basophilism). Bull. John's Hopkins Hosp., 50, 137-144.
DESPRES, J.P., ALLARD, C.A., TREMBLAY, A., TALBOT, J.,
BOUCHARD, C., (1985). Evidence for a regional component
of body fatness in the association with serum lipids in
men and women, Metabolism. 34, 967-973.
DIXON, A.K. (1983). Abdominal fat assessed by computed
tomography: sex difference in distribution. Clin. Radiol.
34, 189-191.
DUCIMETIERE, P., RICHARD, J., CAMBIEN, F., AVONS, P.,
JACQUESON, A. (1985). Relationships between adiposity
measurements and the incidence of coronary heart disease
in a middle-aged male population- The Paris prospective
study I. IN: Metabolic complications of human obesities
J. VAGUE, P. BJORNTORP, B., GUY-GRAND, M. REBUFFE-SCRIVE,
P. VAGUE eds. Excerpta Med. Amsterdam, p. 31-38.

EDWARDS, D.A.W. (1951). Differences in the distinction of subcutaneous fat with sex and maturity. Clin. Sc., 10, 305-315.

EVANS, D., HOFFMANN, R.G., KALKHOFF, R.K., KISSEBAH, A.H. (1984). Relationship of body fat topography in insulin sensitivity and metabolic profiles in premenopausal women, Metabolism, 33, 68-75.

FABSITZ, R., FEINLEIB, M., HRUBEL, Z. (1980). Weight changes in adult twices, Acta Genet. Med. Gemel., 29, 273-279.

FELDMAN, R., SENDER, A.J., SEIGELAUB, A.B. (1969). Difference in diabetic and non diabetic fat distribution patterns by skinfold measurements. Diabetes, 18, 478-486.

Fujioka, S., MATSUZAWA, Y., TOKUNAGA, K., TARUI, S. (1987). Contribution of intra-abdominal fat accumulation to the impairment of glucose and lipid metabolism in human obesity. Metabolism, 36, 54-59.

GARCON, D., CALAF, R., GULIAN, J.M., CASTAY M., MEIGNEN J.M., NEGRIN J.F., THOMAS M., VAGUE J. (1983). A comparative study of epinephrine lipolysis in human deltoid and trochanter adipose tissue. Horm. Metabol. Res. 15, 356-357.

de GENNES, J.L., TURPIN, G., TRUFFERT, J. (1974). Blood lipid regulation in various types of human lipodystrophy in: the Regulation of adipose tissue mass - J. VAGUE and J. BOYER eds. Excerpta Med. Amsterdam, p. 332-340.

GOLDRICK, R.B., McLOUGHLIN, G.M. (1970). Lipolysis and lipogenesis from glucose in human fat cells of different sites. Effects of insulin, epinephrine and theophylline. J. Clin. Invest. 49, 1213-1223.

HAFFNER, S.M., STERN, M.P., HAZUDE, H.P., PUGH, J., PATTERSON, J.K. (1987). Do upper body and centralized obesity measure different aspects of regional body fat distribution? Relationship to non insulin dependent diabetes mellitus, lipid and lipoproteins. Diabetes, 36, 43-51.

HARTZ, A.J., RUPLEY, D.C.jr., KALKHOFF, R.D., RIMM, A.A. (1983). Relationship of obesity to diabetes: influence of obesity level and body fat distribution. Preventive Med., 12, 351-357.

HARTZ, A.J., RUPLEY, D.C., RIMM, A.A. (1984). The association of girth measurements with disease in 32, 856 women. Amer. J. of Epidemiology, 119, 71-80.

HIRSCH, J., FARQUHAR, J.W., AHRENS, E.H., PETERSON, M.L., STOFFEL, W. (1960). Studies of adipose tissue in man. A microtechnique for sampling and analysis. Am. J. Clin. Nutr. 8, 499-506.

JOOS, S.K., MUELLER, W.H. (1984). Diabetes alert study: weight history and upper body obesity in diabetic and non diabetic Mexican American adults. Annals of Human Biology, 11, 167-171.

KALKHOFF, R.K., HARTZ, A.H., DUPLEY, D., KISSEBAH, A.H., KELBER, S. (1983). Relationship of body fat distribution to blood pressure, carbohydrate tolerance, and plasma lipids in healthy obese women. J. Lab. Clin. Med., 102, 621-627.

KISSEBAH, A.H., VYDELINGUM, N., ADAMS, P.W., WYNN, V. (1979). Morphology and metabolism of fat cells in females with gynoid or android obesity. In: Diabetes and Obesity - J. VAGUE and Ph. VAGUE eds. Excerpta Med. Amsterdam, p. 148-152.

KISSEBAH, A.H., MURRAY, A., MURRAY, R., HARTZ, A., VYDELINGUM, N., RIMM, A., KALKHOFF, R. (1980). Relationship of body fat distribution to glucose tolerance and clinical diabetes in obese women. Clin. Res., 28, 520 (abstract).

KISSEBAH, A.H., VYDELINGUM, N., MURRAY, R., EVANS, D.V., HARTZ, A.J., KALKHOFF, R.K., ADAMS, P.W. (1982). Relation of body fat distribution to metabolic complications of obesity. J. Clin. Endocrinol. Metab. 54, 254-260.

KISSEBAH, A.H., EVANS, D.J., PEIRIS, A., WILSON, C.R. (1985) Endocrine characteristics in regional obesities: role of sex steroids. In: Metabolic complication of human obesities - J. VAGUE, P. BJORNTORP, B. GUY-GRAND, M. REBUFFE-SCRIVE, P. VAGUE eds. Excerpta Med. Amsterdam, p. 115-129.

KROTKIEWSKI, M., BUTRUK, E., ZEMBRUSKA, Z. (1966). Les fonctions cortico-surrénales dans les divers types morphologiques d'obésité. Le Diabète , 14, 229-233.

KROTKIEWSKI, M., BJORNTORP, P., SJOSTROM, L. (1983). Impact of obesity on metabolism in men and women, J. Clin. Invest . 72, 1150-1162.

KROTKIEWSKI, M., BJORNTORP, P. (1985). The effect of physical training in obese women and men and in women with apple-and pear-shaped obesity. In: Metabolic complications of human obesity - J. VAGUE, P. BJORNTORP, B. GUY-GRAND, M. REBUFFE-SCRIVE, P. VAGUE eds. Excerpta Med. Amsterdam, p. 259-264.

LAFONTAN, M., DRANG-TRAN, L., BERLAN, M. (1979). Alpha-adenergic antilipolytic effect of adrenaline in human fat cell of the thigh; comparison with adrenaline responsiveness of different fat deposits. Europ. J. Clin. Invest. 9, 261-266..

LAFONTAN, M., MAURIEGE, P., GALITZKY, J., BERLAN, M. (1985). Adrenergic regulation of regional adipocyte metabolism In: Metabolic complications of human obesities - J. VAGUE P. BJORNTORP, B., GUY-GRAND, M. REBUFFE-SCRIVE, P. VAGUE eds. Excerpta Med. Amsterdam, p. 161-172.

LANGERON, L. (1952). De l'obésité gynoïde à l'obésité androïde, Presse Med., 60, 389-390.

LAPIDUS, L., BENGTSSON, C., LARSSON, B., PENNERT, K., RYBO, E., SJOSTROM, L. (1984). Distribution of adipose tissue and risk of cardiovascular disease and death: a 12 year follow up of participants in the population study of 1462 women in Gothenburg, Sweden. British Med. J., 289, 1257-1261.

LARSSON, B., SVARDSUDD, K., WELIN, L., WHILHELMSEN, L., BJORNTORP, P., TIBBLIN, G. (1984). Abdominal adipose tissue distribution, obesity, and risk of cardiovascular disease and death: 13 year follow up of participants in the study of 792 men born in 1913. British Med. J., 288, 1401-1404.

LARSSON, B. (1985). Obesity and prospective risk for associated diseases. In: Metabolic complications of human obesities - J. VAGUE, P. BJORNTORP, B. GUY-GRAND, M. REBUFFE-SCRIVE, P. VAGUE eds. Excerpta Med. Amsterdam, p. 21-29.

LISTER, J., TAANER, J.M. (1955). The physique of Diabetics The Lancet 2, 1002-1004.

MARANON, G. (1927). Adiposidad abdominal climatérica. Ses. Inst. Patol. Med. Hosp. Gen. 2, 129-132.

MARANON, G., RICHET, C. (1940). Estudios de fisiopatologia hipofisaria. Ed. Sud Americana Buenos-Aires.

MORGAGNI, G.B. (1719). Adversaria anatomica omnia. Josephus Cominus, Patavii- and (1766) De Sedibus et Causis Morborum per Anatomen Indagatis, Libri Quinque. Tipographia Academica, Lovanii.

MOUROUX, D., NICOLINO, J. (1986). Apport de l'échotomographie dans l'étude de la surcharge graisseuse et son incidence dans les complications métaboliques chez la femme. Sem. Hop. Paris 62, 3591-3595.

MUELLER, E.H. (1985). The biology of human fat patterning. In: Human body composition and fat distribution - N.G. NORGAN ed. Loughborough, U.K. p, 160-174.

MUELLER, W.H., DEUTSCH, M.I., MALINA, R.M., BAILEY, D.A., MIRWALD, R.L. (1986). Subcutaneous fat topography: age changes and relationship to cardiovascular fitness in Canadians, Human Biology, 6, 955, 973.

OHLSON, L., LARSSON, B., SVARDSUD, K., WELIN, L., ERIKSSON, H., WILHELMSEN, L., BJORNTORP, P., TIBBLIN, G. (1985). The influence of body fat distribution in the incidence of diabetes mellitus, 13.5 years of follow up of the participants in the study of men born in 1913. Diabetes, 34, 1055-1058.

OKER, C. (1969). Discussion, in Physiopathology of Adipose Tissue, J. VAGUE and R.M. DENTON eds. Excerpta Med. Amsterdam, p. 395.

OSTMAN, J. ARNER, P., ENGFELDT, P., KAGER, L. (1979). Regional differences in the control of lipolysis in human adipose tissue. Metabolism, 28, 1198-1205.

PENDE, N. (1939). Trattado di Biotipologia umana e sociale Vallardi - Milano.

RAISON, J., GUY-GRAND, B. (1985). Body fat distribution in obese hypertensives. In: Metabolic complications of human obesities - J. VAGUE, P. BJORNTORP, B. GUY-GRAND, M. REBUFFE-SCRIVE, P. VAGUE eds. Excerpta Med. Amsterdam, p. 67-75.

REBUFFE-SCRIVE, M., BJORNTORP, P. (1985). Regional adipose tissue metabolism in man. In: Metabolic complications of human obesities - J. VAGUE, P. BJORNTORP, B. GUY-GRAND, M. REBUFFE-SCRIVE, P. VAGUE eds. Excerpta Med. Amsterdam, p. 149-159.

REBUFFE-SCRIVE, M., ELDH, J., HAFSTROM, L.O., BJORNTORP, P. (1986a). Metabolism of mammary, abdominal and femoral adipocytes in women before and after menopause. Metabolism 35, 792-797.

REBUFFE-SCRIVE, M. (1986b). Regional differences in adipose tissue metabolism in relation to sex steroid hormones Med. Thesis Univ. Vasastadens Bokbinderi AB. Göteborg.

SCHTEINGART, D.E., CONN, J.W. (1969). Cortisol secretion, turnover and metabolism in obesity in Physiopathology of adipose tissue - J..VAGUE and R. DENTON eds. Excerpta Med. Amsterdam, p. 178-191.

SEIDELL, J.C., BAKX, J.C., DE BOER,E. DEURENBERG, P., HAUTVAST, J.G.A.J. (1985). Fat distribution of overweight persons in relation to morbidity and subjective health. Internat. J. of Obesity, 9, 363-374.

SELTZER, C.C. (1969) Genetics and Obesity. In: Physiopathology of adipose tissue - J. VAGUE and R. DENTON, eds. Excerpta Med. Amsterdam, p. 325-334.

SHELDON, W. (1940). Varieties of human physique, Harpor. New York.

SICARD, J., REILLY, J.P. (1913). Dissociation des fonctions de pilosité par dyssécrétion endocrinienne. Bull. mém. Soc. Hop. Paris, 708-716.

SIGAUD, C. (1914). La forme humaine, Legrand. Paris.

SIMS, E.A.H. (1985). The characterization of obesity and the importance of fat distribution. Blood pressure and physical activity in the Hánes I survey. In: Metabolic complications of human obesities - J. VAGUE, P. BJORN-TORP, B. GUY-GRAND, M. REBUFFE-SCRIVE, P. VAGUE eds. Excerpta Med. Amsterdam, p. 39-48.

SJOSTROM, L., TYLEN, U., KVIST, H., HALLGREN, P., WILLIAM-OLSSON, T., (1983). Determination of adipose tissue volume and distribution by a new computed tomography technique, IV Internat. Congress on Obesity, New-York.

SJOSTROM, L., KVIST, H., TYLEN, U. (1985). Methodological aspects of measurements of adipose tissue distribution. In: Metabolic complications of human obesities - J. VAGUE P. BJORNTORP, B. GUY-GRAND, M. REBUFFE-SCRIVE, P. VAGUE eds. Excerpta Med. Amsterdam, p. 13-19.

SKAMENOVA, B., PARIZKOVA, J. (1963). Hodnoceni disproporcionalniho (pavouciho) a difuzniho typu otylosti merenim celkového a podkozniho tuku. Cas. Lék. ces. 102, 142-146.

SKERLJ, B., BROZEK, J., HUNT, E.E. (1953). Subcutaneous fat and age changes in body build and body form in women. Amer. J. Phys. Anthropol. 11, 577-600.

SPARROW, D., BORKAN, G.A., GERZOF, S.G., WISNIEWSKI, C., SILBERT, C.K. (1986). Relationship of fat distribution to glucose tolerance. Results of computed tomography in male participants of the normative aging study. Diabetes, 35, 411-415.

STUNKARD, A.J., SORENSEN, T.I., HANIS, C.H., TEASDALE, T. W., CHAKRABORTY, R., SCHULL, W.J., SCHULSINGER, F. (1986) An adoption study of human obesity, N. England J. Med. 314, 193-198.

SZATHMARY, E.J.E., HOLT, N. (1983). Hyperglycemia in Dogrib Indians of the Northwest territories Canada: association of obesity to diabetes: influence of obesity level and body fat distribution. Prev. Med. 12, 351-357.

TOKUNAGA, K., MATSUZANA, Y., ISHAKAWA, K., TARUI, S. (1983). A novel technique for the determination of body fat by computer tomography. Int. J. Obesity, 7, 437-445.

VAGUE, J. (1947a) La différenciation sexuelle, facteur déterminant des formes de l'obésité. Presse Méd. 55, 339-340.

VAGUE, J. (1947b) Les obésités. Etude biométrique. Biol. Méd. 36, 1-47.

VAGUE, J. (1949). Le diabète de la femme androïde. Presse Méd. 57, 835-837.

VAGUE, J. (1953). La différenciation sexuelle humaine. Ses incidences en pathologie. Masson ed. Paris.

VAGUE, J. (1956). The degree of masculine differentiation of obesities: a factor determining predisposition to diabetes, atherosclerosis, gout and uric calculous disease. Amer. J. Clin. Nut. 4, 20-34.

VAGUE, J. (1960). La différenciation sexuelle de la femme et sa prédisposition au diabète. In: Prenatal Care - B.N. ten Berge ed. Noordhoof Groningen, 83-101.

VAGUE, J., CODACCIONI, J.L., TEITELBAUM, M., VAGUE, Ph., BERNARD, P.J., BOYER, J., FONDARAI, J. (1964). Clinical and biological peculiarities of diabetogenic obesities. 2nd Internat. Congress Endocrinol. London - Excerpta Med. Amsterdam, p. 977-980.

VAGUE, J., VAGUE, Ph., BOYER, J., CLOIX, M.C. (1971). Anthropometry of obesity, diabetes, adrenal and beta-cell functions. Diabetes. Proceed of the 7th Congress of the Internal. Diab. Fed. Buenos-Aires, Excerpta Med. Amsterdam, p. 517-525.

VAGUE, J., RUBIN, Ph., JUBELIN, J., VAGUE, Ph. (1973). Le nombre et le volume des adipocytes dans les régions deltoïdienne et rétro-trochantérienne. Bull. Acad. Nat. Med. Paris, 157, 297-310.

VAGUE, J., RUBIN, Ph., JUBELIN, J., DESCHAMP, P., HACHEM, A., COMBES, R., RAMAHANDRIDONA, G. (1974a). Deltoid-trochanter ratio of number and volume of adipocytes in diabetic and non diabetic obese subjects. European Assoc. Study Diabetes - Diabetologia (abstract) 10, 390.

VAGUE, J., RUBIN, Ph., JUBELIN, J., LAM VAN, G., AUBERT, F. WASSERMANN, A.M., FONDARAI, J. (1974b). Regulation of the adipose mass: histometric and anthropometric aspects. In: The regulation of the adipose tissue mass - J. VAGUE and J. BOYER eds. Excerpta Med. Amsterdam, p. 296-310.

VAGUE, J., RUBIN, Ph., COMBES, R., HACHEM, A., FLEURIGANT, I. (1976). Effet de la testostérone sur la masse musculaire, la masse grasse, le nombre et le volume des adipocytes deltoïdiens et trochantériens. Ann. Endocrin. 37, 499-500.

VAGUE, J., COMBES, R., TRAMONI, M., ANGELETTI, S., RUBIN, Ph., HACHEM, A., PEREZ, D., LANSADE, M.F., ZIRAS, C. RAMAHANDRIDONA, G. JOUVE, R., SAMBUC, R., JUBELIN, J. (1979). Clinical features of diabetogenic obesity. In: Diabetes and Obesity - J. VAGUE and Ph. VAGUE eds. Excerpta Med. Amsterdam, p. 127-147.

VAGUE, J. (1983a). Different forms of human obesity. In: Biochemical pharmacology of obesity - P.C. CURTIS-PRIOR, ed. Elsevier Amsterdam, p. 13-66.

VAGUE, J., VAGUE, Ph., TRAMONI, M., VIALETTES, B. (1983b). Clinical features of diabetogenic and atherogenic obesity. Tohoku J. Exp. Med. 141. (supp.), 147-159.

VAGUE, J., MEIGNEN, J.M., NEGRIN, J.F., THOMAS, M., TRAMOni, M., JUBELIN, J., (1984a). Androgènes, oestrogènes et cortisol dans la physiopathologie du tissu adipeux. Sem. Hop. Paris 60, 1389-1393 et 1465-1476.

VAGUE, J., MEIGNEN, J.M., NEGRIN, J.F., THOMAS, M., TRAMONI, M, JUBELIN, J. (1984b) Volume and number of deltoid and trochanter adipocytes... 7th Internat. Congress Endocr. (abstract). Excerpta Med. Amsterdam, p. 1466.

VAGUE, J. (1984c). Naît-on ou devient-on obèse? Gazette Med., 91, 53-61.

VAGUE, J., VAGUE, Ph., JUBELIN, J., BARRE, A. (1987). Fettsuchtformen und Stoffwechselstörungen. in 93. Tagung Deutsch. Gesell.f.Inn.Med.Springer.Berlin.inpress

VAGUE, J. (1984c) Accao das hormonas esteroides sobre o tecido adiposo umano. Coimbra médica, 5, 4, 209-226.

VAGUE, J., MEIGNEN, J.M., NEGRIN, J.F. (1984d). Effects of testosterone and estrogens on deltoid and trochanter adipocytes in two cases of transsexualism. Horm. Metabol. Res. 16, 380-381.

VAGUE, J., MEIGNEN, J.M., NEGRIN, J.F., THOMAS, M., TRAMONI, M., JUBELIN, J. (1985a). Le diabète de la femme androïde, 35 ans après. Sem. Hôp. Paris, 61, 1015-1025.

VAGUE, J., VAGUE, Ph., MEIGNEN, J.M., JUBELIN, J., TRAMONI, M. (1985b). Android and gynoid obesities. Past and present. In:Metabolic complications of human obesities. J. VAGUE, P. BJORNTORP, B., GUY-GRAND, M. REBUFFE-SCRIVE, P. VAGUE, eds. Excerpta Med. Amsterdam, 3-12.

VAGUE, J. (1985c). Accion de las hormonas esteroides sobre el tejido adiposo humano. Relacion con la obesidad diabetogena. Rev. Soc. Argent. Diab. 19, 8-25.

VAGUE, J., VAGUE, Ph., MEIGNEN, J.M., JUBELIN, J., TRAMONI, M. (1986). Obésités androïde et gynoïde. Passé et présent. Méd. et Nut. 22, 11-22.

WITHERS, R.F.J. (1964). Problems in the genetics of human obesity, Engen. Rev. 56, 81-90.

VAGUE, Ph. (1966). L'insulinémie dans le diabète et les obésités. Thèse Méd., Marseille.

VAGUE, Ph., BOEUF, G., DEPIEDS, R., VAGUE, J. (1969). Plasma insulin levels in human obesity. In: Physiopathology of Adipose Tissue. J. VAGUE and R.M. DENTON eds. Excerpta Med. Amsterdam, 203-225.

VAGUE, Ph., RAMAHANDRIDONA, G., VIALETTES, B., LASSMANN, ALTOMARE, E. (1979) Insulin secretion at the different stages of diabetes. In: Diabetes and Obesity. J. VAGUE and Ph. VAGUE eds. Excerpta Med. Amsterdam, 203-213.

VAGUE, Ph., VALLO de CASTRO, J., VAGUE, J. (1985). Association between adipose tissue distribution and non insulin dependent (type II) diabetes mellitus. In: Metabolic complications of human obesities. J. VAGUE, P. BJORNTORP, B. GUY-GRAND, M. REBUFFE-SCRIVE, Ph. VAGUE eds. Excerpta Med. Amsterdam, 77-84.

Fat Distribution During Growth and Later Health Outcomes
pages 43–61 © *1988 Alan R. Liss, Inc.*

MEASUREMENT OF FAT DISTRIBUTION

Lars Sjöström

Department of Medicine I, Sahlgren's Hospital,
University of Göteborg, S-413 45 Göteborg

CLASSICAL TECHNIQUES

During the last century a number of techniques have been developed in order to measure adipose tissue distribution. Circumferences at different parts of the body seem to have been first registered by Groddeck (1899). Groddeck observed that the waist circumference changed much more than the femoral one during weight reduction.

In the beginning of this century photographs were used to classify people in different somatotypes. Thus in 1921 Kretchmer claimed that there was a relationship between body build and traits of character and some 30 years later Sheldon (1950) developed these ideas further and introduced a score system to describe the degree of endo-, meso- and ectomorphism.

Since the beginning of the 40:ies, several authors have used radiological techniques to measure subcutaneous adipose tissue thickness (Stuart et al, 1940, 1942; Reynolds, 1944; Tanner, 1952; Hammond, 1955; Garn, 1956). Accurate methods based on electrical conductivity were introduced in the 50:ies (Bauereisen and Paerisch, 1953; Booth et al, 1966) but have never been widely used, probably due to their invasive character.

Ultrasonic techniques to measure the adipose tissue thickness were introduced in the 50:ies for measurements in

cattle (Temple et al, 1956). Booth et al (1966) introduced
ultrasonic methods for measurements of human adipose tissue.
In the beginning of the 70:ies we used ultrasound to describe the adipose tissue distribution in young (Sjöström et
al, 1972) and middle-aged women (Krotkiewski et al, 1975).
The local fat cell number was also characterized by considering the number of fat cells in perpendicular cylinders with
a base of 1 mm². This adipocyte number was possible to
calculate by measuring the subcutaneous thickness with ultrasound, by sizing the fat cells in biopsies from the same
region and by taking the non-fat cell volume at different
adipocyte sizes into account (Sjöström et al, 1972).

Skinfold measurements on a large scale started in the
50:ies (Vague, 1947; Vague, 1953; Keys an Brozek, 1953;
Garn, 1956; Edwards, 1959; Parizkova, 1963) but the technique had been introduced by Richér already in 1890. Most
calipers used for skinfold measurements are constructed to
give a constant pressure independent of the gap between the
shanks. Nevertheless variable skin elasticity, different
subcutaneous tissue mobility, different compression times
and individual skillness might influence the results. Therefore numerous studies have been undertaken to validate the
skinfold techniques by other methods. Skinfold measurements
do correlate significantly both versus x-ray (Garn, 1956;
Vague, 1969), conductivity and ultrasonic (Booth et al,
1966) measurements. However, if a high individual precision
is needed, skinfolds should be used with care since for a
given radiological or ultrasonic measurement the skinfolds
can vary up to 20 mm (Booth et al, 1966; Vague, 1969). On
the other hand, the correlation is considerably higher between ultrasonic and conductivity measurements indicating
that these two techniques have lower errors than the skinfold method (Booth et al, 1966).

By combining skinfold and circumference measurements
valuable information about the relation between adipose and
lean tissues have been obtained. This combination was introduced by Jean Vague who calculated the transsectional
area of adipose tissue and muscle from circumferences, and
skinfolds in the brachial and femoral regions (Vague, 1947,
1953, 1969). The adipo-muscular ratio is larger in females
than in males both in the brachial and the femoral regions
and at all ages except in the youngest.

By dividing the brachial adipo-muscular ratio by the

femoral one an index of upper adipose tissue distribution is obtained (Vague, 1969). This brachial/ femoral adipo-muscular ratio (B/F AMR) is much higher in men than women indicating a preponderance of adipose tissue in the upper part of the body in men and in the lower part of the body in women. It should be observed, however, that since the B/F AMR is a ratio of a ratio this variable reflects brachial and femoral AT distribution only to the extent that there is a fixed ratio between the muscular area in the femoral and brachial regions independent of age, sex and the total mass of muscles. This constancy has not been proven but the ratio between femoral and brachial muscle areas varies probably much less than the ratio between brachial and femoral adipose tissue areas. Therefore, a high value of B/F AMR should certainly reflect upper adipose tissue distribution more than it reflects a lower muscular distribution.

Recently transsectional adipose tissue and muscle areas of the arm have been reported from the NHANES, a population study in the USA including about 13700 subjects (Bishop, 1984). As in Vagues studies women have more fat and less muscles than men. There are also quite large changes of these variables with age. The fat/muscle ratio of the mid upper arm is some 10% higher in the American than in the French population.

TECHNIQUES BASED ON COMPUTED TOMOGRAPHY

During the 80:ies computed tomography (CT) has been used for measurements of adipose tissue. NMR is not yet generally available but as soon as it is, it will be preferable to computed tomography since the patients are not radiated.The mathematical procedures will be very similar for CT and NMR.

In 1982 and 1983 studies were published which assessed the visceral and subcutaneous trunk adipose tissue from single scans (Borkan et al, 1982; Dixon, 1983). Tokunaga (1983) as well as we (Sjöström et al, 1983, 1985, 1986a, 1986b; Sjöström, 1987; Kvist et al, 1986, 1987a, 1987b) have described methods to calculate the total adipose tissue volume. Tokunaga divided the body into 11 cylinders and for each cylinder the adipose tissue area of a mid-scan was multiplied with the height of the cylinder. Borders and mid-positions of the cylinders were determined from external landmarks (Tokunaga, 1983). We have chosen a different approach described below.

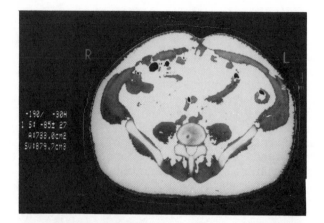

Fig. 1A

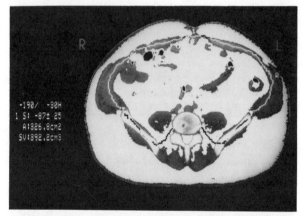

B

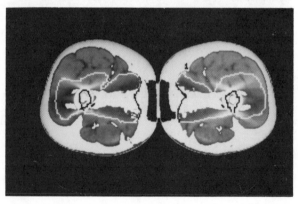

C

Accuracy and Reproducibility of the CT technique

We examine the adipose tissue area of 22 transsectional scans. The subject is lying on his back with his arms stretched over his head. The position of the scans are defined in a strict relation to the skeleton.

The accuracy of the CT technique is dependent on at least four conditions:
1. The AT area of scans must be correctly determined
2. Distances between scans must be correctly determined
3. Correct mathematical models must be used
4. The AT area must change linearly between examined scans

These conditons are of the same importance for regional and total AT volume determinations.

The value obtained of the adipose tissue (AT) area of a scan is dependent on the attenuation borders chosen for AT (fig. 1 A, B). The mean attenuation varies slightly between scans and between subjects and the attenuation limits are influenced by partial volume phenomena along borders on

---

Fig. 1. Determination of Adipose Tissue Areas

Panel A. The total AT area of a scan is obtained by circumscribing the whole scan with a light pen on the terminal screen. The area full-filling the attenuaton condition -190 to -30 HU is shown in white. By changing the lower attenuation border $\pm$10 HU the AT area is changed approx. $\pm$0.2%. By changing the upper attenuation border $\pm$10 HU the AT area is changed approx. 5%.

Panel B. The visceral AT area of a scan is obtained by circumscribing the visceral area and by asking the computor about the area within the circle which fullfills the attenuation condition of AT(-190 to -30 HU).

Panel C. An example of correction for beam hardening in the femoral region. The medial parts of the femoral muscles have attenuations lower than -30 HU. By circumscribing typical muscle areas and examine the area within the circumscriptions having attenuations between -190 and -30 H an area is obtained which should be subtracted from the uncorrected AT area of the scan. The black area indicates AT which due to beam hardening has attenuations below -190 HU. The black area must be added to the uncorrected AT area of the scan. As judged from double examinations the error of these semi-manual corrections is $\pm$0.5% while the corrections as such may constitute up to 20% of the true AT area.

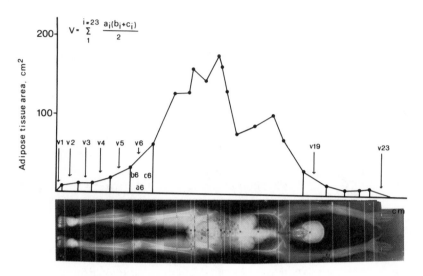

$$V = \sum_{1}^{i=23} \frac{a_i(b_i+c_i)}{2}$$

Fig. 2. Determination of the adipose tissue volume with computed tomography. One of three mathematical algorithms which all give almost identical results (r>0.9999, cf. Kvist et al 1986, 1987a). For explanations, see text. (Reproduced from Kvist et al 1986 with permission).

other tissues (Kvist et al, 1986, 1987a). Particularly in the femoral part of the body, beam hardening effects of the skeleton may sometimes cause muscle to be falsely registered as adipose tissue and adipose tissue as air (Kvist et al, 1987a). These errors must be corrected for by semi-manual procedures (fig. 1 C). In spite of these difficulties it is still evident that CT-determinations of AT is a procedure associated with less assumptions than any other body fat or AT method. From a number of in vivo and phantom experiments we have found it appropriate to chose -30 HU as the upper attenuation limit and -190 HU as the lower limit (Kvist et al, 1986, 1987a).

The distances between the scans are automatically determined by the tomograph with a precision of 0.1 mm. In our calculations these distances are rounded to the nearest mm.

We have tested three different mathematical algorithms (Sjöström et al, 1983, 1985, 1986a; Kvist et al, 1986, 1987a). They all assume that the adipose tissue area is changing linearly between examined scans.

In the first model the adipose tissue area is plotted on the y-axis and the distances between the scans on the x-axis (Fig. 2). Since cm^2 times cm is equal to cm^3 the surface between two scans in such a plot represents the adipose tissue volume between the scans. The 23 partial volumes are summed up to give the total adipose tissue volume.

In the second model the subcutaneous adipose tissue volume between two scans is calculated as the difference between two truncated cones, i.e. the total body volume minus the non-subcutaneous volume between scans. The non-subcutaneous area of a transsectional scan is obtained as the difference between the total area and the subcutaneous area. The visceral adipose tissue is calculated as truncated cones.

The third mathematical model is a simplification of the second one in the sense that the subcutaneous tissue is considered as a series of truncated cones and not as differences between cones.

The three mathematical models give results which are almost identical ($r > 0.9999$) (Kvist et al, 1986, 1987a).

A final factor of importance for the accuracy of the method is the linear change in adipose tissue area between the scans. That this change is linear enough is proven by the fact that calculations of total adipose tissue volumes from 9 selected scans give a very high correlation versus results based on 22 scans ($r = 0.999$). On the other hand it is not enough to base the calculations on 4 scans if a high accuracy is needed in each individual case (Sjöström et al, 1986a; Kvist et al, 1986).

The reproducibility of the method is also very high. From complete double-determinations the error was calculated to be less than 0.6% (Sjöström et al, 1986a). This high reproducibility is of particular value in energy balance experiments. An error of 0.6% means that we can detect a change in adipose tissue volume being less than 0.5 l in a subject having 40 l AT. Since the total volume of AT is calculated as the sum of several partial volumes the error of the method is not larger for regional determinations than for total adipose tissue determinations.

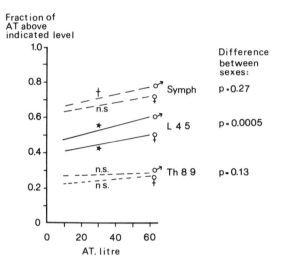

Fig. 3. Fractions of total AT in the upper and lower part of the body at three different levels of separation. To the right, p-values are given for differences between sexes with respect to the fraction of AT located above the indicated level. Symbols at regression lines give the significance of the slope: *, p<0.05; †, p<0.10; ns, non significant. Calculations based on 17 men and 12 women.

Regional Adipose Tissue Determinations with CT

CT is an ideal technique to describe regional adipose tissue distributions. We are often talking about upper and lower forms of AT distribution and that women are characterised by fat preferentially located in the lower parts of the body. The question is then if a border exists which separates the female lower type of AT distribution from the more masculine upper type of AT distribution. If the disc between the thoracic vertebrae 8 and 9 is chosen as the level of separation, then the fraction of AT located above this level is not significantly different between the sexes (Fig. 3). By moving the border between the upper and lower part of the body downwards step by step, we have found that the L 4-5 level separates males and females optimally. With this border, males have on an average 53% of the fat in the upper part of the body while women have 46%, only. This dif-

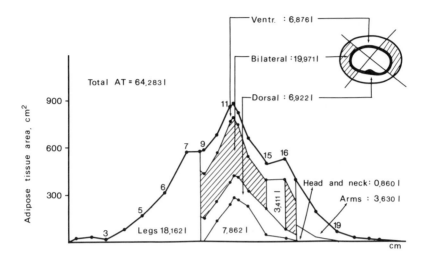

Fig. 4. Exampel of regional determinations of AT. Note that the bilateral subcutaneous AT between Th 8-9 and the lower border of the sternoclavicular joint is 3.4 litres.

ference is highly significant (p <0.0005). Furthermore, with increasing degrees of obesity, both sexes store significantly larger fractions of adipose tissue in the upper part of the body. If the border of separation is pushed further downwards the difference between the sexes disappear again.

As illustrated in fig. 4 CT permits a much more detailed analysis of the adipose tissue distribution than just a division in upper and lower. As a matter of fact, almost any fraction of the AT can be determined. One important exception exists, however. Although attempts have been made to delimit the retroperitoneal AT area of scans by using the kidneys as landmarks (Ashwell, 1986), this does not help to

separate intraperitoneal porta-drained AT from extra peritoneal cava-drained fat. This limitation is due to the fact that CT is not able to detect peritoneum and to the fact that extraperitoneal fat inside the muscle-wall exists also above and below the kidney level and on the lateral and ventral aspects of the trunk.

Table 1 gives the fractions of AT in different regions of men (Kvist et al, 1987a) and women (Kvist et al, 1986). On an average women have 49% of the subcutaneous AT located in the trunk. The corresponding figure for men is about 41%. As compared to men, women have only slightly larger fractions of AT in legs and arms (ns). In both sexes, the fraction of subcutaneous trunk AT is increasing and the fraction of leg AT is decreasing with increasing amounts of AT (Kvist et al, 1986, 1987a).

The most striking difference between the sexes is found with respect to the visceral AT depot (Table 1, fig. 5). In

Table 1. Fractions of AT (%) in different regions of the body (x $\pm$ SD).

	Published data	
	Men[§]	Women[§§]
n	17	8
	%	%
Subcutaneous		
legs	29.0 $\pm$ 7.3	31.8 $\pm$ 5.6
trunk	41.4 $\pm$ 7.4	48.6 $\pm$ 5.1
arms	6.8 $\pm$ 1.0	7.6 $\pm$ 1.2
head and neck	1.4 $\pm$ 1.0	1.8 $\pm$ 0.2
Visceral	20.9 $\pm$ 7.0	10.3 $\pm$ 1.8
	Total experience, May 1987	
	Men	Women
n	24	19
	%	%
Subcutaneous	79.1 $\pm$ 7.1	91.9 $\pm$ 3.1
Visceral	20.9 $\pm$ 7.1	8.1 $\pm$ 3.1
visceral, range	9.1 - 33.5	3.7 - 14.4

[§] Kvist et al 1987 a
[§§] Kvist et al 1986

men, the subcutaneous and visceral depots occupy on an average 79 and 21%, respectively. In women, the corresponding
figures are 92 and 8%. In men, the absolute amount of visceral AT increases linearly with increasing total amounts of
AT (fig. 5, left upper panel). In women, available information indicates that the visceral fat is fairly constant (1-2
litres) in the total AT range 10-30 litres (fig. 5, left
lower panel). Above 30 litres of total AT, the absolute
amounts of visceral AT increases with a slope comparable
with that one in men. Difference in age did not explain this
pattern since lean and obese women were of comparable age.
Although not being a causal evidence, it may be of interest
to point out that in our cross-sectional study (n = 1000)
women were able to put on some 30 kg BF more than men before
they reached comparable degrees of metabolic aberrations
(Krotkiewsky et al, 1983).

The relative amounts of visceral AT ranges between 4 and
14% in women and between 9 and 34% in men (table 1). In none
of the sexes the fraction of visceral fat changes systematically with increasing total amounts of AT (fig. 5, right
panels).

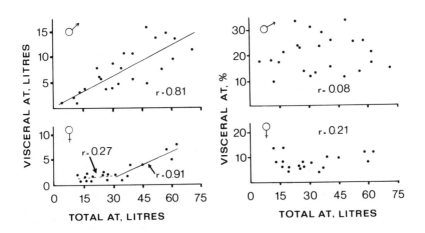

Fig. 5. Relationships between absolute as well as relative amount of
visceral AT and the total AT volume in men (n=24) and women (n=19).

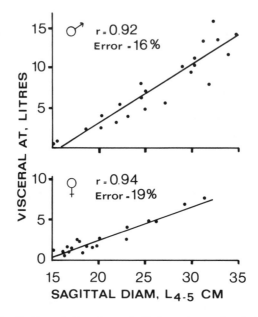

Fig. 6. Prediction of the visceral AT from the sagittal diameter at
the L4-5 level.
Upper panel, men: y = 0.726x - 11.3; r = 0.92; Error 16%.
Lower panel, women: y = 0.406x - 5.70; r = 0.94; Error 19%.

Anthropometric Predictions of the Visceral AT Volume.

Both in cross-sectional (Krotkiewski et al, 1983) and
longitudinal (Larsson et al, 1984; Lapidus et al, 1984) studies relationships have been found between the waist/hip
circumference ratio, metabolic disturbances and cardiovascular disease. Relationships have also been demonstrated
between metabolic disturbances and visceral/total AT area
ratios in abdominal CT-scans (Shuman, 1986; Sparrow, 1986).
These circumstances indicate that the visceral AT may be
related to cardiovascular risks. Since CT is expensive and
less well suited for epidemiological studies it seems important to construct equations which predict the visceral AT
volume from anthropometric measurements.

In a recent report we have examined the predictive power
of a large number of anthropometric measurements (Kvist et

al, 1987b). Equations predicting the CT-measured visceral AT volume were obtained from 17 males and 10 women (primary materials). These equations were then cross-validated in another 7 males and 9 females. One of the better measures and definitely a very simple one was the sagittal diameter of recumbant subjects at the L 4-5 (=crista iliaca) level. With this predictor the error was about 20% in both sexes both in the primary and in the cross-validation materials. The error was not reduced by adding weight, height or any weight-forheight index to the equations. In fig. 6 the relationships between the visceral AT volume and the sagittal diameter are shown for the pooled primary and cross-validation materials.

CT-predictions of the Visceral AT Volume

If the visceral AT area of one abdominal scan is available the predictions of the visceral AT volume can be improved

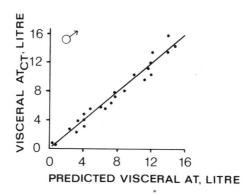

Fig. 7. Relationship between measured and predicted visceral AT volumes in men. Prediction of the visceral AT volume (y) from the visceral AT_{CT} area (cm^2) at the L 3-4 level (x_1) and from weight (kg)/height (m) (x_2).

Predictive equation of men:

$$y = 0.0238x_1 + 0.115x_2 - 4.04$$
$$R^2 = 95.7\%; \text{ Error} = 8.2\%$$

Corresponding equation of women:

$$y = 0.0220x_1 + 0.0410x_2 - 1.03$$
$$R^2 = 97.6\%; \text{ Error} = 7.7\%$$

considerably (errors 11 and 14% in women and men, respectively). By adding weight/height to the equations the errors
are reduced below 9% in both sexes both in the primary materials and the cross-validation materials (Kvist et al,
1987b). Fig 7 shows the relationship between measured and
predicted visceral volumes of the pooled male materials.

Ratios and visceral AT

Visceral/total and visceral/subcutaneous AT area ratios of
single abdominal CT scans have been reported to be associated with metabolic disturbances. Therefore, the relationships between these ratios and the visceral AT volume have
been examined (Kvist et al, 1987b). In table 2 results from
the L 3-4 level are shown but the same type of findings were
obtained from the L 4-5 level. Contrary to the visceral AT
area, the visceral/total and the visceral/subcutaneous area
ratios are no predictors of the absolute amount of visceral
AT. However, the ratios are excellent predictors of the
relative amount of visceral fat (table 2). Together with

Table 2. Correlations between absolute as well as relative amounts
of visceral AT and selected variables.

	Visceral AT, litres		Visceral AT, % of total AT	
	men	women	men	women
n	24	19	24	19
	r	r	r	r
Measurements at the				
L 3-4 level:				
Visceral AT area	0.95***	0.98***	0.72***	0.61**
Visceral/total AT area ratio	0.40	0.25	0.86***	0.73***
Visceral/subcut AT area ratio	0.40	0.14	0.87***	0.60**
Sagittal diameter	0.92***	0.94***	0.44	0.33
Waist circumf.	0.88***	0.85***	0.36	0.19
Waist/hip circumf. ratio	0.77***	0.83***	0.59**	0.48*

*, $p < 0.05$; **, $p < 0.01$; *** $p < 0.001$

metabolic studies quoted above these findings indicate that the relative rather than the absolute amount of visceral AT is statistically related to cardiovascular risks.

As compared to the sagittal diameter or the waist circumference the waist/hip circumference ratio seems to be a less powerful predictor (in men: $p < 0.05$ as judged from comparison of absolute means of residuals) of the absolute amount of visceral AT (table 2). Still the waist/hip ratio predicts the visceral AT volume significantly. The ratio also predicts the relative amount of visceral AT, although at a lower significance level. Contrary to the visceral AT volume, the relative amount of visceral AT seems to be better predicted by the waist/hip ratio than by the waist circumference (table 2). It is interesting to note that both in men (Larsson et al, 1984) and women (Lapidus et al, 1984) the waist/hip ratio was a better prospective predictor of cardiovascular disease than the waist circumference. Again these circumstances indicate that the relative rather than the absolute amount of visceral AT is statistically related to cardiovascular risks. A causal relationship remains to be proven.

CONCLUSIONS

1. AT volume and distribution are determined with a higher reproducibility and accuracy with CT than with classical techniques.

2. The sexes are best separated at the L 4-5 level with respect to upper and lower AT distribution.

3. On an average the visceral AT constitutes 8% of the total AT in women and 21% in men.

4. Women seem to be protected from visceral fat accumulation and metabolic aberrations up to a moderate degree of obesity (30 litres AT).

5. The visceral AT volume can be predicted from the sagittal diameter at the L 4-5 level with an error of 20%.

6. The visceral AT volume can be predicted from weight/height and the visceral AT area of one abdominal scan with an error of 8%.

7. The visceral/total AT area ratio correlates with relative but not with absolute amounts of visceral AT.

8. The waist/hip circumference ratio seems to be better correlated to absolute than relative amounts of visceral AT.

9. The waist circumference correlates with absolute but not with relative amounts of visceral AT.

10. Cardiovascular risks seem to be statistically related to relative but not to absolute amounts of visceral AT. Causal relationships remain to be proven.

ACKNOWLEDGEMENTS

This review is based on a number of studies performed in valuable cooperation with Calle Bengtsson, Badrul Chowdhury, Ulla Grangård, Henry Kvist, Leif Lapidus, Bo Larsson and Ulf Tylén.

REFERENCES

Ashwell M, McCall SA, Cole TJ, Dixon AK (1986). Fat distribution and its metabolic complications: interpretations. In: Human body composition and fat distribution. Ed. N.G. Norgan. Euro-Nut Workshop London dec 1985, pp 227-242.
Bauereisen E, Paerisch M (1953). Die Dickemessung des Unterhautfettgewebes beim Menschen. Z ges exp Med 120:389.
Bishop CW (1984). Reference Values for arm muscle area, arm fat area, subscapular skinfold thickness, and sum of skinfold thicknesses for American adults. J Parent Ent Nutr 8: 515-522.
Booth RAD, Goddard BA, Paton A (1966). Measurement of fat thickness in man: a comparison of ultrasound, Harpenden calipers and electrical conductivity. Brit J Nutr 20:719.
Borkan GA, Gerzof SG, Robbins AH (1982). Assessment of abdominal fat content by computed tomography. Am J Clin Nutr 36:172-77.
Dixon AK (1983). Abdominal fat assessed by computed tomography: sex difference in distribution. Clin Radiol 34: 189-91.
Edwards DAW (1959). Observations on the distribution of subcutaneous fat. Clin Sci 9:259.

Garn SM (1956). Comparison of pinch-caliper and X-ray measu-
rements of skin plus subcutaneous fat. Science 124:178.
Groddeck (1899). Über Messen und Wägen in der ärzlichen Thä-
tigkeit. Wiener Medizinische Presse 43:1759.
Hammond WH (1955). Measurement and interpretation of subcu-
taneous fat, with norms for children and young adult
males. Brit J prev soc Med 9:201.
Keys A, Brozek J (1953). Body fat in adult man. Physiol Rev
33:245.
Kretchmer K (1921). Körperbau und Charakter. Springer Verlag
Berlin.
Krotkiewski M, Sjöström L, Björntorp P, Smith U (1975).
Regional adipse tissue cellularity in relation to metabo-
lism in young and middle-aged women. Metabolism 24:703.
Krotkiewski M, Björntorp P, Sjöström L, Smith U (1983).
Impact of obesity on metabolism in men and women - impor-
tance of regional adipose tissue distribution. J Clin
Invest 72:1150-1162.
Kvist H, Sjöström L, Tylén U (1986). Adipose tissue volume
determinations in women by computed tomography. Technical
considerations. Int J Obesity 10:53-67.
Kvist H, Sjötröm L, Tylén U (1987a). Adipose tissue volume
determinations with CT in men. Submitted to Int J Obesity.
Kvist H, Chowdhury B, Grangård U, Tylén U, Sjöström L
(1987b). Predictive equations of total and visceral adipo-
se tissue volumes derived from measurements with computed
tomography in adult men and women. Submitted to Am J Clin
Nutr.
Lapidus L, Bengtsson C, Larsson B, Pennert K, Rybo E,
Sjöström L (1984). Distribution of adipose tissue and risk
of cardiovascular disease and death: a 12 year follow up
of participants in the population study of women in
Gothenburg, Sweden. Br Med J 289:1261-1263.
Larsson B, Svärdsudd K, Welin L, Wilhelmsen L, Björntorp P,
Tibblin G (1984). Abdominal adipose tissue distribution,
obesity and risk of cardiovascular disease and death: a 13
year follow up of participants in the study of men born in
1913. Br Med J 288:1401-4.
Parizkova J (1963). La morphologie du tissu gras. Probl
actuels Endocr Nutr 7:271.
Reynolds EL (1944). Differential tissue growth in the leg
during childhood. Child Develop 15:181.
Richer P (1890). Du role de la graisse dans la conformation
exterieure du corps humain. Nouv Iconogr Salpet 3:20.

Sheldon WH (1950). Les Varietis de la Constitution Physique de l'homme. Presses Universitaires de France, Paris.

Shuman WP, Newell Morris LL, Leonetti DL, Wahl PW, Moceri VM, Moss AA, Fujimoto WY (1986). Abnormal body fat distribution detected by computed tomography in diabetic men. Invest Radiol 21:483-7.

Sparrow D, Borkan GA, Gerzof SG, Wisniewski C, Silbert CK, (1986). Relationsip of fat distribution in glucose tolerance. Results of computed tomography in male participants of the normative aging study. Diabetes 35:411-415.

Sjöström L, Smith U, Krotkiewski M, Björntorp P (1972). Cellularity in different regions of adipose tissue in young men and women. Metabolism 21:1143.

Sjöström L, Tylén U, Kvist H, Hallgren P, William-Olsson T. Determination of adipose tissue volume and distribution by a new computed tomography technique. The IV International Congress on Obesity 1983 in New York.

Sjöström L, Kvist H, Tylén U. (1985). Methodological aspects of measurements of adipose tissue distribution. In: The Metabolic Complication of Human Obesities. Eds. J. Vague, P. Björntorp, B. Guy-Grand, M. Rebuffé & P. Vague. Elsevier. pp. 13-19.

Sjöström L, Kvist H, Cederblad Å, Tylén U (1986a). Determination of the total adipose tissue volume in women by computed tomography. Comparisons with ^{40}K and tritiuim techniques. Am J Physiol 250:E736-E745.

Sjöström L, Kvist H, Lapidus L, Bengtsson C, Tylén U (1986b). Weight-height indices and adipose tissue distribution - measurements and health consequences. In: Human body composition and fat distribution. Ed. N.G. Norgan. Euro-Nut Workshop London dec 1985, pp 189-198.

Sjöström L (1987). New Aspects of weight-for-height indices and adipose tissue distribution in relatin to cardiovascular risk and total adipose tissue. In: Recent Advances in Obesity Research V. Eds. E Berry, SH Blondheim, HE Eliahou and E Shafir. John Libbey, London. pp 66-76.

Stuart HC, Hill P, Shaw C (1940). Growth of bone, muscle and overlying tissues as revealed by studies of roentgenograms of the leg area. Monograph, Society of Research in hild Development, Vol. 26. Child Development Publications, Evanston, III.

Stuart HC, Kuhlmann D (1942). Studies of the physical characteristics of childred in Marseilles, France in 1941. J Pediat 20:424.

Tanner JM (1952). The effect of weight training on physique. Amer J Phys Anthrop 10:427.

Temple RS, Stonaker HH, Howry D, Posakony G, Hazaleus MH (1956). Ultrasonic and conductivity methods for estimating fat thickness in live cattle. Proc W Sect Amer Soc An Prod 7:477.

Tokunaga K, Matsuzawa Y, Ishikawa K, Tarui S (1983). A novel technique for the determination of body fat by computed tomography. Int J Obesity 7:437-45.

Vague J (1947). La différenciation sexuelle, facteur déterminant de formes de l'obésité. Presse méd 30:339.

Vague J (1953). La Différenciation Sexuella Humaine. Ses Incidences en Pathologie. Masson et Cie., Paris.

Vague J (1969). Physiology of Adipose Tissue. Excerpta Medica Foundation, Amsterdam.

Fat Distribution During Growth and Later Health Outcomes
pages 63–84 © 1988 Alan R. Liss, Inc.

SUBCUTANEOUS FAT DISTRIBUTION DURING GROWTH

Robert M. Malina and Claude Bouchard

Department of Anthropology, University of Texas,
Austin, Texas 78712 (R.M.M.), and Physical
Activity Sciences Laboratory, Laval University,
Ste-Foy, Quebec G1K 7P4, Canada (C.B.)

INTRODUCTION

Changes in the absolute and relative fat content of
the body begin prenatally and continue through postnatal
life. The distribution of fat in the body also changes,
but information on changes in the contribution of internal
(visceral or deep) and subcutaneous (outer) fat to fat mass
(FM) during growth is lacking. Variation among individuals
is probably considerable. While changes in the distribution of internal fat within the body during growth are not
known, skinfold thicknesses and fat widths on radiographs
have been used to document changes in the distribution of
subcutaneous fat. Both types of measurements include subcutaneous tissue plus skin. Computerized axial tomography
is very useful for the study of both internal and subcutaneous fat distribution. However, it requires a radiation
dose and application of CT procedures to large samples of
clinically normal children is unlikely at present.

In an early study, Reynolds (1950) reported an increase in the relative contribution of subcutaneous fat on the
trunk to the sum of fat widths at six radiographic sites
between 6 and 17 years of age. The increase occurred more
in males than females. In a factor analysis of skinfold
thicknesses in children between 2 and 18 years of age,
Hammond (1955) identified a factor which differentiated
between subcutaneous fat on the trunk and on the limbs.
Hammond also indicated different age-associated changes in
arm and trunk fat in boys, but not in girls during the
second decade.

Principal component analysis has recently been used to study the pattern of fat distribution during growth (Mueller and Reid, 1979; Ramirez and Mueller, 1980; Mueller and Wohlleb, 1981; Mueller, 1982; Cronk et al., 1983b; Deutsch et al., 1985; Baumgartner et al., 1986). Such analyses result in two major, and perhaps other components, depending on the specific skinfolds and the number of skinfolds which are included in the analysis. The first component relates to overall fatness, while the second distinguishes between subcutaneous fat on the extremities and trunk. The trunk-extremity component tends to decrease with age in males but not in females. A third component may differentiate between fat on the upper and lower extremities when the appropriate skinfolds are available.

Since the trunk-extremity and upper-lower extremity components are affected by overall fatness, the more recent analyses by Deutsch et al. (1985) and Baumgartner et al. (1986) have controlled for overall subcutaneous fatness by analyzing residuals of the regression of specific skinfolds (log transformed) on the mean skinfold thickness (log). The resulting components distinguish between trunk and extremity, between upper and lower trunk, and between arm and leg skinfold thicknesses, but the general fatness component is lost. The components relating to fatness on the upper and lower trunk and on the arm and leg vary, however, by sex and between Blacks and Whites. The trunk-extremity component also varies with maturity status in males but not in females.

Ratios based on triceps and subscapular skinfold · thicknesses have also been used to define relative fat distribution during growth (Bogin and MacVean, 1981; Frisancho and Flegel, 1982; Bailey et al., 1985). Analyses limited to two skinfolds, however, provide an incomplete and perhaps misleading view of fat distribution.

In order to provide a comprehensive overview of changes in the distribution of subcutaneous fat during growth, several perspectives are considered. These include the distribution of subcutaneous fat relative to FM; the distribution of subcutaneous fat on the extremeties and trunk, on the upper and lower aspects of the trunk, on the upper and lower extremities, and within the upper and lower extremities; and maturity-associated variation in fat distribution.

PROCEDURES

Data for this overview are derived primarily from three sources. The first is a cross-sectional sample of 501 French Canadian youth from the Quebec area, 260 boys and 241 girls 9 through 18 years of age. The data include densitometric estimates of FM and six skinfold thicknesses: triceps, biceps and medial calf on the extremities, and subscapular, suprailiac and abdominal on the trunk. The second is the mixed-longitudinal sample of children from the Harpenden Growth Study (Tanner, 1965, 1968; Tanner et al., 1981). The data include fat widths measured on standardized radiographs of the arm, calf and thigh. The arm and thigh were positioned laterally, and the calf was positioned antero-posteriorly for standardized radiographs (Tanner, 1965). Measurements of anterior and posterior arm and thigh subcutaneous fat widths, and medial and lateral calf subcutaneous fat widths permit evaluation of variation within segments of the upper and lower extremities. Except for the triceps and biceps skinfolds, skinfold data are generally not available for different aspects of limb segments. Sample sizes in half-yearly age groups vary from 40 to 183 for arm and calf measurements and from 23 to 122 for thigh measurements. Numbers of boys and girls below 5 years of age, and numbers of girls above 15 years of age are smaller.

Skinfold thicknesses for the mixed-longitudinal sample of children from the Denver area enrolled in the Child Research Council growth study were also used (R. W. McCammon, unpublished data reported in Malina and Roche, 1983). Age- and sex-specific half-yearly medians from 4.0 to 18.0 years of age are available for 10 skinfold thicknesses, including five on the extremities: triceps, biceps, forearm, medial thigh and medial calf, and five on the trunk: pectoral, subscapular, midaxillary, suprailiac and paraumbilical.

The three samples include boys and girls, and cover a broad age range during growth, excluding the first three years of life during which there are significant changes in subcutaneous fat. Data on subcutaneous fat distribution for this age group, however, are not extensive. The data are either limited to the triceps and subscapular skinfolds, or to skinfolds on one region of the body. Since changes in subcutaneous fat occur rather rapidly during the first two years of life, observations for narrow age inter-

vals are necessary. Half-year or whole-year age categories
are too broad to evaluate changes. An exception is the
data for a mixed-longitudinal sample of 1,119 clinically
normal Guatemalan children from four villages in which
mild-to-moderate undernutrition was endemic (Malina et al.,
1974). Skinfold thicknesses were measured at seven sites:
triceps, biceps, subscapular, midaxillary, anterior and
lateral thigh, posterior calf, at 15 specific age intervals
between 15 days and 7 years of age. Two trunk (subscapular
and midaxillary) and two extremity (triceps and posterior
calf) skinfolds were used to evaluate changes in subcutaneous fat distribution during infancy and early childhood.

There is no consensus as to which methods best define
and describe subcutaneous fat distribution during growth
(Roche et al., 1986). This survey thus utilizes ratios
based on skinfold thicknesses and fat widths measured on
standardized radiographs. Although ratios have limitations
(e.g., they assume the variables change in a linear manner
during growth), they are relatively simple and are useful
in surveys. Age- and sex-specific medians were computed
for subcutaneous fat measurements, sums of skinfold thicknesses, and various ratios in the samples from Quebec and
Harpenden. Sums of skinfolds in various combinations and
ratios of the sums were calculated from medians for the
Denver and Guatemalan samples.

ABSOLUTE AND RELATIVE FAT MASS (FM)

Absolute and relative FM increase gradually during
childhood in both sexes. After about 8 or 9 years of age
in girls, both increase at a more rapid pace which continues through adolescence. In boys, absolute FM increases
slowly with age through adolescence, and there does not
appear to be a significant decline at this time. Relative
fatness also increases in boys until the adolescent growth
spurt, when it gradually declines. Relative fatness
reaches its nadir in boys at about 16 or 17 years of age,
and then rises into young adulthood. The decline in relative fatness is due to the rapid growth of fat-free mass at
this time, while growth in FM is much slower. FM thus contributes a lesser percentage to body weight at this time.
There is, however, significant alteration in fat distribution during male adolescence.

Changes in body composition during adolescence are related to the timing of the growth spurt, which is most often viewed in the context of peak height velocity (PHV). Serial data for densitometric estimates of FM for 40 Czechoslovak boys followed from 10.7 through 17.7 years (Parizkova, 1976) indicate an increase of about 0.8 kg/yr at PHV and about 0.7 kg/yr if viewed for the year before and the year after PHV. Relative fatness declines by about -0.4%/yr for the years just before and after PHV. Estimates for cross-sectional data pooled from several sources indicate a gain of about 0.7 kg/yr in girls between 11 and 13 years and in boys between 13 and 15 years, while estimates for relative FM are +0.7%/yr in girls and -0.5%/yr in boys for these ages (Malina and Bouchard, unpublished).

FAT MASS AND SUBCUTANEOUS FAT

Estimates of FM in the two compartment model do not differentiate between internal and subcutaneous fat, and do not indicate regional variation in the distribution of fat. The ratio of the sum of a variety of skinfolds taken on several trunk and extremity sites to FM may provide an indirect estimate of the contribution of subcutaneous fat to FM (Figure 1). FM and subcutaneous fat increase with age from 9 through 18 years in girls, and from 9 through 13 in boys. FM changes only slightly between 14 and 17 years of age in boys, while subcutaneous fat declines gradually.

There is no sex difference in the ratio of the sum of six skinfolds to FM between 9 and 14 years of age. The ratio declines with age from 9 through 18 years in girls and from 9 through 13 years in boys. It subsequently increases with age in boys. FM apparently increases at a faster rate than subcutaneous fat during childhood; hence, the ratio declines. This trend continues through adolescence in girls. In contrast, the ratio tends to increase in boys after 14 years of age, which suggests a change in the relationship between subcutaneous fat and FM at this time. Similar trends are apparent in cross-sectional samples of Czechoslovak (Parizkova, 1977) and United States (Young et al., 1968; Forbes and Amirhakimi, 1970) children. The ratios, however, are calculated from reported means, and include different extremity and trunk skinfolds.

Changes in extremity and trunk skinfolds relative to FM are shown in Figure 2. There is no difference between

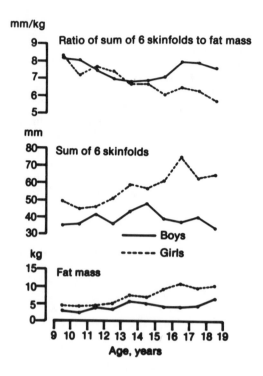

Figure 1. Medians for subcutaneous fat and fat mass, and the ratio of the two in Quebec youth.

the ratios of extremity or trunk skinfolds to FM in girls, especially after 12 years of age. The trend thus suggests that FM increases with age more than subcutaneous fat in girls, and that increases in subcutaneous fat on the extremity and trunk during childhood and adolescence are reasonably similar. In males, on the other hand, the ratio of trunk skinfolds to FM declines to about 13 years of age and then increases, while the ratio of extremity skinfolds to FM declines from 10 through 18 years of age. These trends thus suggest that males have proportionally more subcutaneous fat on the trunk relative to FM, and proportionally less subcutaneous fat on the extremities relative to FM during adolescence.

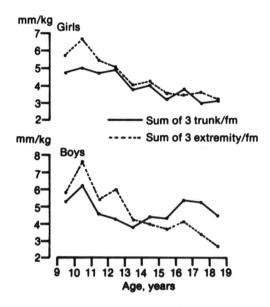

Figure 2. Median ratios of trunk and extremity skinfolds to fat mass in Quebec youth.

SUBCUTANEOUS FAT ON THE EXTREMITIES AND TRUNK

Subcutaneous fat thickness is greater on the extremities than on the trunk during infancy and early childhood. The ratio of trunk to extremity skinfolds decreases from 15 days to 6 months of age in Guatemalan infants as a function of two different trends. During the first three months of life, subcutaneous fat is gained more rapidly on the extremities than on the trunk, but over the next three months, fat thickness declines on the trunk but not on the extremities. Between 6 months and 4 years of age, the ratio of trunk to extremity skinfolds is rather stable, but then increases to 7 years of age as relatively more subcutaneous fat is lost on the extremities than on the trunk.

The sum of five extremity skinfolds is greater than that of five trunk skinfolds at all ages in Denver children, with the exception of 18 years in boys (Figure 3). Sex differences are greater for the sum of extremity skinfolds than for the sum of trunk skinfolds, especially

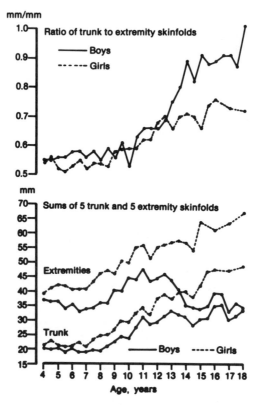

Figure 3. Sums and ratios of trunk and extremity skinfolds in Denver children (based on medians for each skinfold).

during adolescence. Thicknesses of both extremity and trunk skinfolds are reasonably stable between 4 and 7 years. After this age, both increase more or less linearly to 18 years in girls. In boys, on the other hand, trunk skinfolds increase to about 13 years, decline slightly through 14 years, and then increase in thickness through late adolescence. Extremity skinfolds increase to about 11 years and then decline after 12.5 years of age.

The ratio of trunk to extremity skinfolds is rather stable in both sexes during childhood and begins to rise after 8 to 9 years of age in girls and 9 to 10 years in boys. The ratio increases with age through male adolescence, but changes little after 12 or 13 years of age in girls. The rise in the ratio in males reflects two trends. Initially, more fat is gained on the trunk than on the extremities between about 10 and 13 years of age; hence, the ratio increases. This probably reflects the "preadolescent fat wave", which may be primarily a feature of subcutaneous fat on the trunk. Subsequently, subcutaneous fat thickness declines considerably on the extremities, while it declines to a slight degree and then increases slowly on the trunk. Thus, males have proportionally more subcutaneous fat on the trunk during adolescence. In girls, trunk fat also increases more than extremity fat prepubertally, i.e., between 8 and 12 years of age, but after this age, both trunk and extremity fat appear to accumulate at a reasonably similar pace.

Corresponding trends based on medians for three trunk and three extremity skinfolds in Quebec youth are shown in Figure 4. Age trends in the sums of skinfolds and ratios are similar to those for Denver children. The sum of extremity skinfolds is greater than that of trunk skinfolds in both sexes between 9 and 13 years. After this age there is no difference in the sums of extremity and trunk skinfolds in girls, while extremity skinfolds are thinner than trunk skinfolds in boys between 14 and 18 years. This trend is different from that observed in Denver children and probably reflects the skinfolds comprising the sums. A thigh skinfold was not measured in Quebec youth, while it contributes significantly to the increase in the sum of extremity skinfolds in the Denver youth.

The ratios of trunk to extremity skinfolds for the Denver (Figure 3) and Quebec (Figure 4) samples thus indicate a trend towards the accumulation of relatively more trunk subcutaneous fat in boys during adolescence. This trend is accentuated by a reduction in subcutaneous fat on the extremities at this time. Proportionally more trunk fat accumulates in girls during early adolescence, but subcutaneous fat on both the trunk and extremities subsequently increases at a similar pace. Hence, the ratio of trunk to extremity fat does not change appreciably as female adolescence progresses.

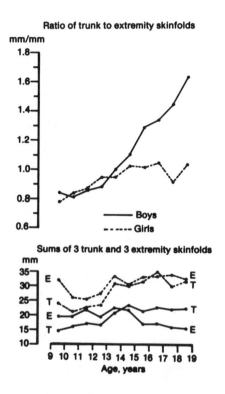

Figure 4. Median sums and ratios of trunk and extremity skinfolds in Quebec youth.

SUBCUTANEOUS FAT ON THE UPPER AND LOWER TRUNK

The sums of two upper trunk skinfolds (subscapular and pectoral) and two lower trunk skinfolds (paraumbilical and suprailiac), and their ratios in Denver children are shown in Figure 5. Sex differences are rather constant for both upper and lower trunk skinfolds during childhood. Between 11 and 18 years of age, the sum of the two upper trunk skinfolds changes only slightly in both sexes, while the sum of the two lower trunk skinfolds increases, more so in girls than in boys.

The ratio of upper to lower trunk skinfolds declines with age in both sexes. There are no sex differences in the ratio prior to adolescence, but after 13 years of age,

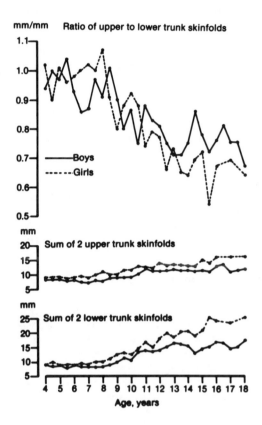

Figure 5. Sums and ratios of upper and lower trunk skinfolds in Denver children (based on medians for each skinfold).

the ratio is generally higher in boys. The decline in the ratio from childhood through adolescence in girls suggests that girls gain more in lower than in upper trunk subcutaneous fat during growth. Ratios calculated from the data of Young et al. (1968) for teen age and young adult females indicate a similar decline. The decline in the ratio in boys during childhood suggests that males also gain more in lower trunk subcutaneous fat at this time. However, during male adolescence, the ratio is more variable, perhaps reflecting differences in upper and lower trunk subcutaneous fat relative to the timing of the growth spurt.

The lower trunk skinfolds show a temporary decline
near the time of the height spurt in boys (approximately 14
years), while the upper trunk skinfolds do not. This is
consistent with longitudinal observations for approximately
280 Belgian boys. When the subscapular (upper trunk) and
suprailiac (lower trunk) skinfolds are related to PHV in
Belgian boys, different trends are evident. Estimated
velocities for the subscapular skinfold remain positive
through the growth spurt and do not vary relative to PHV.
Velocities for the suprailiac skinfold, in contrast, peak
about one year before PHV and then decline around the time
of PHV. The velocities for this lower trunk skinfold,
though declining, are still positive at PHV, but become
negative about 2.0 years after PHV (Beunen et al., 1988).
In a smaller sample of southwestern Ohio children (about 29
of each sex), on the other hand, mean increments for the
subscapular skinfold are negative just before and after PHV
in boys and just after PHV in girls (Cronk et al., 1983a).

SUBCUTANEOUS FAT ON THE UPPER AND LOWER EXTREMITIES

The sums of two upper extremity skinfolds (triceps and
forearm) and two lower extremity skinfolds (medial thigh
and medial calf), and their ratios in Denver children are
shown in Figure 6. The skinfolds were selected to represent the proximal and distal segments of the upper and
lower extremties. Girls gain more subcutaneous fat on the
lower than the upper extremity during growth. Boys appear
to gain more fat on the lower extremity during childhood,
but lose similar amounts on the upper and lower extremities
during adolescence. However, the loss of upper extremity
fat appears to occur earlier than the loss of lower extremity fat during male adolescence.

The ratio of upper to lower extremity subcutaneous fat
declines with age in boys and girls from 4 to 13 years and
there is no sex difference in the ratio. Thus, both sexes
gain more in lower extremity than in upper extermity subcutaneous fat during childhood and early adolescence. After
13 years, the ratio is reasonably stable in girls, which
suggests that girls gain proportionally in upper and lower
extremity fat at this time. On the other hand, the ratio
is more variable but generally lower in boys after 13 years
of age. The latter probably reflects variation in upper
and lower extremity subcutaneous fat loss relative to the
timing of the growth spurt. Among Belgian boys, velocities

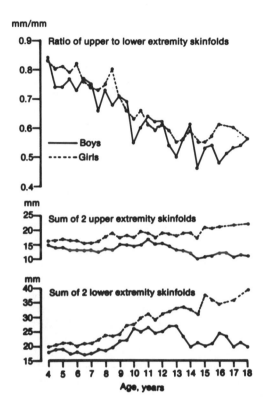

Figure 6. Sums and ratios of upper and lower extremity skinfolds in Denver children (based on medians for each skinfold).

of the triceps skinfold are positive until one year before PHV, and then become negative, reaching a maximum negative velocity about 1.5 years after PHV. Velocities subsequenly increase and eventually become positive. In contrast, velocities of the medial calf skinfold, though declining prior to PHV, approach zero at PHV, and then become negative, reaching a maximum negative velocity about 3.0 years after PHV (Beunen et al., 1988). Among British boys, the maximum negative velocity of upper arm subcutaneous fat (anterior + posterior fat widths) occurs coincidentally with PHV, while the maximum negative velocity of calf subcutaneous fat (medial + lateral fat widths) occurs about one-half of a year after PHV (Tanner et al., 1981).

VARIATION WITHIN THE UPPER AND LOWER EXTREMITIES

Anterior and posterior arm fat widths and the ratios of widths in children of the Harpenden Growth Study are shown in the upper part of Figure 7. There is no sex difference in the ratio of anterior to posterior arm fat during early childhood, but after 6 years of age, the ratio is higher in girls. The ratio declines from 4 to 8 years of age in boys, changes little to 15 years of age, and then declines in late adolescence. Although both anterior and posterior arm fat decline in thickness between 4 and 8 years, the decline is relatively greater on the anterior aspect of the arm; the ratio thus declines at this time. From 8 to 13 years of age, anterior and posterior arm fat change little in thickness, while both decline in thickness between 13 and 15.5 years of age. Changes in anterior and posterior arm fat are generally similar in magnitude so that the ratio of the two fat widths does not change appreciably between 8 and 15 years. In late adolescence, however, the ratio declines since posterior arm fat increases slightly while anterior fat is rather stable.

Among girls, the ratio of anterior to posterior arm fat is rather stable between 5 and 11.5 years, and then declines through adolescence. Girls gain slightly, though consistently, in both anterior and posterior arm fat during childhood; hence, the ratio is rather stable at this time. During adolescence, however, more subcutaneous fat accumulates on the posterior than the anterior aspect of the arm and the ratio thus declines.

Corresponding data for anterior and posterior thigh fat widths are shown in the lower part of Figure 7. Sex differences in thigh fat widths during childhood tend to be larger than those for arm fat widths, but are especially greater than those for arm fat in later adolescence. The ratio of anterior to posterior thigh fat increases in early childhood, and is reasonably stable between 7 and 11 years of age in both sexes. The ratio then declines to about 13 years in girls and to 16.5 years of age in boys.

Both anterior and posterior thigh fat decrease in thickness during early childhood, but the decline occurs

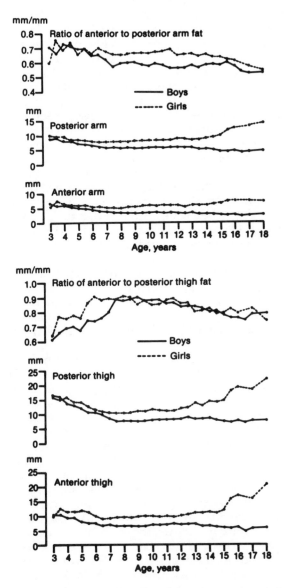

Figure 7. Median fat widths on the arm and thigh, and ratios of the widths in Harpenden children.

more posteriorly than anteriorly. Hence, the ratio increases at this time. Girls have relatively more anterior
than posterior thigh fat than boys between 4 and 7 years,
so that the ratio is higher in girls at this time. The
decline in thickness of posterior thigh fat continues to
7.5 years in boys, while the thickness of anterior fat is
rather stable. Hence, the ratio increases to 7.5 years in
boys, and there is no sex difference. During middle childhood, fat accumulates at about the same pace on both the
anterior and posterior aspects of the thigh, and the ratio
is rather stable. More fat accumulates posteriorly than
anteriorly between 11 and 13 years of age in girls, and the
ratio gradually declines at this time. After 13 years of
age, the ratio is once again rather stable in girls as posterior and anterior fat accumulate at about the same pace.
In boys, on the other hand, the ratio declines systematically from 11 through 16 years as the thickness of subcutaneous fat decreases more anteriorly than posteriorly.

Changes in medial and lateral calf fat widths are
shown in Figure 8. The ratio of lateral to medial fat is
greater in boys at all ages. The ratio increases during
early childhood in boys as lateral fat widths do not change
appreciably and medial fat widths decline in thickness.
The ratio changes slightly between 6 and 10.5 years of age,
and then declines systematically to 18 years. The rather
stable ratio in middle childhood reflects the negligible
changes in medial and lateral calf fat widths at this time.
Between 10 and 16 years of age, it appears that fat accumulates, though slightly, more on the medial aspect than on
the lateral aspect of the calf. Between 16 and 18 years,
fat thickness declines on both aspects of the calf, but the
decrease is slighlty greater on the lateral than on the
medial aspect of the calf. Thus, the ratio in males declines initially apparently as a result of slightly greater
accumulation of medial fat in early and mid-adolescence,
and then as a result of a slightly greater decrease in
lateral fat in later adolescence. The changes in medians,
however, are quite small. Lateral calf fat widths are, on
the average, greater than medial fat widths at all ages
between 3 and 15.5 years, i.e., the ratio is above 100.
Medial fat widths become slightly larger in late adolescence. In contrast, females gain more fat medially than
laterally after 6 years of age, and especially after 15
years of age. The ratio thus declines systematically with
age. Medial fat widths are, on the average, thicker than

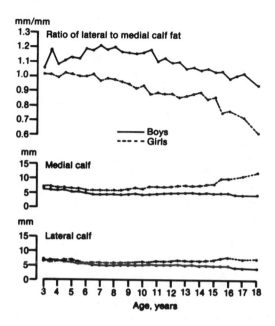

Figure 8. Median fat widths on the calf and ratios of the widths in Harpenden children.

lateral fat widths after 7 years of age.

The late adolescent accumulation of calf fat in girls is apparently a continuation of the trend established during the adolescent spurt. During the growth spurt in stature in girls, velocities of total calf fat widths (medial + lateral) are, on average, consistently positive. They decline about one-half of a year before and one-half of a year after PHV, but are still positive. Subsequently, velocities increase considerably to rates that are twice as large as those before PHV (Tanner et al., 1981).

MATURITY-ASSOCIATED VARIATION

Changes in the distribution of subcutaneous fat are related to the growth spurt and sexual maturity. Baumgartner et al. (1986), for example, noted an increase in the trunk-extremity principal component with stage of sexual maturation in males, but not in females. This trend re-

flects the simultaneous decrease in extremity skinfold
thicknesses and increase in trunk skinfold thicknesses as
males progress through sexual maturation.

The relationship among subcutaneous fat distribution,
FM and menarcheal status in the Quebec sample is shown in
Table 1. Girls were grouped as pre- and post-menarcheal,
and within each group, they were subdivided as younger and
older. It is assumed that the older pre-menarcheal (12.3
years) and the younger post-menarcheal (13.5 years) girls
are closer to menarche than the younger pre-menarcheal
(10.4 years) and older post-menarcheal (16.3 years) girls
respectively. Mean ages at menarche in the younger and
older subsamples are 12.2 ± 0.10 and 13.1 ± 0.09 years respectively. Although the data are cross-sectional, several
trends are apparent. First, the decline in the ratio of
subcutaneous fat to FM from the younger to older pre-
menarcheal girls suggests a relatively greater accumulation
of FM as menarche approaches, but not in subcutaneous fat.
This would imply a gain in internal fat at this time.
Second, when menarche occurs, there is no change in the
ratio of subcutaneous fat to FM, but there is a gain in FM
and subcutaneous fat, and a change in the distribution of
subcutaneous fat. Proportionally more fat accumulates on
the trunk than the extremities. Third, after menarche
occurs, girls gain in FM and subcutaneous fat, and have
proportionally more FM than subcutaneous fat, while the
relative distribution of subcutaneous fat on the trunk and
extremities changes only slightly.

The younger and older post-menarcheal girls can be
viewed as maturing at early and average ages. The two
groups do not differ in the relative distribution of subcutaneous fat on the trunk and extremities, but both have
more subcutaneous fat than the pre-menarcheal girls. These
observations are consistent with the results of Deutsch et
al. (1985). Early and late maturing 12 and 17 year old
girls differed only in overall subcutaneous fatness, and
not in the distribution of subcutaneous fat. Corresponding
data for 14 year old boys, in contrast, indicated relatively more subcutaneous fat on the trunk in early than in late
maturers.

Table 1. Fat mass and subcutaneous fat in pre- and
post-menarcheal girls from the Quebec sample (medians)

	Fat Mass (kg)	Sum of 6 Skinfolds (mm)	Sum of 6/ Fat Mass (mm/kg)
Pre-menarcheal:			
Younger (n=50)	6.9	48.9	7.70
Older (n=32)	7.1	46.3	6.83
Post-menarcheal:			
Younger (n=38)	8.7	61.4	6.96
Older (n=97)	11.0	67.2	6.17
	Sum of 3 Trunk (mm)	Sum of 3 Extremity (mm)	Trunk/ Extremity (mm/mm)
Pre-menarcheal:			
Younger	21.9	26.9	0.77
Older	20.7	25.5	0.83
Post-menarcheal:			
Younger	29.6	30.6	0.94
Older	32.7	35.0	0.97

SUMMARY

Assuming that the ratio of the sum of six skinfolds to
FM provides an estimate of the contribution of subcutaneous
fat to FM, FM increases at a faster rate than subcutaneous
fat during childhood in both sexes. This trend continues
through adolescence in girls, but the relationship between
subcutaneous fat and FM changes during male adolescence.
Relative to FM, males have proportionally more subcutaneous
fat on the trunk and proportionally less subcutaneous fat
on the extremities.

The ratio of trunk to extremity skinfolds declines
during infancy and is rather stable during childhood. Subsequent changes in the ratio indicates sex differences in
subcutaneous fat distribution at puberty. Males accumulate
relatively more fat on the trunk during adolescence, which
is accentuated by a reduction in subcutaneous fat on the
extremities at this time. Proportionally more subcutaneous
fat accumulates on the trunk during early adolescence in
girls, but subcutaneous fat on both the trunk and extremities then increases at a similar pace.

Girls gain more in lower than in upper trunk subcutaneous fat from childhood through adolescence. Boys also

gain more in lower trunk subcutaneous fat in childhood, but there is variation in upper and lower trunk fat which is related to the timing of the adolescent growth spurt.

Both sexes gain more in lower extremity than in upper extremity subcutaneous fat during childhood and early adolescence. During adolescence, girls gain proportionally in upper and lower extremity fat, while there is variation in upper and lower extremity fat loss relative to the timing of the growth spurt in boys.

Changes in anterior and posterior subcutaneous fat on the arm and thigh are generally similar during childood in both sexes. Girls gain proportionally more in posterior arm fat during adolescence. Girls also gain proportionally more in posterior thigh fat in early adolescence, but both anterior and posterior thigh fat subsequently accumulate at a similar pace. During male adolescence, both anterior and posterior arm fat decrease in thickness, while anterior thigh fat decreases more than posterior thigh fat. In late adolescence, arm fat increases relatively more posteriorly.

Females gain proportionally more subcutaneous fat on the medial aspect of the calf during growth and especially in late adolescence. Males, on the other hand, have proportionally more fat on the lateral aspect of the calf from childhood until late adolescence.

Changes in the ratio of subcutaneous fat to FM suggest a relatively greater accumulation of internal fat as menarche approaches. Early and late maturing girls do not differ in subcutaneous fat distribution, while early maturing boys have relatively more subcutaneous fat on the trunk than late maturing boys.

The preceding trends are based on group data. Given individual variation in subcutaneous fatness and amount of visceral fat, the apparent changes during growth may not occur in the same way in all individuals.

ACKNOWLEDGEMENTS

We thank Professor James M. Tanner of the Department of Growth and Development, Institute of Child Health, University of London, for generously providing the data on radiographic fat widths for children in the Harpenden

Growth Study. We also thank Professor Gaston Beunen of the
Institute of Physical Education, Catholic University of
Leuven, for generously providing the data for Belgian boys.
We gratefully acknowledge the assistance of Mr. Claude
Leblanc with computations for the Quebec data and of Mr.
Johan Lefevre with computations for the Belgian data.

REFERENCES

Bailey SM, Gershoff SN, McGandy RB, Nondasuta A, Tanti-
wongse P (1985). Subcutaneous fat remodelling in South-
east Asian infants and children. Am J Phys Anthropol
68:123-130.

Baumgartner RN, Roche AF, Guo S, Lohman T, Boileau RA,
Slaughter MH (1986). Adipose tissue distribution: the
stability of principal components by sex, ethnicity and
maturation stage. Human Biol 58:719-735.

Beunen G, Malina RM, Van't Hof MA, Simons J, Ostyn M,
Renson R, Van Gerven D (1988). "Physical Growth and
Motor Performance of Belgian Boys: A Longitudinal Study
between 12 and 19 Years of Age." Champaign, IL: Human
Kinetics Publishers (in press).

Bogin B, MacVean RB (1981). Nutritional and biological
determinants of body fat patterning in urban Guatemalan
children. Human Biol 53:259-268.

Cronk CE, Mukherjee D, Roche AF (1983a). Changes in triceps and subscapular skinfold thickness during adolescence. Human Biol 55:707-721.

Cronk, CE, Roche AF, Kent R, Eichorn D, McCammon RW
(1983b). Longitudinal trends in subcutaneous fat
thickness during adolescence. Am J Phys Anthropol
61:197-204.

Deutsch MI, Mueller WH, Malina RM (1985). Androgyny in fat
patterning is associated with obesity in adolescents and
young adults. Ann Human Biol 12:275-286.

Forbes GB, Amirhakimi GH (1970). Skinfold thickness and
body fat in children. Human Biol 42:401-418.

Frisancho AR, Flegel PN (1982). Advanced maturation associated with centripetal fat pattern. Human Biol 54:717-
727.

Hammond WH (1955). Measurement and interpretation of
subcutaneous fat, with norms for children and young adult
males. Br J Prev Soc Med 9:201-211.

McCammon RW, Unpublished data from the Child Research
Council, Denver, Co. In Malina RM, Roche AF (1983):

"Manual of Physical Status and Performance in Childhood," New York: Plenum, pp 315-420.

Malina RM, Habicht JP, Yarbrough C, Martorell R, Klein RE (1974). Skinfold thickness at seven sites in rural Guatemalan Ladino children birth through seven years of age. Human Biol 46:453-469.

Mueller WH (1982). The changes with age of the anatomical distribution of fat. Soc Sci Med 16:191-196.

Mueller WH, Reid RM (1979). A multivariate analysis of fatness and relative fat patterning. Am J Phys Anthrop 50:199-208.

Mueller WH, Wohlleb JC (1981). Anatomical distribution of subcutaneous fat and its description by multivariate methods: how valid are principal components? Am J Phys Anthropol 54:25-35.

Parizkova J (1976). Growth and growth velocity of lean body mass and fat in adolescent boys. Pediat Res 10:647-650.

Parizkova J (1977). "Body Fat and Physical Fitness." The Hague: Martinus Nijhoff.

Ramirez ME, Mueller WH (1980). The development of obesity and fat patterning in Tokelau children. Human Biol 52:675-687.

Reynolds EL (1950). The distribution of subcutaneous fat in childhood and adolescence. Mon Soc Res Child Dev 15 (2):serial no 50.

Roche AF, Baumgartner RN, Guo S (1986). Population methods: anthropometry or estimations. In Norgan NG (ed): "Human Body Composition and Fat Distribution," Wageningen: Stichting Nederlands Instituut voor de Voeding (Euro-Nut Report 8), pp 31-47.

Tanner JM (1965). Radiographic studies of body composition. In Brozek J (ed): "Human Body Composition," Oxford: Pergamon Press, pp 211-236.

Tanner JM (1968). Growth of bone, muscle and fat during childhood and adolescence. In Lodge GE (ed): "Growth and Development of Mammals," London: Butterworth, pp 3-18.

Tanner JM, Hughes PCR, Whitehouse RH (1981). Radiographically determined widths of bone, muscle and fat in the upper arm and calf from age 3-18 years. Ann Human Biol 8:495-517.

Young CM, Sipin SS, Roe DA (1968). Body composition of pre-adolescent and adolescent girls. I. Density and skinfold measurements. J Am Dietet Assoc 53:25-31.

Fat Distribution During Growth and Later Health Outcomes
pages 85–102 © 1988 Alan R. Liss, Inc.

SEX DIFFERENCES IN FAT PATTERNING IN CHILDREN AND YOUTH

Francis E. Johnston

Department of Anthropology
University of Pennsylvania
Philadelphia, PA   19104-6398

Although the description of variation in the patterning of subcutaneous fat distribution reaches some 50 years back into the literature, the increase in interest in the past 10 years has been enormous. Not only is this variation of concern to those who deal with human morphology, it is also significant to researchers and clinicians in the health sciences as well. It requires only a cursory examination of recent journals and books to see just how completely the topic has been incorporated into the interests of those who study body composition and its implications for human health.

Despite the foregoing, there are still a number of areas in which we have but little knowledge of fat patterning and its significance. One of these areas concerns the growing years, when children and youth move through those developmental changes which culminate in adulthood. It is known that there are significant correlations of fatness levels of either children or adolescents and of those same individuals as adults. Garn (1985) has noted that, from 5 years of age on, skinfold thickness is correlated with the thickness some two decades later. However these correlations, even while significant, are rather low, ranging from 0.2 in children throuth 0.4 in adolescents, and have no real predictive power in individuals.

The same holds true for overweight in childhood as a risk factor for later obesity. While the relative risk falls between 1.0 and 2.0, the majority of overweight one-year olds display normal levels of fatness as adolescents and adults (Johnston, 1985).

Even less is known of both the existence and extent of fat patterning during the growing years, to say nothing of its persistence in individuals into adulthood. In one of the earliest papers on the subject, Garn (1955) demonstrated the maintenance of patterns of fat deposition in adult men following food restriction. Figures 1 and 2 illustrate this phenomenon in 78 obese women who had undergone a controlled evaluation of diet and behavior therapy in promoting weight loss (Johnston et al, 1987; Wadden et al, 1987). Patterns were elicited from extraction of principal components from a matrix of body circumferences, after adjusting for initial

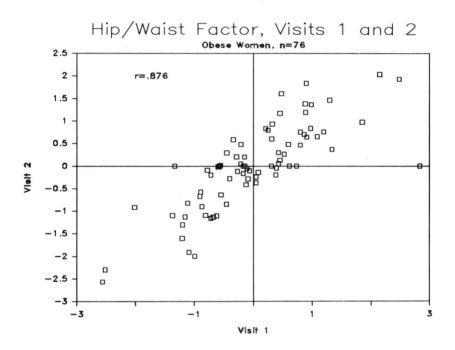

Figure 1. Individual scores for the upper/lower trunk component in obese women before and after weight loss.

fatness. Figure 1 shows the relationship between the pre- and post-treatment scores for the component differentiating between upper and lower body obesity. Even while losing an average of 12.2 kg of weight and 8.9 kg of fat, the correlation of the upper/lower score was .878. Figure 2 presents the scattergram for the other significant principal component,

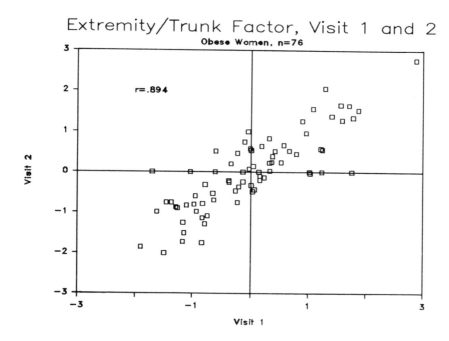

Figure 2. Individual scores for the extremity/trunk component in obese women before and after weight loss.

a trunk/extremity pattern. The correlation is 0.894.

Thus, while it seems that the patterning of subcutaneous adipose tissue over the body is, among adults at least, an individualized characteristic that is resistant to marked reductions in weight, the extent of any tracking of the patterns through childhood and adolescence into the adult years is less clear. Equally uncertain is the timing of appearance of adult patterns. Do they become visible in childhood and persist throughout growth or do they arise during adolescence along with the other changes in body composition which occur at that time?

The remainder of this paper will focus upon fat patterning during the years of growth. In particular, the emphasis will be upon differences between males and females in the expression and development of fat patterns during development.

SEX DIFFERENCES IN FATNESS DURING GROWTH

Differences between males and females in fatness levels during growth represent one of the clearest examples we have of human sexual dimorphism. In contrast to other measurements such as height and weight, females show consistently greater values for fatness at all ages than do males. Significant differences exist even at birth. In a sample of 196 newborns, Johnston and Beller (1976) found that the mean thickness of the triceps skinfold was significantly greater in females than in males. The female subscapular mean was also greater than that of males, but the difference was not statistically significant.

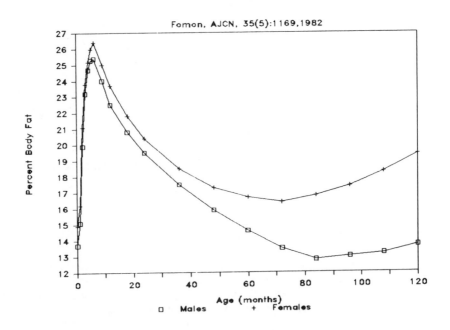

Figure 3. Percentage body fat of reference boys and girls (data from Fomon).

Figure 3 gives the percentage body fat of reference

children, by sex, from birth through 10 years of age (Fomon, 1982). The pattern of change, as indicated by the means, is the same for boys and girls, with an initial rise in relative fatness, followed by a steady decline into mid-childhood; the subsequent rise signals the entry into the adolescent years. At the same time there is a consistent sex difference, females being fatter at every age. The differences range from about 1% in the first year of life to 6% by age 10. Not only do these results persist into adolescence, they intensify near the end of that age period. The percent body fat of females displays a modest increase from 9 to 18, but the sexual dimorphism is heightened by a dramatic decrease in males, beginning at 12 and amounting to almost 50% (Forbes, 1972).

The pattern of sexual dimorphism in whole body fatness is paralleled by data on skinfold thicknesses. Females show greater thickness at virtually every site with sex differences becoming accentuated in upper and lower limb skinfolds in adolescence, again due to the decrease in those of males (Malina and Roche, 1983).

THE DELINEATION OF FAT PATTERNS DURING GROWTH

Where studied, the delineation of fat patterns of children and youth has utilized the same analytic methods as have studies among adults. Two general spproaches have been followed. The first employs essentially a bivariate approach with relationships between individual dimensions, such as ratios of skinfolds and/or circumferences. This approach is methodologically the more simple and uses individual measurements which are more easily grasped than are the constructs yielded by multivariate analyses. Multivariate approaches utilize the relationships among variables to develop clusters which, in theory, yield more information than do univariate or bivariate analyses.

Multivariate analyses based upon a sufficient number of variables and upon large enough samples suggest, that among adults, there are two basic components of adipose tissue distribution: a component which contrasts trunk and extremity fat deposition, and another which contrasts upper and lower trunk fat deposition (Mueller and Wohllweb, 1981; Baumgartner et al, 1986). These components are detected whether or not the investigators use skinfolds or circumferences

(Mueller and Malina, 1987; Johnston et al, 1987). Furthermore, Mueller and Stallones (1981) have suggested that as
few as two skinfolds may be used to represent the trunk/ex-
tremity component, while other investigators have used the
waist and hip circumferences to predict the upper/lower body
component. In a recent paper, Baumgartner and his colleagues
(1986) have analyzed the stability of these principal components across sex, race, and maturation stage. They caution
that, while particular patterns may be statistically significant in specific data sets, stability across a range of
samples seems to exist only for the trunk/extremity pattern.

SEX DIFFERENCES IN FAT PATTERNING IN NEONATES

Fat patterning has not been studied yet in early infancy and truly appropriate data sets may not exist at this
time. Table 1 presents the variance in triceps/subscapular

Table 1. Variance of differences of standard scores of sub-
scapular-triceps skinfold in neonates and teenagers. (Standardized to mean of 50 and s.d. of 10, within group, sexes
combined.)

Group	Male		Female	
	n	Var	n	Var
Neonates	96	39.25	100	51.52
Teenagers	222	33.32	103	48.80

patterning in two samples, one neonatal and the other adolescent. The neonatal sample consisted of 196 infants examined
in the nurseries of two Philadelphia hospitals within 4 days
after birth. The infants were black, white, and Puerto Rican
(Johnston and Beller, 1976). The teenage sample, presented
as an age contrast, was composed of 12 to 17 year olds from
Philadelphia and Minneapolis. Within each sample, skinfold
thicknesses were standardized to means of 50 and standard
deviations of 10, sexes combined. Following the suggestion
of Mueller and Stallones (1981), the standard score for triceps was subtracted from the score for subscapular as an
index of extremity/trunk patterning. While it is true that
the triceps and subscapular sites may not the best for char-

acterizing the extremity/trunk pattern, data on leg skinfolds of infants are rare.

The variances of the differences in the standard scores of neonates are just as great as they are in 12 to 17 year olds. Furthermore, the variances of females are higher than are those of males; however, the sex differences are not statistically significant. Thus, looking at relative values, (standard scores), the intensity of trunk/extremity patterning in newborns is as great as it is in teenagers; furthermore, there is no difference in degree of patterning between male and female neonates.

Table 2. Race-adjusted means and standard errors of measures of fat patterning in neonates.
(n - 96 males, 100 females)*

Measure	Males	Females
Subscapular - Triceps **	0.766	-0.735
Centripetal Fat Ratio ***	0.485	0.475

* Sex differences not significant
** Differences in standard scores
*** (Subscapular) / (Subscapular + Triceps)

Table 2 presents data from the neonatal sample on two measures of trunk/extremity patterning. The first is the mean difference between the standard scores of subscapular and triceps and the second is usually referred to as the centripetal fat ratio. As with other investigators, the ratio has been calculated using the raw unstandardized skinfold thicknesses, There is no difference between males and females in either the difference between standard scores or in the centripetal fat ratios, the probability levels falling between .10 and .15. However, the direction of the differences suggests that newborn males have more fat at the subscapular site and less at the triceps than do females.

Measures of fat patterning in a sample of 326 youth from 12 to 17 years, from Philadelphia and Minneapolis may be seen in Figure 4. The figure shows the mean differences

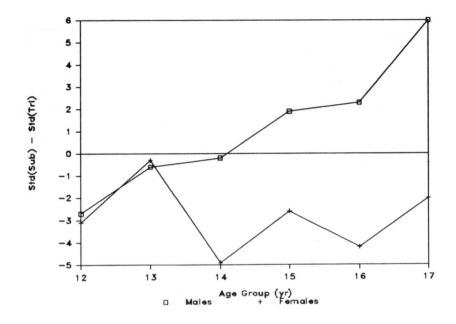

Figure 4. Triceps/subscapular patterning in 12-17 year olds.

in the standard scores (mean=50, SD=10) of the subscapular
and triceps skinfolds by age group and by sex. The standard
scores were calculated for each skinfold with age and sex
combined. The changes and differences in extremity/trunk
fat patterning in this age range are well known and have been
discussed by many other investigators. Males show a steady
redistribution of fat, as relatively more is stored on their
trunks and relatively less on their extremities. No clear
pattern is seen in females; the fluctuation in female means
probably represents the fact that their sample size in 103,
less than half that of the males, distributed over 6 age
groups. The age-adjusted sex difference in triceps/subscap-
ular patterning is significant at the probability of less
than .0001. These data, along with those of other investigators, indicate that sex differences in trunk/extremity fat
patterning develop during the teenage period. Males increasingly store relatively less fat on their arms than their

trunks, while females display a general continuity of pattern.

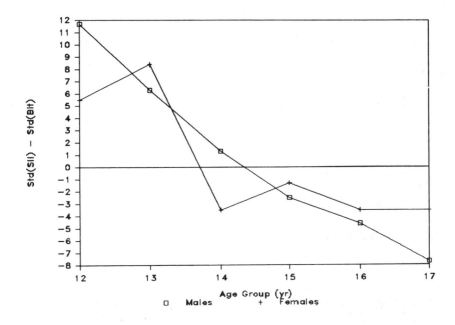

Figure 5.   Upper/lower trunk patterning in 12-17 year olds.

        Figure 5 presents an analysis of upper/lower trunk pat-
terning in the 12-17 year old sample. For a measure of upper
trunk fatness the thickness of the suprailiac skinfold was
used. For the lower trunk, the bitrochanter breadth was
employed. Bitrochanteric breadth was chosen because, in a
subsample of the subjects where both measurements were available, the age-adjusted correlation of bitrochanteric breadth
and hip circumference was +0.86. As before, measurements
were standardized to means of 50 and standard deviations of
10, age and sex combined.

        Again there is less regularity in the female curve per-
haps due to their smaller numbers. However, in both sexes,
there is a relative redistribution of fat from the upper to
the lower body with increasing age. The differences between
the sexes, adjusted for age, are not significant. However,

in the 15, 16, and 17 year groups, the mean differences are greater in females than males, suggesting greater lower body patterning in the latter half of the teens.

The data on fat patterning presented so far deal with neonates and adolescents and, where comparable information is available, are consistent with that information. For patterning during childhood, we may examine the 1951 longitudinal analysis by Reynolds of 88 males and 88 females from the Fels Institute study (Reynolds, 1951). He measured fat thickness on 8 radiographs per examination over an average of 6 examinations per subject spanning the age range of 6 through 17 years, a total of 1066 examinations and over 8500 x-rays. Figure 6 presents the mean relative fat breadth at the waist; each mean is expressed as a percentage of the sum of six breadths for an individual taken at the calf, trochanter, waist, chest, forearm, and deltoid sites.

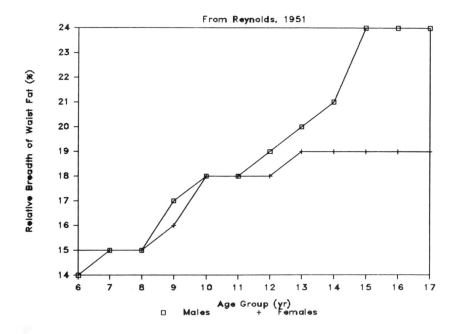

Figure 6. Mean fat breadth at the waist as a percentage of the total breadth at 6 sites (radiographic data, taken from Reynolds, 1951).

Relative waist fat shows no sex difference until age 10. However, from 10 through 17, female means level off, while those for males continue to increase until 15. In other words, during childhood and adolescence, fatness in males becomes steadily concentrated in the abdominal region, at the expense of fat in the extremities. 'In females, there is an increase in the percentage of waist fat, but only up to the adolescent years, when the mean relative breadth levels off.

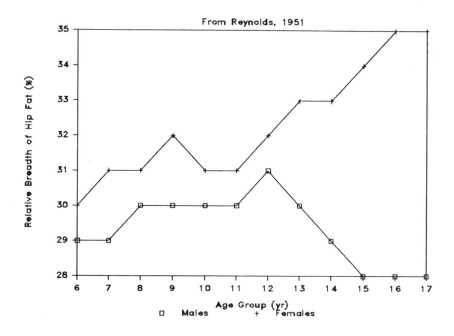

Figure 7. Mean fat breadth at the trochanters as a percentage of the total breadth at 6 sites (radiographic data, taken from Reynolds, 1951).

Figure 7 presents Reynolds' data for relative fat at the trochanter level. The picture differs from the previous one for the waist. Females have higher relative breadths of hip fat than do males from 6 years on. The relative breadths in females increase steadily through 18 years as increasingly more fat becomes concentrated there. Male relative breadths increase through childhood decreasing from 12-15, and then leveling off.

As figures 8 and 9 indicate, these data are generally consistent with waist/hip ratios of means from an early 16-state survey (O'Brien, 1941, reported by Martin, 1953) as well as from Cycle II of the US Health Examination Survey (Malina, 1973).

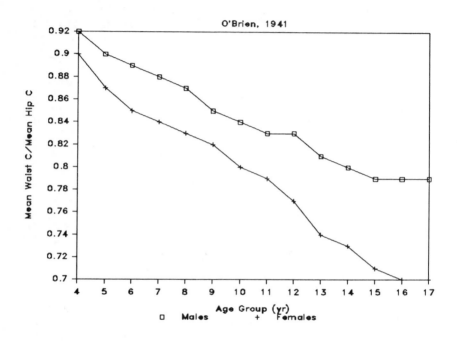

Figure 8. Waist/hip ratios, derived from means. of American children and youth in the 1930's (data from O'Brien, 1941).

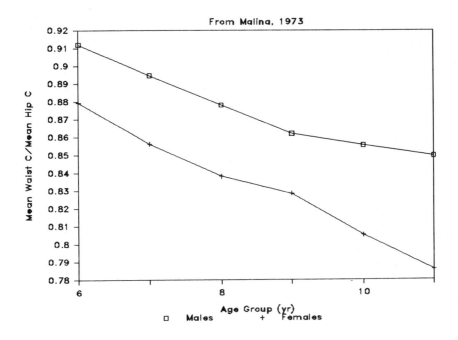

Figure 9. Waist/hip ratios, derived from means, of American children in the 1970's (data from HES, Cycle II, Malina 1973).

Summarizing the above, the tendency for concentration of fat in the abdomens of males and the hips of females is seen at least as early as 4 years, with this sex difference becoming marked during adolescence. Thus sexual dimorphism in waist and hip fat is related both to growth gradients in childhood and to intensification of these gradients during adolescence.

Sex differences in the development of trunk/extremity patterning are not seen during childhood to any great extent. However, the loss of fat in the extremities of males during adolescence results in the sexual dimorphism noted among adults. Figure 10 presents the centripetal fat ratios in two samples of teenagers. The first sample, labelled white, consists of the Philadelphia and Minneapolis youth already described. The second sample is mixed longitudinal and is

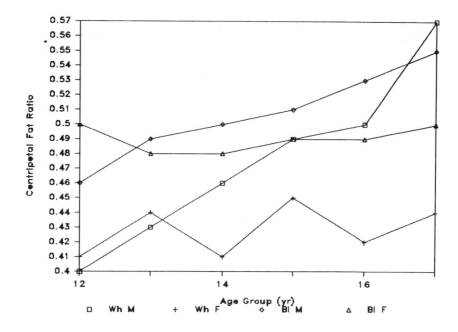

Figure 10. Centripetal fat ratios in black and white adolescents (black data from Valleroy, 1987).

comprised of black youths analyzed by Valleroy (1987) consisting of 862 examinations of males and 789 of females.

Similar patterns of sexual dimorphism are seen in both the black and white samples. Centripetal fat ratios increase in males throughout adolescence as a result of the decrease in triceps skinfold thickness. The ratios change little if at all in females. This provides further evidence that sex differences in trunk/extremity patterning is primarily an adolescent phenomenon.

The data of Figure 10 raise another issue relative to sex differences in trunk/extremity patterning. Except for 17 years in males, mean centripetal ratios are higher in blacks than in whites of the same age and sex; i.e. there is more fat on the subscapular, relative to the triceps, in blacks. Bogin and Sullivan (1986) recently published their analysis of triceps and subscapular patterning in Guatemalan children of upper and lower SES. They found that patterning was dependent upon socioeconomic status. Upper SES children showed greater sexual dimorphism in triceps/subscapular patterning, after adjusting for overall fatness, than did lower SES children. Furthermore, lower SES children had greater subscapular fat deposits, relative to the triceps, than did upper SES children.

If we assume a socioeconomic difference between the black and white samples, then Bogin and Sullivan's findings may be relevant to the race differences seen in Figure 8. The black sample has greater deposits of fat on the triceps, as represented by higher centripetal ratios than do whites of the same age and sex. And, from 13 on, the sexual dimorphism in whites is greater than that of blacks. Since there are ethnic differences in the black/white comparison as well, we cannot rule out possible genetic factors. However, regardless of the cause, sexual dimorphism in fat patterning is affected by mechanisms which operate across populations as well as within individuals. This phenomenon needs to be examined further, especially with reference to upper/lower trunk patterning. Since upper/lower body fatness is related in adults to disease risk, the possibility that socioeconomic factors may affect the degree of patterning could have important implications for public health.

DISCUSSION

Two generally consistent patterns of subcutaneous fat distribution have been described in the literature. The first contrasts fat on the trunk and on the extremity and the second contrasts fat deposited on the upper and on the lower trunk. In adults, fat patterns, especially those associated with gender, are increasingly implicated in study of disease risk, in particular with increasing degrees of obesity (e.g., Vague, 1956; Kissebah, et al, 1982; Lapidus et al, 1984; Larsson, 1984).

The genesis of adult fat patterning lies in the growing years of childhood. However, because the interest in the health implications of differential deposition of subcutaneous fat is relatively recent, studies which analyze and describe the development and persistence of fat patterns through the

growing years and into adulthood are lacking. From the neonatal data presented here, it seems that there is as much
individual variability in fat deposition at different sites
as there is among adolescents, even after correcting for
initial fatness. This suggests that individual infants
differ in relative fat deposition. However, no firm
conclusions can be drawn as to sex differences.

In summary, then, the fat patterns identified in adults
extend back into the years of childhood. Sex differences
in trunk/extremity fatness appear primarily at adolescence
as males lose extremity fat. Differences in upper/lower
trunk patterning are found as early as 4 years, becoming
more marked at adolescence as males show an increase in
abdominal fat and females in fat thickness at the hip.
Since these patterns are, in adults, indicators of risk,
investigations which seek to understand the development of
that risk must begin with understanding the role of growth
in populations and individuals in contributing to adult
patterns of fat deposition.

REFERENCES

Baumgartner RN, Roche AF, Guo S, Lohman T, Boileau RA,
    Slaughter MH (1986). Adipose tissue distribution: the
    stability of principal components by sex, ethnicity, and
    maturation stage. Hum Biol 58:719-736.
Bogin B, Sullivan T (1986). Socioeconomic status, sex, age,
    and ethnicity as determinants of body fat distribution for
    Guatemalan children. Am J Phys Anthropol 69:527-536.
Fomon SJ, Haschke F, Zeigler EE, Nelson SE (1982). Body
    composition of reference children from birth to age 10
    years. Am J Clin Nutr 35:1169-1175.
Forbes GB (1972). Growth of lean body mass in man. Growth
    36:325-338.
Garn SM (1955). Relative fat patterning: an individual
    characteristic. Hum Biol 27:77-89.
Garn SM (1985). Continuities and changes in fatness from
    infancy through adulthood. Curr Prob in Pediat 15:3-47.
Johnston FE (1985). Health implications of childhood obesity.
    Ann Int Med 103:1068-1072.
Johnston FE, Beller A (1976). Anthropometric evaluation of
    the body composition of black, white, and Puerto Rican
    newborns. Am J Clin Nutr 29:61-65.
Johnston FE, Hamill PVV, Lemeshow S (1974). Skinfold thick-

ness in a national probability sample of US males and
females 6 through 17 years. Am J Phys Anthropol 40:321-324.
Johnston FE, Wadden TA, Stunkard AJ, Pena M, Wang J, Pierson
R, Van Itallie T (1977). Body fat deposition in adult
obese women. Part I Patterns of fat distribution. Am J
Clin Nutr, in press.
Kissebah AH, Vydelingum N, Murray R (1982). The relation of
body fat distribution to metabolic complications of obesity.
J Clin Endocrin Metab 45:254-260.
Lapidus L, Bengstonn C, Larsson B, Pennert K, Rybo E,
Sjostrom L (1984). Distribution of adipose tissue and
risk of cardiovascular disease and death: a 12 year follow-
up of participants in the population study of women in
Gothenburg, Sweden. Brit Med J 289:1257-1261.
Larsson B, Svardsudd K, Welin L, Wilhelmsen L, Bjorntorp P,
Tibblin G (1984). Abdominal adipose tissue distribution,
obesity, and risk of cardiovascular disease and death: 13
year followup of participants in the study of men born in
1913. Brit Med J 288:1401-1404.
Malina RM (1973). Selected body measurements of children
6-11 years old. United States DHEW Pub (HSM) 73-1605.
Washington DC: US Govt Print Off.
Malina RM, Roche AF (1983). "Manual of Physical Status and
Performance in Childhood, Vol 2, Physical Performance."
New York: Plenum.
Martin WE (1953). Basic body measurements of school age
children. Off of Educ, US Dept Health, Educ, Welfare.
Washington DC: US Govt Print Off.
Mueller WH, Stallones L (1981) Anatomical distribution of
subcutaneous fat: skinfold site choice and construction of
indices. Hum Biol 53:321-336.
Mueller WH, Wohlleb JC (1981). Anatomical distribution of
subcutaneous fat and its distribution by multivariate
methods: how valid are principal components? Am J Phys
Anthropol 54:25-36.
Mueller WH, Malina RM (1987). Relative reliability of circumferences and skinfolds as measures of body fat distribution. Am J Phys Anthropol 72:437-440.
O'Brien RG, Girschick MA, Hunt EP (1941). Body measurements
of American boys and girls for garment and pattern construction. Bur Home Econ, Misc Pub No 366. Washington DC:
US Dept Agric.
Reynolds EL (1951). The distribution of subcutaneous fat in
childhood and adolescence. Monog Soc Res Child Dev 15(2).
Vague J (1956). The degree of masculine differention of
obesities: a factor determining predisposition to diabetes,

atherosclerosis, gout, and uric calculus disease. Amer J Clin Nutr 4:20-34.

Valleroy LA (1987). Blood pressure and body size, body composition, and subcutaneous fat in black American adolescents. PhD Diss in Anthropology, U of Penna, Philadelphia.

Wadden TA, Stunkard AJ, Johnston FE, Wang J, Pierson RN, Van Itallie TB, Costello E, Pena M (1987). Body fat deposition in adult obese women. Part II Changes in fat distribution accompanying weight reduction. Am J Clin Nutr, in press.

Fat Distribution During Growth and Later Health Outcomes
pages 103–125 © 1988 Alan R. Liss, Inc.

INHERITANCE OF HUMAN FAT DISTRIBUTION

Claude Bouchard

Physical Activity Sciences Laboratory,
Laval University, Ste-Foy
Quebec, G1K 7P4   Canada

This paper will attempt to delineate the contribution of the genotype in human fat distribution. Two
kinds of genetic effects will be primarily considered,
namely the additive genetic effect and the geno-
type-environment interaction (GxE) effect. The additive
genetic effect will be estimated from family data encom-
passing several kinds of biological relatives and relatives by adoption. The GxE effect will be studied under
the influence of short-term and long-term exposure to
overfeeding using several pairs of young adult male
identical twins.

Several phenotypes will be considered in this
paper. First, a review of our research on the additive
genetic effect and the GxE effect for total body fat will
be presented. Second, the same genetic effects will be
considered for several commonly used and newly derived
indicators of fat distribution. Third, the size of the
additive genetic effect will be estimated for the main
principal component scores obtained from six individual
skinfolds so that one can also have an idea about the
role of the genotype in subcutaneous fat patterning. In
these cases, the analyses will be reported for the data
unadjusted and adjusted for total fatness.

TOTAL BODY FAT

In an attempt to understand the importance of the
genetic effects in total body fat, the following pheno-

types are retained: body mass, body mass index (weight in kg divided by height in m²), percent body fat, fat mass in kg and the sum of 6 skinfolds (biceps, triceps, medial calf, subscapular, suprailiac and abdominal) as a surrogate variable for total subcutaneous fat. These phenotypes were measured in a maximum of 1698 individuals from 409 families of French descent from the Quebec city area (Bouchard, 1985, Bouchard and Tremblay, 1985, Bouchard et al., 1985).

One indication about the role of heredity is provided by the comparison of correlations computed in sets of foster midparent - adopted child versus those in sets of midparent - natural child. Such data are presented in table 1 for the variables of interest. They suggest that body mass and subcutaneous fat are little affected by genes inherited from the biological parents while the percent fat and fat mass correlation pattern is more compatible with a significant biological inheritance component.

TABLE 1. Midparent-child correlation for body weight and total fatness[a]

Variable	Foster midparent-Adpted child (N = 154 units)	Midparent-Natural child (N = 622 units)
Body weight	0.24*	0.34**
Body mass index	0.29**	0.30**
Percent fat $(\log_{10})$[b]	0.14	0.37**
Fat mass[b]	0.20*	0.36**
Sum 6 skinfolds $(\log_{10})$	0.36**	0.31**

[a] Adapted from Bouchard, 1985, Bouchard et al., in press. Scores were adjusted for age and gender effects by generation.

[b] For those variables, N is 111 and 242 units, respectively

* $P \leq 0.05$;   ** $P \leq 0.01$

Genetic epidemiologist have developed several methods to estimate the additive genetic effect from data gathered on several kinds of biological relatives and relatives by adoption. One approach is to use a path analysis procedure specially designed to estimate the biological inheritance component and other relevant parameters for quantitative traits such as body fat. We have applied one of these methods, the BETA path analysis model (Cloninger et al., 1979), to data that were gathered in our laboratory in 9 kinds of relatives. Some of the results have been summarized in table 2. Briefly, data indicate that although the total transmissible variance between generation is quite significant ($37\% \leq t^2 \leq 55$), most of this transmission is not genetics. Data indicate that the genetic effect reaches about 10% for BMI, 20% for body fat but almost zero for subcutaneous fat.

Let us now turn our attention to a special genetic effect, one that is often known as the genotype (G) and environment (E) interaction effect or GxE. The GxE effect results from the fact that all individuals (or genotypes) do not respond similarly to changes in E. In the present report, we ask whether such a GxE component exists for body fat when energy balance is systematically manipulated. In other words, are there innate differences in the sensitivity to a positive or a negative energy balance. We believe there are as suggested by the study briefly reviewed below.

In our laboratory, Poehlman et al. (1986) submitted 6 pairs of male MZ twins (i.e. only a maximum of 6 genotypes were tested) to a 1000 kcal/day overfeeding stress for a period of 22 consecutive days. Data indicate that adaptation to caloric affluence in terms of fat deposition differs between genotypes but is significantly similar in members of the same MZ pair (table 3). Subjects gained weight and fat with overfeeding, but there were considerable inter-individual differences in the changes observed. However, these changes were not randomly distributed as indicated by the presence of significant genotype-overfeeding interactions. Intrapair resemblance in the response to overfeeding was consistently high as revealed by the intraclass coefficients.

TABLE 2. Total transmissible variance and its additive genetic component for several indicators of total fat mass [a) b)]

	Transmissible variance (t^2)	Biological inheritance (h^2)	Cultural inheritance (b^2)	$X^2(p)$
Body weight	.37	.14	.21	10.2 (< 0.01)
Body mass index	.40	.09	.28	2.62 (< 0.50)
Percent fat	.55	.22	.31	2.07 (< 0.50)
Fat mass	.48	.15	.32	2.77 (< 0.25)
Sum of 6 skinfolds	.37	.02	.35	6.84 (< 0.05)

a) t^2, h^2 and b^2 were obtained with the BETA path analysis model. Only the data of the full solution model are reported.

b) Adapted from Bouchard, 1985, Bouchard et al., in press.

For instance, the 0.90 intraclass correlation for changes in percent fat implies that about 90% of the variance in the response is between genotypes, while only about 10% of the variance can be found within pairs. These data suggest that fat deposition in response to caloric affluence is largely determined by the genotype. In other words, there is a GxE effect when exposed to a positive energy balance and some individuals are more at risk than others to deposit fat.

FAT DISTRIBUTION

To evaluate the relative importance of inherited characteristics on body fat distribution, several analytical strategies will be used. The absolute size of various skinfolds, the ratio of trunk to extremity skinfolds, and the ratio of subcutaneous fat to total fat mass will be considered. The effects of age, gender and heaviness or fatness on these markers of fat distribution are described in table 4 for children and adolescents and table 5 for adults. These data clearly show that when age, gender and fatness or heaviness are controlled, the individual differences in absolute skinfold values are rather small. This is particularly true when one considers the residuals of age, gender and the sum of all six skinfolds. In this case, only about 15 to 20 percent of the variance in children and 20 to 30% of the variance in adults are unaccounted for. While these unexplained variances are still quite important by themselves, they nevertheless reveal that the problem of fat distribution needs to be considered in the context of the total level of fatness of the individual.

There are also two important ratios in tables 4 and 5, namely the ratio of the trunk skinfolds (sum of subscapular, suprailiac and abdominal) to the extremity skinfolds (sum of triceps, biceps and medial calf), and the ratio of subcutaneous fat (sum of 6 skinfolds) to total fat mass in kg. The trunk to extremity skinfolds ratio (T/E) is quite influenced by age, gender and level of fatness in both generations, but slightly more in the adults. However, the ratio of subcutaneous fat to total fat mass is affected by age, gender and total fatness only in the sample of adults (about 25% of the variance).

TABLE 3. Analysis of variance and intraclass correlation for body fat changes following short-term overfeeding[a]

Variable	Effect of overfeeding F ratio [b]	Genotype-overfeeding interaction F ratio	Intrapair resemblance in response
Body weight	49.4**	4.6*	0.64
Body mass index	79.0**	0.8	0.13
Percent fat	3.8	18.4**	0.90
Fat mass	6.2*	16.3**	0.88
Sum 9 skinfolds	46.1**	7.7*	0.77

a) An extra 1000 kcal/day for 22 consecutive days in 6 pairs of male MZ twins. Adapted from Poehlman et al., 1986.

b) The effects of overfeeding and the genotype-overfeeding interaction were assessed with a two-way analysis of variance for repeated measures on one factor. Intraclass coefficient computed with changes caused by overfeeding.

* $P \leq 0.05$; ** $P \leq 0.01$

TABLE 4. Effects of age, gender and indicators of heaviness or fatness on variation in skinfolds in the children and adolescents (N ≤ 973)

	Age and gender [a]	Age, gender and BMI	Age, gender and sum skinfolds
Triceps	27[b]	62	84
Biceps	18	54	82
Medial calf	22	55	79
Subscapular	14	59	82
Suprailiac	7	47	76
Abdominal	9	53	85
Trunk/extremity skinfolds	41	47	48
Sum skinfolds/fat mass	3	4	4

a) Age + gender + (age x gender) + age^2
b) R^2 x 100

TABLE 5. Effects of age, gender and indicators of heaviness or fatness on variation in skinfolds in the adults (N ≤ 725)

	Age and gender[a])	Age, gender and BMI	Age, gender and sum skinfolds
Triceps	46[b])	68	82
Biceps	32	60	76
Medial calf	47	61	70
Subscapular	3	55	76
Suprailiac	4	44	72
Abdominal	3	46	77
Trunk/extremity skinfolds	54	58	60
Sum skinfolds/fat mass	21	22	25

a) Age + gender + (age x gender) + age^2
b) R^2 x 100

Table 6 presents the foster midparent-adopted child versus the midparent-natural child correlations for the skinfolds and other indicators of fat distribution. (Bouchard, 1985, Bouchard and Tremblay, 1985). With data adjusted only for sex and gender, the pattern of correlation suggests that absolute amount of subcutaneous fat in a given region of the body is not significantly associated with biological inheritance. However, the trunk to extremity ratio and the sum of skinfolds to total fat mass ratio exhibit a different pattern, one suggestive of a genetic effect (Bouchard et al. in press).

Similar data for the amount of fat in the lower trunk area without adjustment and with adjustment for BMI and total subcutaneous fat are presented in table 7. Correlations for both the abdominal skinfold taken individually and the sum of abdominal plus suprailiac skinfolds are identical whether adjusted only for age and gender or adjusted for age, gender and BMI. A different pattern emerges, however, when subcutaneous lower trunk fat is adjusted for age, gender and total subcutaneous fat. Thus, the foster midparent-adopted child correlation decreases while the midparent-natural child correlation remains constant or increases slightly. These data seem to suggest that the amount of fat in the abdominal or lower trunk area given the total amount of subcutaneous fat is partly determined by inherited characteristics.

The same correlations have been computed for the T/E ratio and another describing regional subcutaneous fat distribution. These correlations without and with adjustment for BMI and total subcutaneous fat are presented in table 8. The unadjusted data (residuals of age and gender) were indicative of a significant genetic effect for the amount of fat deposited in the trunk in contrast to that in the extremities. Controlling for BMI or total subcutaneous fat does not modify the correlation pattern. Thus, sets of biologically related individuals (midparent natural child) have a correlation of about 0.35 while the correlations in the biologically unrelated individuals (foster midparent-adopted child) reach about 0.18. This pattern fits well with our previous reports

TABLE 6. Midparent - child interclass correlation
for skinfold measurements[a]

Variable	Foster midparent - Adopted child (N = 154 units)	Midparent - Natural child (N = 622 units)
Triceps	.32**	.29**
Biceps	.31**	.30**
Medial calf	.24*	.31**
Subscapular	.38**	.35**
Suprailiac	.36**	.47**
Abdominal	.33**	.25**
Extremity skinfolds	.31**	.31**
Trunk skinfolds	.38**	.34**
Trunk/extremity skinfolds	.26**	.42**
Sum skinfolds/fat mass[b]	.11	.30**

a) After $\log_{10}$ transformation, scores were adjusted for
age and gender effects by generation (Adapted from
Bouchard, 1985, Bouchard and Tremblay, 1985, and
Bouchard et al, in press).
b) Number of sets in this case is 111 and 242, respectively.
* $P \le 0.01$; ** $P \le 0.001$

demonstrating a significant genetic effect in regional
fat distribution (Bouchard, 1985, Bouchard and Tremblay,
1985, Bouchard et al., 1985, Bouchard et al. in press).

Data for the absolute skinfold values adjusted only
for age and gender were available in 9 kinds of relatives
by descent or by adoption (Bouchard, 1987). The BETA
path analysis model was applied to the correlations
obtained in these relatives (Table 9). The total
transmissible variance in skinfold residuals of age and
gender varies from a low of 28% (abdominal) to a high of
55% (suprailiac). However, most of this transmission is
cultural and it does not appear to be closely associated
with the genotype.

TABLE 7. Midparent-child interclass correlations for indicators of body fat in the lower trunk area[a]

Variable	Foster midparent-Adopted child (N = 154 units)	Midparent-Natural child (N = 622 units)
Abdominal skinfold (AS)	.33**	.25**
AS adj. BMI	.26**	.25**
AS adj. sum 6 skinfolds	.09	.26**
Abdominal + suprailiac skinfolds (AI)	.37**	.32**
AI adj. BMI	.30**	.32**
AI adj. sum 6 skinfolds	.24*	.40**

[a] Data were adjusted for age and gender and then BMI or the sum of 6 skinfolds as shown previously (see tables 4 and 5).

[b] * $P \leq 0.05$; ** $P \leq 0.01$

Analyzing the skinfold data after adjusting not only for age and gender, but also for heaviness or fatness gives a slightly different picture. For instance, residuals of abdominal skinfolds further adjusted for BMI translate into a biological inheritance component of about 10% while adjustment for age, gender and the sum of six skinfolds yields a h^2 of about 20% (Table 10). One must, however, keep in mind that the unexplained variance in the latter cases was considerably reduced (see tables 4 and 5). In other words, h^2 is increased when total heaviness or subcutaneous fat is taken into account but it is not associated with a significantly larger contribution of total human variation.

Is there a GxE component for fat distribution when energy balance is systematically manipulated? This question was considered in our study of 6 pairs of male MZ twins (i.e. only a maximum of 6 genotypes were tested)

TABLE 8. Midparent-child interclass correlations in
          markers   of   regional   subcutaneous   fat
          distribution[a]

Variable	Foster midparent-Adopted child (N = 154 units)	Midparent-Natural child (N = 622 units)
Trunk/extremity skinfolds (T/E)	.26**	.42**
T/E adj. BMI	.19*	.32**
T/E adj. sum 6 skinfolds	.17*	.36**
Abdomen + suprailiac (AI)/ triceps + calf (TC) skinfolds	.22**	.35**
AI/TC adj. BMI	.20*	.33**
AI/TC adj. sum 6 skinfolds	.19*	.36**

[a] Data were adjusted for age and gender and then BMI or
    the sum of 6 skinfolds as shown above (see tables 4
    and 5)
T/E = Ratio of sum of abdominal, suprailiac and subsca-
    pular skinfolds divided by sum of biceps, triceps and
    medial calf skinfolds.
AI = Sum of abdominal and suprailiac skinfolds
TC = Sum of triceps and medial calf skinfolds
* $P \leq 0.05$;   ** $P \leq 0.01$

who were subjected to a 1000 kcal/day overfeeding stress
for a period of 22 consecutive days. Data indicated that
adaptation to caloric affluence in terms of location of
fat deposition differed between genotypes but was significantly similar in members of same MZ pair (Table 11).
Subjects gained weight and fat with overfeeding, but
there were considerable inter-individual differences in
terms of the regional fat deposition. For instance, the
0.74 intraclass correlation for changes in the ratio of
subcutaneous fat to total fat mass implies that about
three-quarters of the variance in the response were
between genotypes, while only 25% of the variance could
be found within pairs. These data suggest that fat
deposition and the location of fat deposition in response
to caloric affluence are partly determined by the genotype. In other words, there is a GxE effect when exposed

TABLE 9. Components of phenotypic variance with the complete BETA model for individual skinfolds[a]

Variable	Transmissible Variance (t^2)	Biological Inheritance (h^2)	Cultural Inheritance (b^2)	χ^2 (P)
Triceps skinfold	.44	.03	.40	6.91 (< 0.05)
Biceps skinfold	.38	.08	.29	6.31 (< 0.05)
Medial calf skinfold	.40	.08	.31	0.26 (< 0.90)
Subscapular skinfold	.41	.02	.40	6.03 (< 0.05)
Suprailiac skinfold	.55	.18	.34	5.00 (< 0.10)
Abdominal skinfold	.28	.01	.27	8.38 (< 0.02)
Extremity skinfolds	.39	.03	.36	3.19 (< 0.25)
Trunk skinfolds	.39	.05	.34	8.46 (< 0.02)

a) Only the full model solution is presented. From Bouchard, 1987.

TABLE 10. Total transmissible variance and its additive genetic component for the abdominal skinfold without and with adjustment for heaviness or fatness[a]

Variable	Transmissible Variance (t^2)	Biological Inheritance (h^2)	Cultural Inheritance (b^2)	X^2 (P)
Abdominal skinfold (AS)	.28	.01	.27	8.38 (< 0.02)
AS adj. BMI	.41	.12	.29	11.10 (< 0.005)
AS adj. sum skinfolds	.33	.20	.13	2.85 (< 0.25)

a) The BETA path analysis procedure was used to obtain these estimates. Only the full model solution is presented.

to a positive energy balance and some individuals are more at risk than others to deposit fat and to store it in the wrong place.

SUBCUTANEOUS FAT PATTERN

The skinfold data of one of our studies based on 1698 subjects yielding 9 different kind of relatives were analysed by the multivariate technique of principal component analysis. Using 6 skinfold measurements adjusted for age and gender, the first two principal components accounted for 71% and 11% of the variance, respectively, or a total of 82% of the total variance (Table 12). As expected from the work of others, the first principal component represented general subcutaneous fat while the second principal component described a trunk to extremity fat pattern. Adjusting the skinfold data for BMI yielded essentially the same pattern for the first two principal components which accounted then for only a total of 67% of the variance. Adjusting the skinfold data for the sum of the six skinfolds changed the solution considerably. Thus the first two principal components accounted for only 53% of the variance and they described a different reality. In this case, the first principal component represented a trunk to extremity pattern, while the second was primarily a lower trunk component i.e. abdominal vs suprailiac (Table 12).

Midparent-child correlations for the principal component scores are presented in table 13. These data are highly suggestive of a genetic effect for the principal component scores associated with the trunk to extremity subcutaneous fat profile even when the data are adjusted for BMI or for total skinfold thickness. In other words, the pattern of superficial fat deposition among the various fat depots, even when one controls for the size of the adipose organ, is not independent of some genetic characteristics which are unknown at this time.

IMPLICATIONS OF THESE FINDINGS

Obesity in the adult population is associated with higher serum triglycerides, total cholesterol and

TABLE 11. Analysis of variance and intraclass correlation for fat distribution changes following short-term overfeeding[a].

Variable	Effect of Overfeeding (F Ratio)[b]	Genotype-Overfeeding Interaction (F Ratio)	Intrapair Resemblance in response
Trunk skinfolds (mm)	40.7**	5.6*	0.70
Extremity skinfolds (mm)	30.5**	6.9*	0.75
Trunk/extremity ratio	0.34	4.1	0.61
Skinfold (mm)/total body fat (kg)	0.72	6.7*	0.74

a) An extra 1000 kcal/day for 22 days in 6 pairs of MZ twins. Adapted from Poehlman et al., 1986.

b) The effects of overfeeding and the genotype-training interaction were assessed with a two-way analysis of variance for repeated measures on one factor. Intraclass coefficient computed with changes caused by overfeeding.

* $P < 0.05$; ** $P < 0.01$

LDL-cholesterol but lower HDL-cholesterol, higher blood pressure, disturbances in glucose and insulin metabolism, increased cancer risks and higher overall mortality rate. Some of these obesity associated complications are more frequently observed in adult males.

As shown by a variety of recent reports (see two recent symposiums: Vague et al., 1985, Norgan, 1985), adipose tissue topography can also be an independent risk factor related to several metabolic complications and even mortality rate. In this case, research has proceeded in several directions since the early proposal of Vague (see Vague, 1956, Vague et al, 1985a) and the «rediscovery» of the concept of fat distribution in more recent years (Kissebah et al, 1982). From the early visual characterization of the android and gynoid types of obesity, we have evolved to a battery of anthropometric measurements to ratios of circumferences. More recently, ratios of skinfolds, linear combination of weighted skinfolds, Z transforms of skinfolds have also been used to evaluate fat topography and study its relationship to health and disease states. Computerized axial tomography has been incorporated as a research technique to quantify fat distribution, particularly the visceral fat compartment of total abdominal fat.

Concomitantly, scientists have attempted to define the mechanisms that could explain the link between fat topography and the metabolic disturbances or mortality rate (Björntorp, 1984, Kissebah et al, 1985, Landsberg, 1986). A growing understanding of these mechanisms along with several recent reports (Raison and Guy-Grand, 1985, Desprês et al., 1985, in press) has led us to believe that, in addition to total fat mass, the abdominal fat mass is the main factor involved in the fat distribution connection. In addition, along with others, we believe that a case can be made for the size of the visceral fat compartment to be the critical component of the abdominal fat mass connection because of its proximity to the hepatic circulation. In other words, the associations or risks that have been described in the past few years for anthropometric ratios or other non-abdominal indicators of fat topography were perhaps the results of the back-

TABLE 12. Principal component loadings for skinfold data adjusted for age, gender, heaviness or fatness

Loadings for principal components 1 and 2

	Adjusted for age and gender		Adjusted for age, Gender and BMI		Adjusted for age, gender and sum 6 skinfolds	
	1	2	1	2	1	2
Triceps	.42	.32	.45	.37	.52	.08
Biceps	.42	.16	.45	.21	.36	-.09
Medial calf	.37	.68	.35	.60	.50	.01
Subscapular	.42	-.35	.41	-.38	-.23	.25
Suprailiac	.40	-.42	.38	-.43	-.37	-.76
Abdominal	.41	-.34	.41	-.37	-.40	-.58
Eigen value	4.26	0.64	3.01	1.04	1.98	1.21
Proportion of variance	71	11	50	17	33	20

TABLE 13. Midparent-child interclass correlations for
the first two principal components

Variable	Foster midparent- Adopted child (154 units)	Midparent Natural child (622 units)
Principal component adj. for age and gender		
1 (General subcutaneous fat)	0.39**	0.29**
2 (Trunk vs extremity)	0.13	0.31**
Principal component adj. for age, gender and BMI		
1 (General subcutaneous fat)	0.13	0.33**
2 (Trunk vs extremity)	0.15	0.35**
Principal component adj for age, gender and sum skinfolds		
1 (Trunk vs extremity)	0.13	0.36**
2 (Abdominal vs suprailiac)	0.34**	0.44**

* $P \leq 0.05$; ** $P \leq 0.01$

ground covariation between any measures pertaining to fat mass or excess weight. For instance, the relationship observed between upper trunk adiposity or subscapular skinfold thickness and risks of metabolic complications is probably the result of the correlations between upper trunk fat and total fat mass as well as abdominal fat mass. The same is perhaps true, although the link is more complicated, for the waist to hip ratio.

So, if the abdominal or intra-abdominal fat mass is the major component of the fat distribution risk factor, what have we found about the role of heredity in human variation for this fat topography characteristic. First, one must recognize that lower trunk fat is at least moderately correlated with total amount of fat. If one controls for age, gender and total amount of fat, human variation in abdominal fat or lower trunk fat is considerably reduced. We have found that the variance of abdominal fat after adjustment for these three concomitant variables was reduced by as much as 70% to 80% in children and adults as well. In other words, the genetics of abdominal or lower trunk fat is best undertaken on these residual scores which exhibit considerably less variation.

Second, we have no data on the genetics of the size of the intra-abdominal fat compartment. Third, once the effect of total subcutaneous fat has been removed, the additive genetic effect for the size of the abdominal skinfold reaches about 20% of the phenotypic variance. An additive genetic effect of about the same magnitude has been reported before for the trunk to extremity skinfolds ratio and the subcutaneous fat to fat mass ratio (Bouchard, 1985, Bouchard et al., in press). Fourth, we are also reporting a significant genetic effect for the skinfold principal component scores describing a trunk to extremity profile without and with control over total fatness. Fifth, there are good indication that individual differences in the sensitivity of the various fat depot, including the lower trunk area, to accumulate fat under conditions of chronic overfeeding are partly determined by the genotype. However, we need to learn a great deal more about this GxE effect, particularly in terms of its potential significance for the size of the visceral fat compartment.

As for the genetics of fat distribution during growth per se, there is no reason to believe that it will be strikingly different from the general conclusions given above as these studies have been undertaken with children and adults (for the additive genetic effect) and young adults (for the GxE effect). As we have discussed elsewhere for other biological phenotypes (Bouchard, 1986, 1987), the rather low additive genetic effect reported here is sufficient to be of considerable importance for human variation in fat topography. In spite of such a low genetic effect, one finds high-gainers and low-gainers to chronic overfeeding and genetically determined variation in the preferred site of fat deposition. These findings are supported by our more recent research on the role of the genotype in the adaptation to long-term overfeeding using monozygotic twins (Bouchard et al, unpublished results).

ACKNOWLEDGMENTS

Thanks are expressed to Drs Claude Allard, Angelo Tremblay, Marcel R. Boulay, Germain Thériault, Jean-Pierre Després, and Roland Savard who were associated with the research reported in this chapter. Gratitude is also expressed to Louis Pérusse, Guy Fournier, Claude Leblanc and other colleagues of the Physical Activity Sciences Laboratory who were involved in these studies. Research supported by NSERC of Canada, Health and Welfare Canada, FCAR-Quebec and National Institutes of Health, USA.

REFERENCES

Björntorp P (1984). Hazards in subgroups of human obesity. Eur J Clin Invest 14: 239-241.
Bouchard C (1985). Inheritance of fat distribution and adipose tissue metabolism. In: Vague J, Björntorp P, Guy-Grand B, Rebuffé-Scrive M, Vague P (eds). Metabolic complications of human obesities. Amsterdam: Elsevier, pp 87-96.
Bouchard C (1986). Genetics of aerobic power and capacity. In: Malina RM, Bouchard C (eds). Sport and human genetics. Champaign (Il): Human Kinetics, pp 59-88.
Bouchard C (1987). Genetics of body fat, energy expenditure and adipose tissue metabolism. In: Berry EM, Blondheim SH, Eliahou HE, Shafir E (eds). Recent advances in obesity research V. London: John Libbey, pp. 16-25.
Bouchard C, Tremblay A (1985). Genetics of body composition and fat distribution. In: Norgan NG (ed). Human body composition and fat distribution. Euro-Nut report 8, pp. 175-188.
Bouchard C, Pérusse L, Leblanc C, Tremblay A, Thériault G (in press). Heredity, human body fat and fat distribution. Int J Obesity.

Cloninger CR, Rice J, Reich T (1979). Multifactorial inheritance with cultural transmission and assortative mating. II. A general model of combined polygenic and cultural inheritance. Am J Hum Genet 31: 176-198.

Després JP, Allard C, Tremblay A, Talbot J, Bouchard C (1985). Evidence for a regional component of body fatness in the association with serum lipids in men and women. Metabolism 34: 967-973.

Després JP, Tremblay A, Pérusse L, Leblanc C, Bouchard C (in press). Abdominal adipose tissue and serum HDL-cholesterol: association independent from obesity and serum triglyceride concentration. Int J Obes

Kissebah AH, Vydelingum N, Murray R, Evans D, Hartz A, Kalkhoff R, Adams P (1982). Reduction of body fat distribution to metabolic complications of obesity. J Clin Endocrinol Metab 54: 254-260.

Kissebah AH, Evans DJ, Peiris A, Wilson CR (1985). Endocrine characteristics in regional obesities: role of sex steroïds. In: Vague J, Björntorp P, Guy-Grand B, Rebuffé-Scrive M, Vague P (eds). Metabolic complications of human obesities. Amsterdam: Elsevier, pp 115-130.

Landsberg L (1986). Diet, obesity and hypertension: an hypothesis involving insulin, the sympathetic nervous system, and adaptive thermogenesis. Quarterly J Med 61: 1081-1090.

Norgan NG (ed) (1985) . Human body composition and fat distribution. Euro-Nut report 8.

Poehlman ET, Tremblay A, Després JP, Fontaine E, Pérusse L, Thériault G, Bouchard C (1986). Genotype-controlled changes in body composition and fat morphology following overfeeding in twins. Am J Clin Nutr 43: 723-731.

Raison J, Guy-Grand B (1985). Body fat distribution in obese hypertensives. In: Vague J, Björntorp P, Guy-Grand B, Rebuffé-Scrive M, Vague P (eds). Metabolic complications of human obesities. Amsterdam: Elsevier, pp 67-75.

Vague J (1956). The degree of masculine differentiation of obesities, a factor determining predisposition to diabetes, atherosclerosis, gout and uric calculous disease. Am J Clin Nutr 4: 20-34.

Vague J, Björntorp P, Guy-Grand B, Rebuffé-Scrive M, Vague P (eds) (1985). Metabolic complications of human obesities. Amsterdam: Elsevier.

Vague J, Vague P, Meignen JM, Jubelin J, Tramoni M (1985a). Android and gynoid obesities, past and present. In: Vague J, Björntorp P, Guy-Grand B, Rebuffé-Scrive M, Vague P (eds). Metabolic complications of human obesities. Amsterdam: Elsevier, pp 3-11.

Fat Distribution During Growth and Later Health Outcomes
pages 127–145 © 1988 Alan R. Liss, Inc.

ETHNIC DIFFERENCES IN FAT DISTRIBUTION DURING GROWTH

William H. Mueller

School of Public Health, University of Texas Health Science Center, P.O. Box 20186, Houston, Texas 77225

INTRODUCTION

In this paper it will be shown that there are ethnic differences in body fat distribution as assessed by the skinfold method.   The ethnic groups compared were samples of black, white, Japanese and Mexican Americans from national and local surveys in the U.S.A.   In all comparisons, white children tended to have a more peripheral distribution of body fat than the other ethnic groups.   The ethnic differences are evident as early as the preschool period and continue through adolescence. They are apparently independent of fatness level or socio-economic differences between the samples compared. In contrast to the skinfold method, the ratio of waist to hip circumference reflects a sex difference, but not an ethnic difference.   Body circumferences may be reflecting the growth of lean mass and thus not correctly reflect body fat distribution during development.

In comparing three major ethnic groups of the U.S. –black, white, Mexican American, it is shown that black children tend to a centralized pattern (with reduction of both arm and leg fat) relative to white children's values. However, Mexican American children have an upper body fatness, with reduced leg fat only in relation to the values of white children.   Thus there may be different patterns in different ethnic groups, although the possibility that this trend could be due to the greater obesity of Mexican American children (vis a vis black children) cannot be ruled out.

Other masculine-like skeletal characteristics known to predict diabetic status in adults, like the shoulder/hip breadth ratio, do not follow the above cited ethnic differences in fat patterning. Black children have the broadest shoulders and narrowest hips, while both white and Mexican American children have narrower shoulders and broader hips. Thus factors conducing to skeletal androgyny during growth are apparently independent of those factors related to ethnic differences in fat patterning.

The magnitude of the fat patterning difference between ethnic groups is small. The variance in fat patterning accounted for by ethnicity is about 1/3 to 1/2 of that accounted for by sex or maturity status at adolescence. The practical significance of these small but consistent ethnic differences in body fat distribution, remains to be seen. The data support the idea of a genetic mechanism in the development of individual fat patterning differences.

METHODS

Data on national and other surveys were obtained from Roche and Malina (1983) and Malina and Roche (1983). These data were supplemented by information on Mexican American children from our own studies (Mueller et al., 1984, Joos et al., 1984). Skinfold sites available were: Triceps, subscapular, suprailiac and medial calf. All of these sites were not available at all ages, or for all ethnicities. Often only the triceps and subscapular skinfolds could be found. It has been shown that these sites are useful, if somewhat inefficient indicators of centralized fatness when used in combination (Kaplowitz et al., 1987). The waist/hip ratio and the biacromial and bicristal breadths (for skeletal androgyny) were also available in one of the surveys, so these methods could be compared with the results for skinfolds. Bivariate plots were made of the means, for example, subscapular versus medial calf (or the less efficient but sometimes necessary, subscapular versus triceps skinfolds). The bivariate plots were done within reasonable age groups (1-5, 6-11, 12 to 17 years). After it was established that ethnic trends were independent of fatness level, socio-economic status and age group, ratios such as subscapular/triceps skinfolds, waist/hip circumferences, biacromial/bicristal breadths, were used to illustrate further ethnic comparisons. Finally, results from two multivariate analyses of ethnic differences in fat patterning (Mueller, 1982; Baumgartner et al., 1986) are presented to assess the relative importance of ethnicity in explaining variation in fat patterning vis a vis other factors like sex, age or maturity.

RESULTS

We will start with the age group 12 to 17 years, as more skinfold sites are available. In figure 1a are shown mean subscapular against mean medial calf skinfolds in 12 to 17 year old white, black and Mexican American girls. The axis shown from lower left to upper right is the line along which the values of the two sites are equal. This line is not a regression line but is a

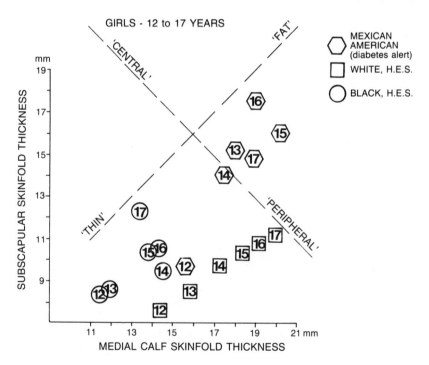

Figure 1a. Bivariate display of mean subscapular and mean medial calf skinfolds in girls 12 to 17 years from three ethnic groups. See text for data sources.

fatness-thinness axis which provides a visual frame of reference. The central-peripheral axis is naturally at right angles to this one. Note first that fatness increases with age in all three groups. White girls are also more peripheral at ages 12 to 17 years, than either black girls, who are generally thinner than white girls, or Mexican American youths, who are generally fatter that white girls. Thus the more central distribution of fat in black and Mexican American children as compared to white youths of this age group, is independent of average fatness levels in the samples.

In figure 1b comparable data are shown for boys 12 to 17 years of age. Note first in boys that centrality in the distribution of fat increases with age in all three groups. This is different from the girls in which there was an increase in fatness with age, but this is an

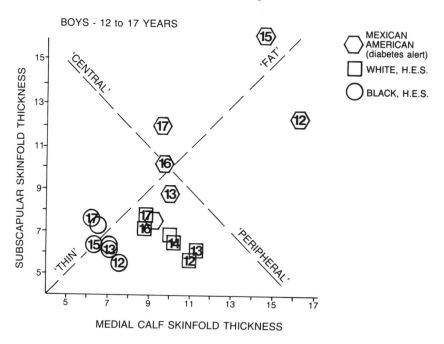

Figure 1b. Bivariate display of mean subscapular and mean medial calf skinfolds in boys 12 to 17 years from three ethnic groups. See text for data sources.

expected trend in boys during adolescence (Deutsch et al., 1985). Note also that black and Mexican American boys are more central in their distribution of fat than white boys. This is consistent with the ethnic related trends seen in figure 1a for girls.

Figure 2 presents the same data on boys 12 to 17 years as in figure 1b, except that black children from two socio-economic (S.E.S) groups have been substituted for those of the Health Examination Survey of figure 1b. The Dallas black children of Schutte et al. (1979), are more centrally distributed in their fat compared to whites, and this is true of both S.E.S. groups. Low income black boys 12 to 17 years are slightly thinner than middle income black boys, but S.E.S. is unrelated

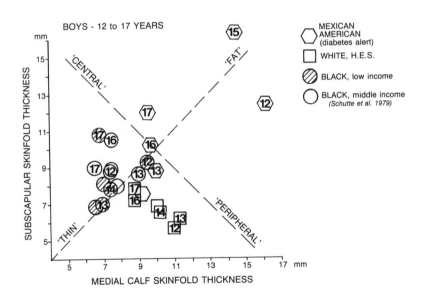

Figure 2. Bivariate display of mean subscapular and mean medial calf skinfolds in boys 12 to 17 years as in figure 1b except that black children from two socio-economic classes are included.

to the tendency to a more central distribution of fat. That is to say, neither the low income or middle income black boys appear to differ in fat patterning. Thus socioeconomic factors do not appear to account for ethnic differences in fat patterning.

The data in Figure 3a present smoothed percentiles for white girls from the Health Examination Survey (H.E.S.) for four skinfold sites. They allow us to explore ethnic differences in fat patterning with a larger number of sites. Superimposed on the percentiles are the medians for Mexican American children (from the

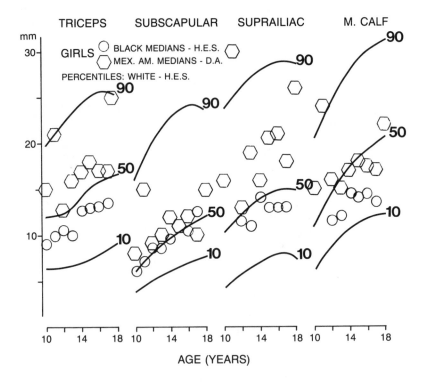

Figure 3a. Medians of four skinfold thicknesses in two ethnic groups of adolescent girls compared to white percentiles. See text for data sources.

Diabetes Alert Study) and black children from the H.E.S. These are the same groups of children shown in figure 1a except there are two additional skinfold sites and the frame of reference for comparison are the white percentiles. Values for Mexican American children are generally between the 50th and 90th percentiles of the white children for triceps, subscapular and suprailiac skinfolds. However, they are generally at or below the 50th percentile for the medial calf site. Thus Mexican American adolescents appear to have an upper body obesity as compared to white adolescents. Black children show a different pattern. They are generally between the 10th and 50th percentiles, at both arm (triceps) and leg (calf) sites. Hence their fat is more centrally distributed.

Figure 3b shows the results of the same surveys in

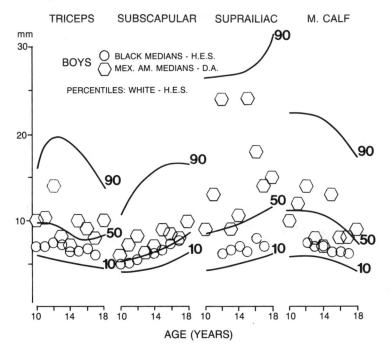

Figure 3b. Medians of four skinfold thicknesses in two ethnic groups of adolescent boys, compared to white percentiles. See text for data sources.

boys. The ethnic trends noted for girls in figure 3a are also evident for boys. However, suprailiac fat at the waist also appears to be reduced in black boys, in comparison to the white children. The data in Figures 3a and 3b suggest that different ethnic groups may have different degrees of upper or centralized obesity, although this could be a result of the different obesity levels in the black and Mexican American children.

In figure 4a we move to 6 to 11 year old girls. In this age group only the subscapular and triceps skin folds were available, and for black and white children only. However, data are available from three different surveys: A survey of private schools in Philadelphia Malina (unpubl.), the Health Examination Survey cycle

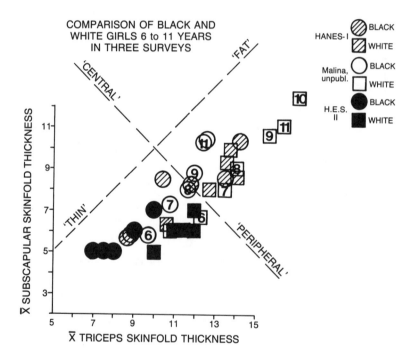

Figure 4a. Bivariate display of mean subscapular and mean triceps skinfolds in girls 6 to 11 years from two ethnic groups. See text for data sources.

II, and the first Health and Nutrition Examination Survey (HANES-I). Note that fatness level differs markedly between the three surveys. Philadelphia children of Malina (unpubl.) (in Malina and Roche, 1983) are the fattest, and children from the H.E.S., cycle II, are the thinnest. Independent of these fatness differences, black children are more centrally distributed in their fat at all the ages shown. However, the ethnic difference in body fat patterning is small compared to age or survey related differences in fatness <u>level</u>. Figure 4b

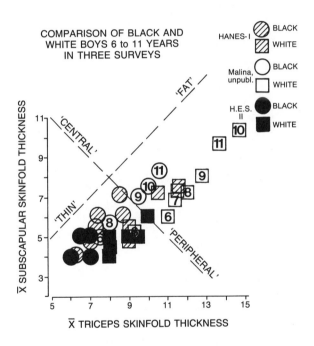

Figure 4b. Bivariate display of mean subscapular and mean triceps skinfolds in boys 6 to 11 years from two ethnic groups. See text for data sources.

gives the same data for boys 6 to 11 years from the same surveys. They confirm the trends seen in the data for the girls.

   Data comparing the same two skinfolds in black and white children aged 1 to 5 years, (sexes combined) are shown in figure 5. Preschool children are much more peripheral in their fat distribution than older children as is evident in the triceps values, which are roughly double those at the subcapular site in figure 5. The more centralized distribution of fat in black preschool children compared to the white children is evident even at these early ages.

   Figure 6 compares ethnic differences (black-white)

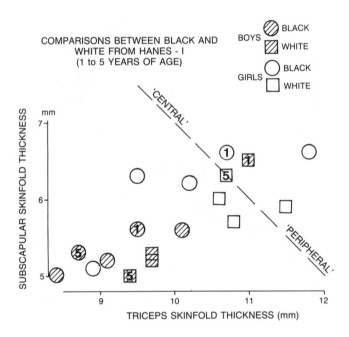

Figure 5. Bivariate display of mean subscapular and mean triceps skinfolds in children 1 to 5 years of age from two ethnic groups. See text for data source.

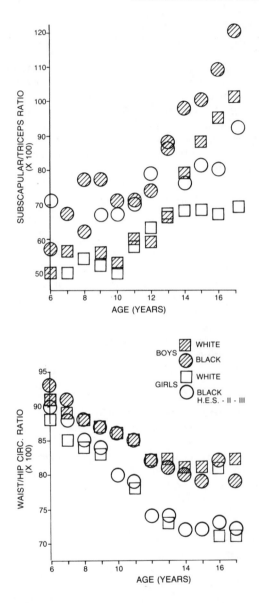

Figure 6. Ethnic and sex differences in the subscapular/triceps skinfold ratio (above) compared to the waist/hip circumference ratio (below) in children 6 to 17 years. See text for data source.

in a skinfold index, the subscapular/triceps ratio (top), with those of the waist/hip ratio (below). The data are from H.E.S. cycles II and III. When looking at the skinfold ratio depicted at the top of figure 6, black children 6 to 17 years are consistently more central in their fat patterning than white children. A sex difference in this index emerges at about 14 years of age, but the ethnic difference remains. In contrast, the ratio of the circumferences at the waist and hip, shown below in figure 6, shows a consistent sex difference but no ethnic difference like that reflected in the skinfold data above. Body circumferences may not accurately reflect fatness in children, as they may be more reflective of muscle or bone development.

The data in figure 7 in part support this view. Four circumferences known to be useful in studying fat patterning in adults (Mueller et al., 1987) are shown in the data from Huenemann et al. (1974). Black, white and oriental adolescent children from California were compared in this survey. To standardize the scales of the four circumferences, black and oriental mean values were subtracted from the white means and divided by the white standard deviation. Note in figure 7, that black and oriental children have smaller circumferences than whites. Both black and oriental youths are expected to have larger arm and waist circumferences relative to hip and thigh circumferences if they are more central in their distribution of body fat than white adolescents. In fact this is reflected only in oriental girls (bottom, figure 7). Thus, once more ethnic differences in fat patterning evident when comparing groups using the skinfold method, are generally not reflected in data using the body circumference method.

Skeletal androgyny is evident in diabetic Mexican Americans as well as a more androgynous distribution of fat (Mueller et al., 1985). This means that individuals with non-insulin dependent diabetes (II) tend to have broader shoulders and narrower hips than non-diabetic individuals of the same sex and age-group. Skeletal androgyny can be studied with the biacromial/bicristal breadth ratio. This ratio is compared in whites, blacks and Mexican Americans ages 6 to 17 years in figure 8.

It does not, however follow the ethnic patterns described earlier for fat patterning. At all ages black children have relatively broader shoulders and narrower hips then the other two ethnic groups, which tend to cluster together. Mexican Americans tend to have the most relatively narrow shoulders of the three groups. Factors contributing to ethnic differences in skeletal androgyny, may be different from those determining ethnic differences in fat patterning.

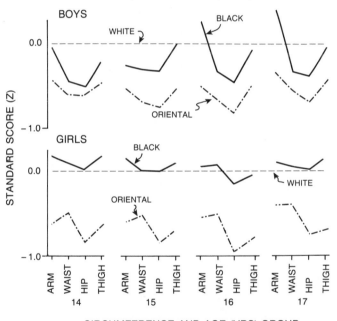

BODY CIRCUMFERENCE PATTERN
PROFILES IN TWO ETHNIC GROUPS (COMPARED TO WHITES)
(Huenemann et al., 1974)

CIRCUMFERENCE AND AGE (YRS) GROUP

Figure 7. Mean body circumference pattern profiles in black and oriental adolescents compared to white values (=0.0). Values are expressed as deviations from white means divided by the white standard deviation in order to have comparable scales for each circumference.

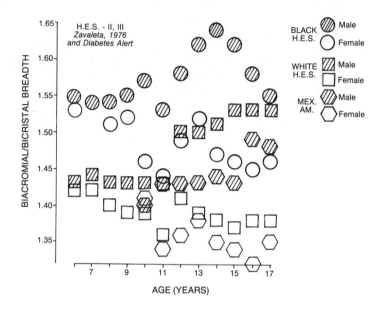

Figure 8. Ethnic and sex differences in skeletal androgyny (biacromial/bicristal breadth ratio) in children 6 to 17 years. See text for data sources.

   Some idea of the magnitude of ethnic differences in fat patterning and the ages during growth at which these first appear are shown in figure 9. In this figure the subscapular/triceps skinfold ratio in Japanese (Kondo and Ito, 1975), black and Mexican American children are compared to a standard ratio of 1.0 in whites. These ratios are anywhere from 10 to 40% higher in the three ethnic groups than in whites, and ethnic differences are evident at an early age. In comparison, the sex difference in this ratio is about 50 to 60% higher in men than women (Mueller, n.d.).

Another way to look at the importance of ethnicity as a factor in fat pattening is to ask how much variance in centralized obesity is explained by ethnicity relative to other factors like sex, age or maturation status during growth. Results of two such studies are shown in

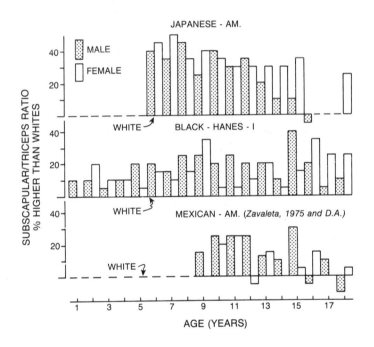

Figure 9. Subscapular/triceps skinfold ratio in three ethnic groups over the growth period, expressed as % higher than white values. See text for data sources.

figure 10.   Both of these studies used principal components   analysis   to   define   a   'component'   of centralized fatness using 5 or more skinfold thicknesses from areas of the body representing both limbs and the trunk (Mueller 1982, Baumgartner et al. 1986).   The figure shows that ethnicity (comparing black and white youths and young adults) accounted for about 5% of the variance in the principal component of central fat distribution.

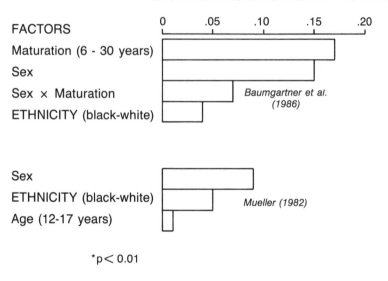

PROPORTION VARIANCE IN CENTRALIZED
FAT PATTERNING EXPLAINED BY FACTORS*

FACTORS

Maturation (6 - 30 years)

Sex

Sex × Maturation

ETHNICITY (black-white)

Baumgartner et al.
(1986)

Sex

ETHNICITY (black-white)

Age (12-17 years)

Mueller (1982)

*p< 0.01

Figure   10.   Proportion   of   variance   in   a   principal component of centralized fatness using multiple skinfold measurements,   explained   by   sex,   maturity,   age   and ethnicity in two studies.

In contrast, sex accounts for from 10 to 15% of variation in central fatness, and maturation status about 17% of variation in the study of Baumgartner et al. (1986) in which subjects ranged in age from 6 to 30 years. Thus the magnitude of the fat patterning difference between ethnic groups is small. Ethnicity accounts for a third to a half of the variance in fat patterning accounted for by sex and maturation status.

CONCLUSIONS

The data on skinfolds show a consistent tendency for white children to have a more peripheral distribution of body fat than Mexican American, Japanese American or black American children. Furthermore these ethnic differences are evident as early as the preschool period. On this point our data compares only black and white children, but Kautz and Harrison (1981) found a more central distribution of body fat in preschool Mexican American children as compared to white children. These differences appear to be independent of how fat the children were in the survey and independent of socio-economic factors. Hence these ethnic trends appear to have a physiological basis, and may point to genetic factors in the distribution of body fat. Body circumferences may not be as useful for studying fat patterning in children as they are in adults, although this methodology needs to be looked at further. Finally we have emphasized data from field surveys, as skinfolds and circumferences are available on various ethnic groups. As yet data from computed tomography or other more technically sophisticated methods are not available to study this question.

REFERENCES

Baumgartner, RN, Roche, AF, Guo, S, Lohman T, Boileau, RA, Slaughter, MH (1986) Adipose tissue distribution: The stability of principal components by sex, ethnicity and maturation Stage, Hum Biol 58:719-735.

Deutsch, MI, Mueller, WH, Malina, RM (1985) Androgyny in fat patterning is associated with obesity in adolescents and young adults. Ann Hum Biol 12:275-286.

Huenemann, RL, Hampton, MC, Behnke, AR, Shapiro, LR, Mitchell, BW (1974) "Teenage Nutrition and Physique." Springfield (IL): Charles C. Thomas.

Joos, SK, Mueller, WH, Hanis, CL, Schull WJ (1984) Diabetes Alert Atudy: Weight history and upper body obesity in diabetic and non-diabetic Mexican American adults. Ann Hum Biol 11:167-171.

Kaplowitz, HJ, Mueller, WH, Selwyn, BJ, Malina, RM, Bailey, DA, Mirwald, RL (1987) Sensitivities, specificities, and positive predictive values of simple indicies of body fat distribution. Hum Biol (in press)

Kautz L, Harrison, GG (1981) Comparison of body proportions of one-year-old Mexican American and Anglo children. Am J Pub Health 71:280-282.

Kondo, S, Eto M (1975) Physical growth studies on Japanese-American children in comparison with native Japanese, in: Horvath, SM, Kondo, S, Matsui, H., Yoshimura, H (eds): "Comparative Studies on Human Adaptability of Japanese, Caucasians and Japanese Americans", Tokyo: University of Tokyo Press, pp. 13-45.

Malina, RM, Roche, AF (1983) "Manual of Physical Status and Performance in Childhood, Volume 2: Physical Performance." New York: Plenum Press.

Mueller, WH (1982) The changes with age of the anatomical distribution of fat. Soc Sci Med 16:191-196.

Mueller, WH (n.d.) The measurement and health implications of body fat patterning. (submitted).

Mueller, WH, Joos, SK, Hanis, CL, Zavaleta, AN, Eichner, J, Schull, WJ (1984) The Diabetes Alert Study: Growth, fatness and fat patterning, adolescence through adulthood in Mexican Americans. Am J Phys Anthrop 64:389-399.

Mueller, WH, Joos, SK, Schull, WJ (1985) Anthropometric differences between age-matched diabetic and non-diabetic Mexican American adults. Am J Phys Anthrop 66:208.

Mueller, WH, Wear, ML, Hanis, CL, Barton, SA, Schull, WJ (1987) Body circumferences as alternatives to skinfold measurements of body fat distribution in Mexican-Americans. Int J Obesity (in press).

Roche, AF, Malina RM (1983) "Manual of Physical Status and Performance in Childhood, Volume 1b: Physical Status",: New York: Plenum Press.

Schutte, JE (1979) "Growth and Body Composition of Lower and Middle Income Adolescent Black Males." Ph.D Thesis Dallas: Southern Methodist University.

Zavaleta, AN (1976) "Densitometric Estimates of Body Composition in Mexican American Boys," PhD Thesis, Austin: University of Texas.

Fat Distribution During Growth and Later Health Outcomes
pages 147–162 © 1988 Alan R. Liss, Inc.

TRACKING IN FAT DISTRIBUTION DURING GROWTH

Alex F. Roche and Richard N. Baumgartner

Department of Pediatrics, Division of Human Biology
Wright State University School of Medicine,
1005 Xenia Ave.,
Yellow Springs, Ohio 45387-1695

INTRODUCTION

Little is known about the extent of tracking in fat patterns during growth. This reflects the lack of suitable data for the analysis of this tracking in children. Relatively few long-term serial studies of children have included measurements of subcutaneous adipose tissue thicknesses at multiple sites. Some of these studies are listed in Table 1. At first glance, there may appear to be a massive compound data set, but this is not so. Pooling is impossible because of variations in the sites selected, in the ages at measurements, and in the calipers used. Also there are ethnic and socio-economic differences both among the studies as listed and within the group of European growth studies. The sample sizes given in Table 1 for most of the studies are the total numbers enrolled; the numbers with serial data for at least 5 years are much smaller. Despite the paucity of data, the existing literature and new analyses allow some tentative conclusions.

The early work on fat patterns in children developed from the recognition of sex, age and maturational differences in the thicknesses of subcutaneous calf adipose tissue. These differences are present for absolute thicknesses and for thicknesses relative to total calf width or calf adipose tissue thickness in adulthood (Stuart et al., 1940; Stuart and Dwinell, 1942; Reynolds, 1944, 1946; Reynolds and Grote, 1948). These studies were extended by Reynolds in his 1950 monograph: "The Distribution of Subcutaneous Fat in Childhood and Adolescence." In this work, Reynolds analyzed data from The Fels Longitudinal Study for 6 sites and showed marked parallelism between site-specific means across age within each sex. He presented serial data for some individuals to illustrate differences in fat patterns; two of these data sets are shown in Figure 1. The data for the boy (Figure 1a) indicate some parallelism among serial values for different sites from 7.5 to 17.5 years

TABLE 1.   Selected Studies with Relevant Serial Data Extending 5
Years or More.

SKINFOLD THICKNESSES

Berkeley Growth Study (N = 67*; 4 sites, Franzen caliper)

European (CIE) Growth Studies (N = 1488*; 4 sites, Harpenden caliper)

Fels Longitudinal Study (N = 111; 3 sites, Holtain caliper)

Guidance Study (N = 630*; 3 sites, Franzen caliper)

Hawk-Brook (N = 621; 4 sites, Holtain caliper)

Melbourne Growth Study (N = 83; 6 sites, Harpenden caliper)

Oakland Growth Study (N = 391*; 3 sites, Franzen caliper)

Tecumseh Study (N = 383; 2 sites, caliper not reported)

Thailand-Bailey Study (N = 1048; 2 sites, caliper not reported)

RADIOGRAPHIC FAT THICKNESSES

Denver Growth Study (N = 334*; 5 sites)

Fels Longitudinal Study (N = 970*; 4 sites)

*Total enrolled; not all have suitable data.

but the changes with age at the forearm site differ from those at the other sites. The data for the girl also show a more definite parallelism with little crossing-over and, therefore, a tendency to retain rank order across age from 6.5 to 13.5 years. Reynolds did not attempt to describe fat patterns numerically nor did he analyze possible tracking of fat patterns. Nevertheless, the data of Reynolds suggest the existence of at least a modest amount of tracking.

Soon after Garn joined to the Fels Research Institute in 1952, he became interested in fat patterns, but most of his early work was based on data from men. Garn and Young (1956) analyzed radiographic adipose tissue thicknesses at the anterior calf and trochanteric sites in children and in adults. In adults, the anterior calf thicknesses tend to decrease while the trochanteric thicknesses increase. Nevertheless, the thicknesses at both these sites decrease in males but increase in females from 12.5 to 17 years in mixed-longitudinal data analyzed cross-sectionally. These findings suggest that the means for anterior calf and

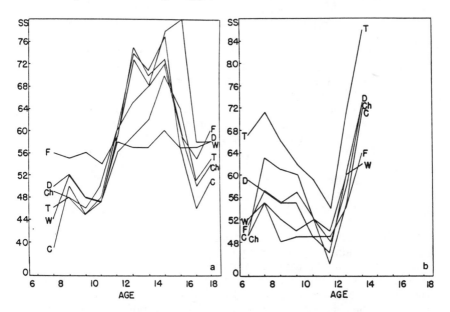

Figure 1. Serial standard scores for radiographic adipose tissue thicknesses (C = calf, Ch = chest, D = deltoid, F = forearm, T = trochanter and W = waist) from Reynolds (1950). The data in "a" are for a boy with "adolescent obesity and regional differences in the distribution of subcutaneous fat." The data in "b" are for "a girl showing marked fluctuations---and---excessive trochanteric fat."

trochanteric adipose tissue thicknesses tend to change in similar ways during adolescence but not during adulthood.

Tracking. The concept of tracking for a measurement implies maintenance of the same rank order among a group of individuals across age (Woynarowska et al., 1985). With acceptance of this concept, the extent of tracking can be determined from age-to-age correlations within sex-specific groups. There are numerous reports of age-to-age correlations for the separate measurements that are included in fat pattern indices but few reports of corresponding correlations for fat pattern indices.

Age-to-age correlations for adipose tissue thicknesses one year apart are high (0.7 to 0.9; Roche et al., 1982). Nevertheless, age-to-age correlations for skinfold thicknesses are generally low when the interval is long, for example, infancy to pubescence (Prader et al., 1974; Wacholder, 1976) and they are only moderate for brief intervals during infancy (Garn, 1958). Hawk and Brook (1979) reported correlations across 15-year intervals beginning at ages ranging from 4 to 14 years (Figure 2a, b). These differ little between the triceps, biceps, subscapular, and suprailiac sites and average about 0.4 in each sex.There is little age trend in the boys, but there are large fluctuations in the correlations for the girls. The latter decrease for intervals beginning at 7 to 9 years, increase for intervals beginning from 9 through 11 years and decrease for intervals beginning from 11 to 14 years. These correlations are generally similar to those found by Bielicki (personal communication) for an interval of 9 years, but are considerably higher than those reported by Garn and LaVelle (1985) between skinfold thicknesses at 1 to 5 years and those 20 years later (Figure 3). The trends in the correlations of Garn and LaVelle, in association with variations in ages at first measurements, are slight but appear similar for the triceps and subscapular sites within each sex.

Roche et al. (1982) reported correlations between values at 16 years and at younger ages for single adipose tissue thicknesses. These correlations are similar for data from trunk sites and for data from extremity sites. Within each group of sites, the correlations are very low when the earlier data are recorded at ages younger than 4 years, but the correlations increase rapidly to about 0.7 for comparisons between values at 8 years and at 16 years and show little subsequent increase. These findings of Roche et al. (1982) are in general agreement with other reports (Whitelaw, 1977; Shukla et al., 1972; Hernesniemi et al., 1974; Zack et al., 1979; Hawk and Brook, 1979; Garn and LaVelle, 1985).

These studies of adipose tissue thicknesses at single sites show there is little tracking during infancy or from infancy to pubescence or

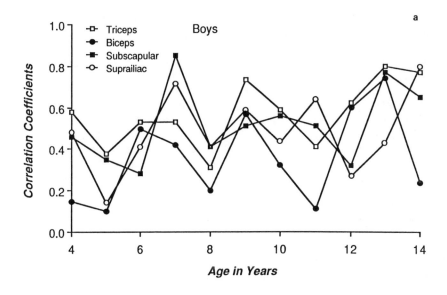

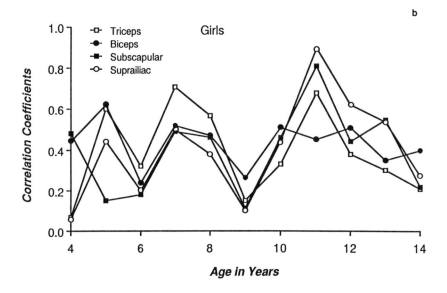

Figure 2. Correlations across 15-year intervals beginning at the ages shown on the x-axis (data from Hawk and Brook, 1979). a: boys and b: girls.

adulthood, but moderate tracking is present when the earlier data are recorded after the age of 4 years. These findings suggest that fat pattern indices, calculated as ratios between selected trunk and extremity thicknesses of adipose tissue, or as principal components derived from adipose tissue thicknesses, are unlikely to show more than moderate tracking during growth.

There are far fewer analyses of tracking in fat pattern indices. Schlüter et al. (1976) published weekly data for skinfold thicknesses at the triceps, subscapular and suprailiac sites in two infants. Logarithms of the ratios of these values have been used to calculate two fat pattern indices. The changes with age differ between these infants for each of these fat pattern indices especially between about 20 and 35 weeks of age (Figure 4a, b). It seems likely that study of a larger sample would show that tracking in these fat pattern indices during this age range is absent or slight.

Analyses of data from The Melbourne Growth Study show generally low correlations between fat pattern indices at 14 years with corresponding values at younger ages (Figure 5a, b). These

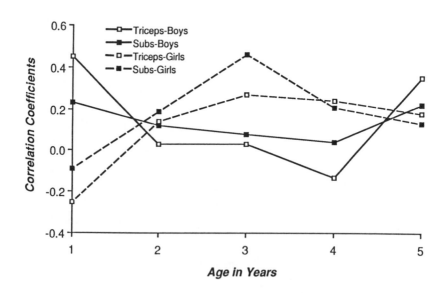

Figure 3. Correlations for triceps and subscapular skinfold thicknesses across 20-year intervals beginning at the ages shown on the x-axis (data from Garn and LaVelle, 1985).

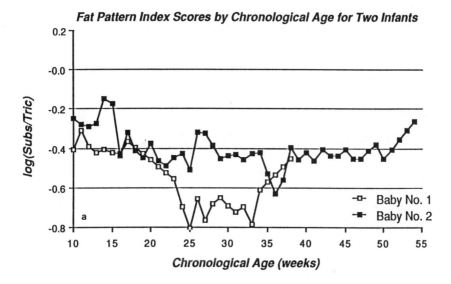

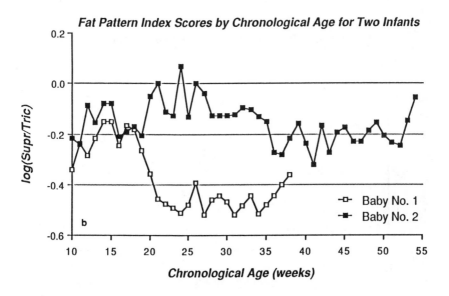

Figure 4. Weekly values for logarithms of ratios of skinfold thicknesses calculated from the data of Schluter et al. (1976) for two infants. a: subscapular/triceps and b: suprailiac/triceps.

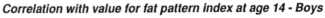

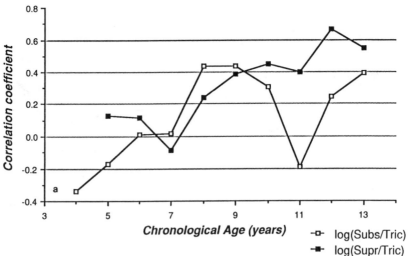

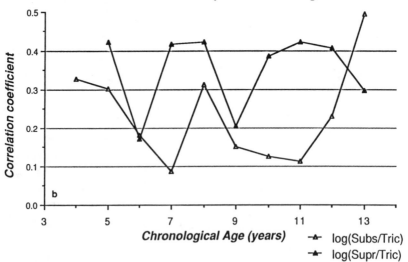

Figure 5. Correlations between indices of fat patterns at 14 years and at younger ages in The Melbourne Growth Study.

correlations for logarithms of the ratios of skinfold thicknesses tend to increase slightly in each sex as older ages at the first examinations are considered but there is considerable variability.

Other age-to-age correlations have been calculated for ratios of logarithms of skinfold thicknesses using data from The Fels Longitudinal Study. These correlations are for 5-year intervals with the first examinations at 7 to 13 years. After adjustments for the ages at the first examinations, the correlations are .60 to .79 with only small differences between the sexes and between the correlations for the subscapular/lateral calf and subscapular/triceps indices of fat patterns. These correlations are considerably higher than those for the 5-year interval from 9 to 14 years in data from the Melbourne Growth Study.

These age-to-age correlations for Fels data are in general agreement with the correlations between slopes fitted to serial Fels data for two indices of fat patterns during 5-year periods. The indices compared are ratios of logarithms of skinfold thicknesses (subscapular/lateral calf vs subscapular/triceps). The correlations are .66 for boys and .68 for girls indicating considerable similarity in the rates of change within individuals. By contrast, the correlations between these indices for all ages combined are 0.82 for boys and 0.92 for girls. The slopes for each of these ratios are correlated with the mean skinfold thicknesses in ways that differ between the sexes (-0.2 to -0.3 for boys; 0.5 for girls). This indicates that tracking, for individuals, may be affected by fatness and by changes in fatness.

In summary, little information is available concerning the tracking of fat pattern indices. It appears that such tracking is slight or absent during infancy but it increases with age and is considerable for 5-year intervals that begin at 7 years or older. Furthermore, it is important to note that the extent of tracking within an individual may be related to changes in total fat mass.

Canalization. Canalization, or homeorrhesis, is the tendency of a trait to proceed to a highly predictable genetically-determined endpoint in adulthood (Waddington, 1957). Values during a growth period are needed to study canalization by establishing the amount of variation, in serial data for individuals, around a "canal" joining the points at the beginning and the end of the period. Canalization, therefore, relates to changes in a serial data set for an individual whereas tracking refers to "parallelism" of the changes among a group of individuals judged from values at the beginning and the end of a period. The best approach to the analysis of canalization is to fit mathematical models to serial data for individuals and to judge canalization from the goodness of fit. The data analyzed in this way must, of course, be descriptors of fat patterns, if the analyses are to be relevant in the present context.

The word "channelization" is used in some literature from the United States. Occasionally, channelization is used synonymously with canalization. For example, Defoe in his "Journal of the Plague Year," written in 1722, noted that "things returned to their own channel again." Sometimes, however, channelization is used to refer to the tendency for serial data from an individual to stay within one channel, defined as a band between adjacent selected percentiles on a growth chart. The latter use is not relevant to fat pattern indices because reference data for these have not been presented in the form of growth charts. The concept of canalization, as described by Waddington, includes strict genetic control, but this aspect has remained inferential and has received little attention. The analysis of canalization requires serial data for individuals with a minimum of about 5 data points per individual. This is in contrast to tracking which can be analyzed if data at paired ages are available for a group.

Canalization has been studied using serial data from The Fels Longitudinal Study for the logarithms of skinfold thicknesses combined as the subscapular/triceps and subscapular/lateral calf ratios. Regressions fitted to these data for 5-year periods have higher R^2 values for the boys than for the girls and the R^2 values tend to increase with age in the boys (p<.001) but not in the girls (Figure 6). These linear

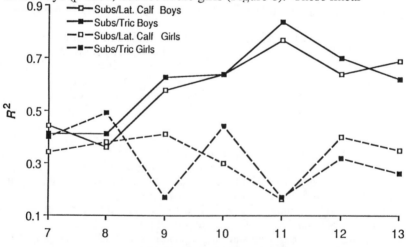

Beginning of 5-Year Periods

Figure 6. R^2 values from linear regressions of ratios based on logarithms of serial skinfold thicknesses for individuals enrolled in the Fels Longitudinal Study.

functions explain about 60% of the variance in the boys and about 30% of the variance in the girls.

Examples of regressions fitted to the data for two boys from the Melbourne Growth Study are shown in Figure 7. These examples were chosen because the trend in Boy No. 1125 (Figure 7a) is almost linear, whereas that for Boy No. 1112 (Figure 7b) is markedly curvilinear. The percentage of the variance explained (R^2) is 12% for Boy No. 1125 and 72% for Boy No. 1112. The rather low percentages of the variance explained indicates the need for more complex models, but these should not be so complex that they cannot be interpreted biologically.

More complex models were used by Cronk et al. (1983a) who analyzed serial changes in biceps, subscapular and paraumbilical skinfold thicknesses using data from The Berkeley, Guidance and Oakland Growth Studies. Longitudinal principal component analyses showed the age changes in the median loadings for Component 1, which describes the general fatness level, differ markedly between the biceps skinfold thicknesses and those on the trunk. The differences between sites in loadings were less marked for Component 2 than for Component 1. Component 2 describes an increase in thickness followed by a decrease, i.e., a fat wave. Component 2 explains more of the variance for the biceps skinfold thickness than for the truncal skinfold thicknesses in each sex. Components 1 and 2, in combination, explain 76.6% to 89.2% of the variance in the three skinfolds, considered separately in each sex (Cronk et al., 1983a). This indicates marked non-linear canalization for single skinfold thicknesses when a complex model is applied that can be readily interpreted biologically. The differences between the patterns of change with age, as described by the longitudinal principal components, between extremity and truncal skinfold thicknesses would be expected from analyses of cross-sectional data. This is in agreement with the well-established age changes that occur in indices of fat patterning derived from skinfold thicknesses (Baumgartner et al., 1986).

Using data from The Fels Longitudinal Study, Cronk et al. (1983b) reported analyses of serial skinfold thicknesses at the triceps and subscapular sites, relative to age at peak height velocity (PHV). There are prepubescent increases and midpubescent decreases for thicknesses at triceps that are much larger in boys than in girls. Corresponding changes do not occur in subscapular skinfold thicknesses in either sex. In each sex, 6-month increments decrease temporarily at about PHV for both triceps and subscapular skinfold thicknesses in each sex; these changes are more marked in boys than in girls. The correlations between the increments in the triceps and subscapular skinfold thicknesses are about 0.5 and do not show a

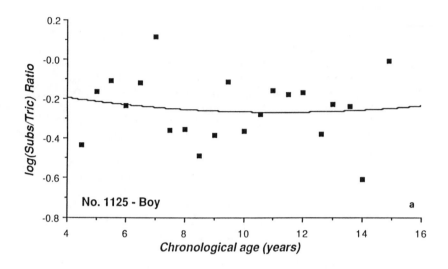

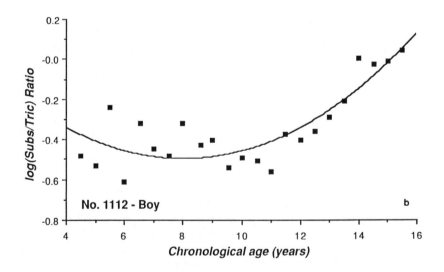

Figure 7. Non-linear regressions fitted to serial log (subscapular/triceps) ratios for two boys in the Melbourne Growth Study. See text for details.

tendency to change with age. These findings are in general agreement with reported analyses of cross-sectional data for subscapular skinfold thicknesses. These analyses do not show decreases and subsequent increases at pubescence in either sex, when the data are analyzed relative to chronological age. These findings of Cronk differ from the cross-sectional literature regarding pubescent changes in triceps skinfold thicknesses relative to chronological age (Johnston et al., 1975; Garn et al., 1981; Johnson et al., 1981; Cronk and Roche, 1982). Finally, it should be noted that analyses of serial data have shown pubescent decreases at other truncal sites in boys (Reynolds, 1950; Heald et al., 1963; McCammon, 1970).

This review directs attention to deficiencies in our knowledge of canalization during growth. Linear regressions do not explain the changes adequately, so more complex models are needed to study the canalization of fat pattern indices. Maturational effects can be omitted from tracking studies, if the ages at the first and last examinations are before and after pubescence, but these effects must be included in studies of canalization.

CONCLUSION

The occurrence of only moderate tracking during growth may be associated with the well-documented change to a more centripetal distribution of subcutaneous adipose tissue in boys but not in girls during pubescence (Baumgartner et al., 1986). The timing of this change is related to the timing of pubescence. Nevertheless, variations in the timing of pubescence do not entirely explain the occurrence of only moderate levels of tracking when the age intervals extend from before pubescence to after pubescence (Hawk and Brook, 1979; Roche et al., 1982; Garn and LaVelle, 1985). Furthermore, if the change to a more centripetal distribution were a major factor, it would be expected that tracking would be considerably more marked in boys than in girls. Reductions in tracking could, however, be due, in part, to interindividual differences in the amounts of circulating gonadal and androgenic hormones during and after pubescence. Alternatively, it could be suggested that the presence of only moderate tracking for fat pattern indices based on skinfold thicknesses reflects errors in the measurement of skinfold thicknesses. This could be true for some data sets but not that of Hawk and Brook (1979) who state that the accuracy of duplicate measurements was much less than 5%. Also, at The Fels Research Institute, the technical errors for skinfold thicknesses at seven sites range from 0.4 to 1.4 mm with coefficients of reliability of 92.4% to 98.9%.

It is difficult to comment broadly on the findings available regarding canalization. Little is known because suitable data are scarce and because better models should be applied.

There is a need to develop a better fat pattern index for application to data recorded during childhood. This might be a ratio with fractional powers selected to maximize the association between childhood values of the index and risk factors for disease in adulthood. Anthropometric data in childhood and risk factor data (eg. blood pressures, plasma lipids) in adulthood would be needed for a sufficient number of individuals. The fat pattern index could be derived from canonical correlations between the childhood anthropometric variables and the adult risk factor variables. The anthropometric variables should include several skinfold thicknesses on the arm, leg and trunk. Circumferences for the trunk and the limbs could be included also. This is the critical need, rather than further analyses of tracking and canalization for simple indices chosen on the basis of the data available. Few existing data sets would allow the construction of such an index but, if this approach were feasible, our understanding of the health implications of particular fat patterns during childhood would be greatly enhanced. Attempts to achieve this understanding should not be delayed until we have the ideal data: an approximate answer to the right question is worth much more than an exact answer to a question of doubtful value.

The extent of tracking or of canalization can be determined only from analyses of existing serial data. If tracking is slight during growth, childhood values for fat pattern indices would have little prognostic importance. If, however, such tracking is marked, childhood values indicating centripetal distributions could cause concern that might lead to changes in management. If canalization is slight, there would be little concern about even marked changes in fat pattern indices but, if canalization is marked then changes that differ from the usual "canals" could cause concern.

ACKNOWLEDGEMENT

This work was supported by Grant HD-12252 from the National Institutes of Health, Bethesda, MD.

REFERENCES

Baumgartner RN, Roche AF, Guo S, Lohman T, Boileau RA, Slaughter MH (1986) Adipose tissue distribution: the stability of principal components by sex, ethnicity and maturation stage. Hum Biol 58:719-735.

Cronk CE, Roche AF (1982) Race- and sex-specific reference data for triceps and subscapular skinfolds and weight/stature^2. Am J Clin Nutr 35:347-354.

Cronk CE, Roche AF, Kent R Jr, Eichorn D, McCammon RW (1983a) Longitudinal trends in subcutaneous fat thickness during adolescence. Am J Phys Anthrop 61:197-204.

Cronk CE, Mukherjee D, Roche AF (1983b) Changes in triceps and subscapular skinfold thickness during adolescence. Hum Biol 55:707-721.

Defoe D (1722) "Journal of the Plague Year." London: E. Nutt.

Garn SM (1958) Fat, body size and growth in the newborn. Hum Biol 30:265-280.

Garn SM, Young RW (1956) Concurrent fat loss and fat gain. Am J Phys Anthrop. 14:497-504.

Garn SM, LaVelle M (1985) Two-decade follow-up of fatness in early childhood. Am J Dis Childh 139:181-185.

Garn SM, Ryan AS, Owen CM, Falkner F (1981) Developmental differences in the triceps and subscapular fatfolds during adolescence in boys and girls. Ecology of Food and Nutrition 11:49-51.

Hawk LJ, Brook CGD (1979) Influence of body fatness in childhood on fatness in adult life. Br. Med. J. i:151-152.

Heald FP, Hunt EE Jr, Schwartz R, Cook CD, Elliott O Vajda B (1963) Measures of body fat and hydration in adolescent boys. Pediatrics 3:226-239.

Hernesniemi I, Zachmann M, Prader A (1974) Skinfold thickness in infancy and adolescence. A longitudinal correlation study in normal children. Helv Paediat Acta 29:523-530.

Johnson CL, Fulwood R, Abraham S, Bryner JD (1981) Basic data on anthropometric measurements-d-and angular measurements of the hip and knee joints for selected age groups 1-74 years of age. U.S. DHHS Publication No. (PHS)81-1669 Series 11, Number 219.

Johnston FE, Dechow PC, MacVean RB (1975) Age changes in skinfold thickness among upper class school children of differing ethnic backgrounds residing in Guatemala. Hum Biol 47:251-263.

McCammon RW (1970) Human growth and development. Charles C Thomas, Springfield, IL.

Prader A, Hernesniemi I, Zachmann M (1974) Skinfold thickness in infancy and adolescence. A longitudinal correlation study in normal children. Compte-Rendu de la XII Reunion des Equipes Chargees des Etudes sur la Croissance et le Developpement de l'Enfant Normal. Centre International de l'Enfance. Paris.

Reynolds EL (1944) Differential tissue growth in the leg during childhood. Child Developm 15:181-205.

Reynolds, EL (1946) Sexual maturation and the growth of fat, muscle and bone in girls. Child Developm 17:121-144.

Reynolds EL (1950) The distribution of subcutaneous fat in childhood and adolescence. Monogr Soc Res Child Developm 15:1-189.

Reynolds EL, Grote P (1948) Sex differences in the distribution of tissue components in the human leg from birth to maturity. Anat Record 102:45-53.

Roche AF, Siervogel RM, Chumlea WC, Reed RB, Valadian I, Eichorn D, McCammon RW (1982) Serial changes in subcutaneous fat thicknesses of children and adults. Monogr Paed No.17. Karger, Basel.

Schluter K, Funfack W, Pachaly J, Weber B (1976) Development of subcutaneous fat in infancy; standards for tricipital, subscapular, and suprailiacal skinfolds in German infants. Eur J Pediat 123:255-267.

Shukla A, Forsyth HA, Anderson CM, Marwah SM (1972) Infantile overnutrition in the first year of life. A field study of Dudley, Worchestershire. Br Med J iv:507-515.

Stuart HC, Dwinell PH (1942) The growth of bone, muscle and overlying tissues in children six to ten years of age as revealed by studies of roentgenograms of the leg area. Child Developm 13:195-213.

Stuart HC, Hill P, Shaw C (1940) The growth of bone, muscle and overlying tissues as revealed by study of roentgenograms of the leg area. Monogr Soc Res Child Developm 5:1-190.

Wachholder A (1976) Poids et taille des enfants, en fonction de l'alimentation precoce, dans l'echantillon de Bruxelles. Compte-Rendu de la XIII Reunion des Equipes Chargees des Etudes sur la Croissance et le Developpement de l'Enfant Normal. Centre International de l'Enfance, Rennes.

Waddington CH (1957) The strategy of the genes. George Allen and Unwin Ltd., London.

Whitelaw A (1977) Infant feeding and subcutaneous fat at birth and at one year. Lancet ii :1098-1099.

Woynarowska B, Mukherjee D, Roche AF, Siervogel RM (1985) Blood pressure changes during adolescence and subsequent adult blood pressure level. Hypertension 7:695-701.

Zack PM, Harlan WR, Leaverton PE, Cornoni-Huntley J (1979) A longitudinal study of body fatness in childhood and adolescence. J Pediat 95:126-130.

Fat Distribution During Growth and Later Health Outcomes
pages 163–173 © 1988 Alan R. Liss, Inc.

METABOLIC DIFFERENCES IN FAT DEPOTS

Marielle Rebuffé-Scrive

Department of Medicine I
University of Göteborg
Sahlgren's Hospital
S-413 45 Gothenburg

INTRODUCTION

Recent research in the field of obesity has clearly indicated the differences in risk between obesity as such, defined in generalized terms, for example BMI, and the distribution of adipose tissue, defined by circumferences, (Groddeck, 1899), or skinfold measurements (Edwards,1956). Generally, abdominally localized adipose tissue is associated with a number of diseases while the distribution of fat to the gluteal-femoral regions is less malignant (Larsson et al, 1980).

These new developments have made it important to examine factors that regulate the distribution of body fat to different parts of the body. This is interesting from at least two viewpoints. First, the adipose tissue itself might be responsible for the pathogenesis of the complicating diseases following abdominal distribution of fat. If this is not the case, then factors regulating adipose tissue distribution are still of interest, because they might lead to new ideas of the pathogenesis of diseases frequently associated with abdominal obesity.

The following will summarize recent studies of this problem. The main focus of these studies have been placed on the role of steroid hormones, which probably play important roles in the regulation of adipose tissue distribution and are involved, in a so far unknown way, in the syndromes of android and gynoid obesity (Vague, 1947). Obviously, in order to direct depot fat from one region to another, or preferentially to one depot at the expense of another, the steroid hormones have to affect the metabolic pathways that are responsible for fat accumulation and mobilization. Therefore, in the following studies, the main pathways for lipid accumulation, lipoprotein lipase (LPL) activity, and lipid mobilization as glycerol release in vitro, have been measured in human adipose tissues. Other methods have been utilized when needed, including checks of the "in vitro" data with "in vivo" measurements.

Studies on regional adipose tissue metabolism have been performed earlier but without definition of the sex and endocrinological status of the patients, preventing any conclusions about specific regional effects of steroid hormones (Kather et al, 1977, LaFontan et al, 1978, Lithell and Boberg, 1978, Smith et al, 1979, Guy-Grand and Rebuffé-Scrive, 1980).

SEX STEROID HORMONES AND METABOLIC DIFFERENCES IN FAT DEPOTS.

Subcutaneous Abdominal and Femoral Fat Depots.

Women
In a first series of examinations the activities mentioned above were measured in a descriptive way in women with various endocrinological status.

During their fertile life women tend to accumulate fat (LPL high), preferentially in the femoral region compared to the abdominal, which is difficult to mobilize (noradrenaline stimulated lipolysis low). This can explain why women have enlarged fat cells in this region.

During pregnancy these phenomenons are even more pronounced while during lactation exogenous triglycerides are not any longer preferentially taken up in the femoral region (femoral LPL activity not higher than abdominal) and lipids are now as easy to mobilize in the femoral as in the abdominal region (high lipolysis in both regions). These changes in metabolism during lactation have lead to the hypothesis that the typical female fat depot, the femoral fat, has a typical female function, as a reserve of energy which can be utilized as energy supply for lactation (Rebuffé-Scrive et al, 1985a).

After menopause, when the ovarian production of sex hormones has considerably decreased or ceased, the typical
increased LPL activity in the femoral region disappears,
and there are no regional differences in LPL activity between abdominal and femoral fat depots. However, in postmenopausal women who received estradiol and progestagen therapy, LPL activity increases in the femoral region. In
comparison with fertile women, postmenopausal women have a
reduced abdominal lipolysis which thus is not different
from the femoral region. The combination of a low abdominal lipolysis and a low femoral LPL can explain the lack
of regional differences in fat cell size between abdominal
and femoral adipocytes, in postmenopausal women. It can
also be concluded that menopause is associated with a
disappearance of the female characteristics of adipose
tissue and that fat will now accumulate without regional
preferences, (Rebuffé-Scrive et al. 1987a).

In conclusion, female sex steroid hormones seem to regulate the accumulation of fat in the gluteal-femoral
regions in women by activating LPL. It is also possible
that they regulate the mobilization of fat in the abdominal region, but this is only speculative.

Lipid accumulation in a certain adipose tissue region
is, however, dependent not only on the amount of lipid in
each fat cell but also on the number of available fat
cells. Recent studies in our laboratory, have indicated
that female sex steroid hormones, particularly progesterone, increase adipose precursor cell differentiation
(Xuefan and Björntorp,1987a). The fact that both the LPL
activity is increased as well as the rate of differentiation of adipose precursor cells might contribute to both
enlargement and increased number of fat cells in the gluteal-femoral regions in women.

The effects of progesterone as well as of other steroid
hormones seem to be mediated via specific cytoplasmic
receptors, which transport the hormone-receptor complex to
the nucleus. Such receptors can be demonstrated in both
mature adipocytes and in adipose precursor cells (Xuefan
et al, 1987b). The affinity of the binding is the same,
but there are more receptors on the precursor cells. These
are, however, data from rat adipose tissue. Receptors of
this type have so far not been possible to demonstrate in
human. This might be due to technical reasons. An alterna-

te explanation is that progesterone receptors are actually missing in human adipose tissue. If this is the case, then obviously progesterone has to act via another mechanism in human adipose tissue. Corticosteroid receptors are present in human adipose tissue (Rebuffé-Scrive et al, 1985b), and it is of interest that progesterone might compete for the corticosteroid receptor.

Insulin is of obvious importance for the regulation of lipid uptake. Therefore, the antilipolytic effect of insulin has been measured in parallel with insulin binding (Rebuffé-Scrive et al, 1987). Although the antilipolytic effect of insulin is higher in the abdominal than in the femoral region, no regional differences in insulin binding are observed between those two depots. It seems thus that insulin effects are responsible for little, if any, of the regional differences in fat accumulation and its metabolic regulation.

Obviously, the measurements presented have been performed in small shreds of adipose tissue "in vitro". This has to be confirmed by studies "in vivo" in order to attain real significance. Such measurements have been performed in our laboratory by administering labelled glucose to subjects (Mårin et al, 1987). The half-life of the labelled glyceride-glycerol is followed by repeated biopsies. The turnover of labelled triglyceride is more rapid in the abdominal than in the femoral region, in excellent agreement with the in vitro data. In order to check the LPL activity, further experiments are currently performed, examining the regional distribution of labelled lipid given orally.

Men
Men have no increased LPL activity in the femoral region like premenopausal women, this activity is even lower than in post-menopausal women, suggesting a possible inhibitory role of testosterone on femoral LPL activity (Rebuffé-Scrive et al,1987a). The lipolytic response to noradrenaline of abdominal adipocytes is high compared to femoral, however, it decreases with age. Whether this is an effect of a decreased level of testosterone and or an age effect is unknown yet. The association between high abdominal lipolysis and low femoral LPL activity can probably explain the lack of regional differences in adipocytes size, at least in younger men. A tentative conclusion here

would be that testosterone inhibits LPL and stimulates lipolysis, producing the leanness of young men , but this is not clear as yet. A major problem here is that hormone substitution experiments with testosterone in men are very difficult to perform.

Polycystic ovarian syndrome (PCO)
 The regional adipose tissue metabolism of women with a PCO syndrome is of particular interest because these women have an abdominal type of fat distribution, an increased level of testosterone, a low level of sex hormone binding globuline (SHBG), and also other similarities with women with android obesity such as hirsutism, diabetes, hypertension, hyperlipidemia. We have studied a group of non obese PCO women and compared them to non obese men and women in order to try to answer the following question: Can the metabolic complications found in these women, as well as android obese women, be explained by disturbances in adipose tissue metabolism or by the hormonal derangement?

  Non obese PCO women have, like men, no increased femoral LPL activity and similar lipolytic response to noradrenaline. Furthermore, they have no regional difference in fat cell size between abdominal and femoral adipocytes, again like men. This is due to the fact that even if non obese, these women have enlarged abdominal adipocytes (Rebuffé-Scrive et al, 1987b). In summary this study has shown that non obese PCO women have an android type of fat distribution and an adipose tissue metabolism similar to that of men.

  The conclusion of this study is not clear as far as the association between adipose tissue function and obesity complications. However, it is of considerable importance that essentially all the metabolic complications can be seen in PCO women without obesity, but with an abdominal distribution of body fat. These results seem to support the idea that abdominal adipose tissue distribution is rather a consequence of the syndrome than a cause to the associated complications.

  We will now examine other fat depots than the abdominal and femoral ones.

Mammary and Intraabdominal Fat Depots

Mammary adipose tissue metabolism has been studied in parallel with abdominal and femoral in pre- and postmenopausal women.

The typical increased LPL activity and fat cell size found in the femoral fat depot of premenopausal women does not exist in the mammary adipose tissue, like in the abdominal depot. Furthermore, the lipolytic response to noradrenaline from mammary adipocytes is higher than from femoral and not different from abdominal. No regional differences, neither in LPL nor in lipolysis, were observed between the three regions studied, in postmenopausal women In conclusion mammary adipocytes metabolism is more like abdominal than femoral (Rebuffé-Scrive et al, 1986).

A very important and neglected part of adipose tissue is the intraabdominal fat depots. It has been suggested that they could play a role for the metabolic complications associated to android obesity (Björntorp 1985). Subcutaneous abdominal, retroperitoneal as well as the intraabominal fat depots drained by the portal vein (omental and mesenteric) have been studied in men and pre and postmenopausal women. Lipolysis was, as previously described, higher in young women than in postmenopausal women or older men in the subcutaneous abdominal fat depot but also in the retroperitoneal depot. On the contrary the lipolytic response to noradrenaline of omental and mesenteric adipocytes was high independently of the sex or the age of the patients. This suggest that other hormones than sex steroid hormones could play a major role in the regulation of the metabolism in these depots, possibly corticosteroid hormones.

It is also noticable in this study that men have larger adipocytes in intraabdominal depots than women, particularly than young women. This might be of importance for the differences in female and male distribution of adipose tissue, women having more fat in the gluteal-femoral regions and men in the abdominal regions.

No main differences were observed in LPL activity among regions or between groups, however, these studies have as yet only been performed in non obese patients (Rebuffé-Scrive et al, 1987c). A similar study on obese patients is currently performed in our laboratory.

CORTICOSTEROID HORMONES AND METABOLIC DIFFERENCES IN FAT DEPOTS.

The role of corticosteroid hormones on adipose tissue metabolism is unclear and complicated, and seem to be very much dependent on the time and dose of exposure to the hormones. (Fain et al, 1965, Krotkiewski et al, 1970, De Gasquet et al,1975, Krotkiewski et al, 1976, Cigolini and Smith, 1979).

Cushing's disease clearly is associated with abdominal obesity. It is therefore very likely that cortisol excess is producing an accumulation of abdominal adipose tissue, but it is not clear how this is accomplished. The following concerns some of our preliminary data on this problem. A first study included healthy women who were given prednisolone 5mg x 3 daily, for one week. Lipolysis and LPL activity were measured in the subcutaneous abdominal and femoral fat depots. Lipolysis stimulated by isoproterenol was increased in the abdominal but also in the femoral region. However, in this study with a moderate dose of corticosteroid hormone, and for a short period of time (only 1 week), no effects of the treatment were observed on LPL activity in neither of the fat depots studied (Rebuffé-Scrive al el, 1987d).

These results obviously do not explain why fat is accumulated in abdominal regions. They might, however, contribute to our knowledge of fat mobilization from the peripheral femoral region.

In another study we have had the possibility to examine subcutaneous abdominal and femoral adipose tissue metabolism in five premenopausal women with Cushing's disease. These women have a doubled abdominal LPL activity whether they are compared to control fertile women ($p < 0.01$) or to android young obese women ($p < 0.05$). These results are preliminary but might explain why women with Cushing's disease have a central distribution of fat.

Finally, we have shown that the synthetic corticosteroid, triamcinolone, binds to human adipose tissue with regional specificity, with an increased binding capacity in omental as compared with subcutaneous abdominal fat depots (Rebuffé-Scrive et al, 1985b). This contributes to the suggestion that corticosteroid hormones might play an important role in the regulation of omental and mesenteric adipose tissue metabolism which, as previously described, do not seem to be regulated by sex steroid hormones. More work is obviously necessary here.

Furthermore, this study has shown that progesterone is an important competitor for cytoplasmic corticosteroid receptors, suggesting interactions between the different steroid hormones for the receptors in adipose tissue (as suggested earlier).

CONCLUSIONS

To sum up, it seems clear that the effects of steroid hormones on adipose tissue are complex. Some features seem reasonably certain, for example, the stimulatory effects of female sex steroid hormones (estradiol and progesterone), on LPL activity, particularly in the femoral region. They might also increase the rate of differentiation of adipose precursor cells. Estrogen is lipolytic in rats (Rebuffé-Scrive 1987c) and possibly in young women, particularly in subcutaneous and mammary fat depots although this is not clear yet. Testosterone might inhibit femoral LPL and stimulate abdominal lipolysis, but this is only tentative. Corticosteroid hormones effects are not clear. They seem, to be lipolytic and to increase LPL activity in subcutaneous abdominal fat. Hypothetically, the later might be more pronounced in the intraabdominal tissues where the receptors density is high. This is however, mainly a speculative picture, weakly supported by data so far.

The complexity of this field makes it likely that the effects of steroid hormones are not entirely specific. Clearly, several hormones might be lipolytic (for example corticosteroids, estrogen and testosterone). Progesterone and testosterone have possibly opposite effects on LPL. There is thus a number of interactions between the steroid hormones. Furthermore, it also seems to be a realistic possibility that the steroid hormones receptors are not entirely specific.

There is a lot of work remaining in this area before we can understand the regulatory mechanisms by steroid hormones on the accumulation and mobilization of fat, and thereby the regulation of adipose tissue distribution.

Acknowledgements
This work has been realized with the kind cooperation of coworkers from Departments of Medicine I, Medicine II, Gynecology, General Surgery, Plastic surgery, Endocrinology of the Sahlgren's Hospital, Göteborg, Sweden, who are gratefully acknowledged.

REFERENCES

Björntorp P (1985). Adipose tissue in obesity. (Willendorf Lecture). In: Recent Advances in Obesity Research:IV. Eds: Hirsch/VanItallie. John Libbey & Co Limited163-170.
Cigolini M, Smith U (1979). Human adipose tissue in culture VIII. Studies on the insulin-antagonistic effect of glucocorticoids. Metabolism 28:502-510.
de Gasquet P, Pequignot-Planche E, Tonnu NT, Diaby FA (1975). Effect of glucocorticoids on lipoprotein lipase activity in rat heart and adipose tissue. Horm Metab Res 7:152-157.
Edwards D.A.W. (1956). Estimation of the proportion of fat in body measurement of skinfold thickness. Amer J Clin Nutr 4:35.
Fain JN, Czech MP. (1974). Glucocorticoid effects on lipid mobilization and adipose tissue metabolism. In: Blaschko H Sayers G.Smith AD eds: Handbook of physiology. Baltimore: Waverby.4:169-178.
Groddeck (1899). Über Messen und Wägen in der ärzlichen Thätigheit. Wiener Medizinische Presse 43:1759.
Guy-Grand B and Rebuffé-Scrive M.(1980). Anatomical and nutritional correlates of lipoprotein lipase of human adipose tissue. Proc.3rd Int Congr.Obesity, Rome, Italy. p.273.
Kather H, Schröder F, Simon B and Schlierf G (1977). Human fat cell adenylate cyclase: regional differences in hormone sensitivity. Eur J Clin Invest 7:595-597.
Krotkiewski M, Krotkiewska J and Björntorp P (1970). Effects of dexamethasone on lipid mobilization in the rat. Acta Endocrinol (Kbh)63:185.
Krotkiewski M, Blohmé B and Björntorp P (1976). The effects of adrenal corticosteroids on regional adipocyte size in man. J Clin Endocrinol Metab 42:91-97.

LaFontan M, Dang-Tran L and Berlan M (1978). Alpha-adrenergic antilipolytic effect of adrenaline in human fat
cells of the thigh: comparison with adrenaline responsiveness of different fat deposits. Eur J Clin Invest
9:261-266.
Larsson B, Svärdsudd K, Welin L, Wilhelmsen L, Björntorp
P, Tibblin G (1984). Abdominal adipose tissue distribution, obesity and risk of cardiovascular disease and
death: 13 year follow-up of participants in the study of
men born in 1913. Br Med J 288:1401-1404.
Lithell H and Boberg J (1978). The lipoprotein-lipase
activity of adipose tissue from different sites in obese
women and the relationship to the cell size. Int J Obesity 2:47-52.
Mårin P, Rebuffé-Scrive M & Björntorp P. (1987). Glucose
uptake in human adipose tissue. Metabolism, in print.
Rebuffé-Scrive M, Enk L, Crona N, Lönnroth P, Abrahamsson
L, Smith U and Björntorp P. (1985a). Fat cell metabolism
in different regions in women. Effect of menstrual cycle, pregnancy and lactation. J Clin Invest 75:1973-1976.
Rebuffé-Scrive M, Lundholm K and Björntorp P (1985b). Glucocorticoid binding to human adipose tissue. Eur J Clin
Invest 15:267-271.
Rebuffé-Scrive M, Eldh J, Hafström LO and Björntorp P.
(1986). Metabolism of mammary, abdominal and femoral
adipocytes in women before and after menopause. Metabolism 35:792-797.
Rebuffé-Scrive M, Lönnroth P, Mårin P, Wesslau C, Björntorp P and Smith U. (1987a). Regional adipose tissue
metabolism in men and postmenopausal women. Int J Obesity, in print.
Rebuffé-Scrive M, Cullberg G, Lundberg P.A, Lindstedt G
and Björntorp P. (1987b). Anthropometric variables and
metabolism in polycystic ovarian disease. Submitted for
publication.
Rebuffé-Scrive M, Andersson B, Olbe L, Björntorp P.
(1987c). Metabolism of adipose tissue in different intraabdominal depots. Submitted for publication.
Rebuffé-Scrive M, Lönnroth P, Andersson B, Björntorp P and
Smith U. (1987d). Effects of short-term prednisolone
administration of the metabolism of human subcutaneous
adipose tissue. Submitted for publication.
Rebuffé-Scrive M. (1987e). Hormones and adipose tissue
metabolism in adrenalectomized and ovariectomized rats.
Acta Physiol Scand 129:471-477.

Smith U, Hammarsten J, Björntorp P and Kral J (1979).
Regional differences and effect of weight reduction on
human fat cell metabolism. Eur J Clin Invest 9:327-332.
Vague J (1947). La differenciation sexuelle-facteur déterminant des formes de l'obesité. La Presse Médicale
30:339-340.
Xuefan X, Björntorp P.(1987a). Effects of sex steroid hormones on multiplication, differentiation and lipid accumulation in adipose precursor cells in primary culture.
Submitted for publication.
Xuefan X, Rebuffé-Scrive M and Björntorp P. (1987b). Cytoplasmic sex hormones binding in rat adipose precursor
cells. Submitted for publication.

Fat Distribution During Growth and Later Health Outcomes
pages 175–191 © *1988 Alan R. Liss, Inc.*

POSSIBLE MECHANISMS RELATING FAT DISTRIBUTION AND
METABOLISM.

Per Björntorp

Department of Medicine I

Sahlgren's Hospital
413 45 Göteborg, Sweden.

Abstract:

Abdominal obesity, as indicated by the waist/hip circumference (W/H) ratio, has been shown to be statistically
associated (independent of BMI) to cardiovascular disease,
stroke, non-insulin dependent diabetes mellitus (NIDDM)
and female carcinomas, while BMI (independent of the W/H
ratio) shows considerably weaker associations except for
NIDDM. Recent studies have shown different strength also
in the associations to the W/H ratio and the BMI (independently from each other) on the one hand, and established
risk factors for the mentioned diseases on the other. The
W/H ratio is thus positively correlated to most of these
risk factors (plasma lipids and fibrinogen, hypertension,
smoking, decreased glucose tolerance, insulin resistance
as well as, for female cancers, irregular menstruations),
while BMI only is associated to plasma triglycerides, as
well as hypertension, and is negative correlated to smoking. Further analyses along these principles revealed
other striking differences suggesting that an increased
W/H ratio is associated with a poor health in general,
particularly in psychosomatic disease and psychiatric conditions, as well as to a relatively poor socioeconomic
adjustment. Earlier and new preliminary studies suggest
that an increased W/H ratio is followed by increased activity in both the sympatho-adrenal, and pituitary-adrenal
axes. These findings are compatible with an increased W/H
ratio being associated with an arousal at the hypothalamic
level.

This in turn might be due to a poor coping to environmental stress. The W/H ratio might be a secondary consequence, or a stabile symptom, of such a chronic arousal syndrome via effects of adrenal corticosteroids on abdominal adipose tissue metabolism. An increased adrenocortical secretion would also help to explain the insulin resistance and the elevated cholesterol levels, while an arousal of the sympathoadrenal axis might explain the hypertension seen in association with elevated W/H ratio. A disturbance of the pituitary-ovarian axis might help to explain irregular ovulations and menstruations, and give a link to endometrial carcinoma, via unopposed estrogen exposure to the cells of the endometrial mucosa. Furthermore, the increased androgenicity might be explained along with these disturbances, although this is as yet entirely hypothetical. BMI seems to be associated mainly with NIDDM and hypertriglyceridemia, an effect perhaps triggered by increased mobilization of free fatty acids from lipolytically sensitive, enlarged abdominal adipose tissues. It is concluded that the distribution factor which might be a stabile symptom of a hypothalamic arousal, should be separated from obesity, defined as an increase of body fat mass, in the analysis of the hazzards of these two conditions. It should be emphasized, however, that the information referred to is obtained from non-selected samples of the population, containing only a limited number of moderately obese and few very obese subjects. Severe, morbid obesity is probably a separate, more malignant condition.

Key words: Obesity, abdominal adipose tissue, BMI, W/H, diabetes mellitus, hyperlipidemia, hypertension, insulin resistance, female carcinomas, cortisol, sympathetic nervous system, stress, coping, arousal, estrogen.

INTRODUCTION

Previous and recent cross-sectional studies have shown consistently that obesity localized to abdominal adipose tissue is associated with disease to a much higher degree than when excess adipose tissue is distributed peripherally, mainly over the hips and buttocks. The concept that abdominal obesity is hazzardous has been considerably strengthened by recent prospective studies. In such studies abdominally localized adipose tissue, has been shown to be a risk factor for cardiovascular disease, stroke,

diabetes mellitus and female carcinomas. It has previously been well-known that these conditions are prevalent
among obese subjects. The prospective studies show, however, that obesity may not always necessarily be involved,
or might be a less powerful "risk factor" than the abdominal distribution of adipose tissue. (For a more detailed
review, see Björntorp,1985).

A natural question in this situation is of course why
abdominal adipose tissue is statistically associated with
the diseases mentioned. Principally, of course, statistical associations tell nothing about cause-effect relationships. They might, however, be useful in providing new
ideas for pathophysiological mechanisms. Adipose tissue in
the abdominal regions might either be causing the disease
in question directly or indirectly, or be a parallel consequence, together with the diseases in question, of an
independent mechanism. There could of course be a combination of these possibilities. These alternatives will be
discussed in the following.

Associations between W/H or BMI and risk factors for
diseases.

The diseases in question have a number of so called
"risk factors" in prospective studies. Such factors are
statistically associated with the development of disease,
and although not necessarily meaning a cause-effect relationship, such factors might help in understanding the
development of disease. Several of the conditions mentioned have "risk factors" in common, for example hypertension for cardiovascular disease, and stroke, insulin
resistance for cardiovascular disease, and non-insulin
dependent diabetes mellitus (NIDDM). In an attempt to find
explanations to the tight associations between abdominal
localization of adipose tissue and the diseases mentioned,
it might therefore be helpful to first examine the relationship between on the one hand such risk factors and, on
the other, obesity in general terms, measured as body mass
index (BMI), or abdominally localized adipose tissue, measured simply as the ratio of the waist and hip circumferences (W/H ratio). As already mentioned, the risk with an
elevated W/H ratio might sometimes be independent of BMI.
It is therefore probably useful to examine the associations between various variables and the BMI or W/H , where
the latter factors have been analysed mutually independent

from each other.

These analyses have basically been performed in two prospective studies of, men (The men born 1913) and of women (The Gothenburg Population Study of Women) which are ongoing in Göteborg, Sweden (Tibblin, 1967, Bengtsson et al, 1973). Both these studies, which were started in the sixties, were designed to elucidate the association bet- ween various factors and long-term morbidity and mortali- ty. An unusual number of observations were registered at the start, making these studies uniquely helpful for ana- lyses of the type that will be described in the following. A more detailed description of results from these studies will be given by Larsson in this symposium.

There are a number of well-established risk factors for cardiovascular disease, stroke, NIDDM and female carci- nomas, the diseases which have so far been found to be predicted by abdominal obesity. For cardiovascular disease such factors are the concentration of plasma lipids, par- ticularly cholesterol, smoking, hypertension, decreased glucose tolerance, as well as increased plasma insulin and fibrinogen. For stroke, hypertension is a well-known risk factor. A very recent analysis of the cohort of men born 1913 has shown that diastolic blood pressure, the death of stroke of the mother, and the W/H ratio are the three only independent risk factors for stroke (Welin et al, 1987). Among less strong risk factors were BMI, and plasma lipids. A similar analysis of risk factors for NIDDM has shown that heredity is again important, as well as blood glucose and lactate (at rest), blood pressure and the W/H ratio as well as BMI (Ohlsson et al,1985). Factors asso- ciated with female carcinomas include obesity, hyperten- sion, NIDDM and elevated blood lipids in cross-sectional studies. This is, however, not the case in a recent pros- pective study, where the W/H ratio, but not BMI, was a prospective risk factor. The small number of end points in this study precluded more detailed conclusions, but it seems clear from other studies that exposure of unopposed estrogen is a strong pathogenetic factor for the develop- ment of for example endometrial cancer (For review, see Simopoulos, 1985).

Most of the mentioned risk factors are possible to ana- lyse in relation to W/H or BMI in the population studies in question, and this has been performed recently in the men (Larsson et al, 1987), and women (Lapidus et al, 1987), showing remarkably consistent results in the both sexes. The W/H ratio, independent of BMI, was associated with all the mentioned risk factors (cholesterol, trigly-cerides, smoking, hypertension, decreased glucose toleran-ce, fibrinogen, and blood lactate) in both men and women. However, BMI, independent of the W/H ratio, correlated only with plasma triglycerides and hypertension, while smoking actually was negatively correlated to BMI. This also was found in both men and women.

Unfortunately, plasma insulin concentration or other direct, indicators of insulin resistance were not measured as prospective variables in the studies in question. In cross-sectional studies, where this has been measured in great detail, an increased W/H ratio has, however, been found to be closely associated to insulin resistance and mechanisms have been suggested, to explain this phenome-non, supported by convincing experimental evidence (Peiris et al,1987). These observations strongly suggest that if plasma insulin concentration had been measured in the prospective studies, it had correlated with the W/H ratio, and perhaps also with the BMI, as has been shown in seve-ral cross-sectional studies (Krotkiewski et al 1983, Kissebah et al 1983,).

W/H ratio and BMI in relation to general health and socioeconomic factors

The amazing persistance of the positive associations to the W/H ratio, in contrast to the much less tight associa-tions to BMI, of various examined obesity-related disea-ses, symptoms and risk factors encouraged further analyses with other diseases and symptoms. These were selected to include conditions which are known to be associated to obesity. It was then first observed that both men and women with high W/H ratio were in general sick more often and during longer periods of time than subjects with a lower W/H ratio. They used hospital facilities more fre-quently such as X-ray, and needed surgical operations more often. In contrast, if anything, a high BMI was followed by less of these phenomena. Of specific diseases it seemed that peptic ulcer, and, in the women, accidents, fractures and even some infectious diseases were more prevalent with elevated W/H, while again this was, if anything, less fre-quent in persons with elevated BMI. Psychiatric disease, and psychological variables were examined in detail in a subgroup of the women only. In contrast to women with high BMI women with elevated W/H ratio were often sleepless and had nightmares and they often felt stressed. These women also frequently used tranquilizers and antidepressants. Of particular interest here was an association between the W/H ratio and general psychological impairment, including periods of depression. Women taking antidepressant drugs showed a marked shift to the right of their distribution of the W/H ratio.

A related phenomenon was probably that women with elevated W/H ratio also used more alcohol and tobacco, while elevated BMI was associated with less use of beer, wine, strong liquor and cigarettes. In men smoking was again found to be positively correlated to the W/H and negatively to the BMI. No significant associations were found to alcohol.

There were also differences in socioeconomic variables, but here the sexes showed different characteristics. While a low social class and low education was associated with an elevated W/H in the men, women with elevated BMI showed these characteristics. Men showed interesting differences in the correlation to other anthropometric variables than BMI and W/H. BMI was positively correlated to lean body mass and frame measurements while in contrast, the W/H ratio was negatively correlated to frame and height. No such correlations were found in women.

Taken together this seems to result in the following picture. Distribution of adipose tissue to the abdominal regions, irrespective of degree of obesity, seems to be associated with poor health in general terms. It appears that it is particularly psychosomatic and psychiatric entities that are involved, at least in women. Such women feel stressed, are suffering from sleep disturbances and are often medicating against such problems. Of particular interest are the suggestions of associations to depressive symptoms and disease. The use of stimulants and the proneness to accidents might be other features of the same general psychological personality of these women. The picture that is emerging seems to be one of a women subjected to a high degree of environmental stress with which she has difficulties to cope, producing a number of psychological, psychosomatic and psychiatric consequences. The men show several similar features. They seem to be socially less well-adjusted, and are often sick in psychosomatic diseases such as peptic ulcer.

Stress and neruoendocrine responses.

These analyses then have brought a number of other observations into the picture, suggesting that socioen-vironmental factors are associated statistically with adi-pose tissue distribution and are involved in psychosocial maladjustment, and as pathogenetic agents.

Such mechanisms are well-known from studies in the experi-mental animal as well as in humans. The studies by Henry have shown that mice stressed by social interactions in colonies show either a dominant, controlled behaviour, a defense reaction, or a defeated, submissive behaviour with a loss of control (Henry and Stephens, 1977). In primates Mason (1968) as well as more recently Kaplan et al (1984) have reported similar but more detailed findings. Conti-nued or frequently repeated stress is associated with ele-vated blood pressure and plasma lipids. In defeated, sub-missive females adrenal cortex is hypertrophied and ovula-tion irregular. Aortic and coronary artery atherosclerosis is also seen. There are thus remarkable similarities bet-ween these primates, which are stressed under highly stan-dardized conditions, and particularly the women with a high W/H ratio. These various forms of stress seem to be followed by specific neuroendocrine responses, the domi-nant stress response is associated with mainly an increase in the activity of the sympathetic nervous system, and an increase in testosterone production in males, while the defeat syndrome is characterized by primarily an increased activity of the pituitary-adrenal cortex axis, producing an excess of adrenal steroid hormones.

Experiments in humans in a laboratory situation have also shown stress responses in both the symatho-adrenal and the pituitary-adrenal axes, resulting in an incresed urinary excretion of both catecholamines and cortisol. Men seem to respond more than women to both physical and psychological stress stimuli (Frankenhaeuser, 1983). In more chronic stress situations there is suggestive eviden-ce for adverse effects on a number of functions of the body, of potential pathogenetic importance. These include peptic ulcer, plasma lipids, cardiovascular disease among a number of other conditions (Wolf and Godell, 1968).

Increased W/H ratio as consequence of a hypothalamic
arousal syndrome.

The observations made in the population studies on the
associations between abdominally localized adipose tissue
and various signs of poor coping to socioenvironmental
stress might be seen in the light of the information
referred to. It is suggested that a common denominator to
the symptoms of poor somatic and psychologic health seen
is a consequence of a poor coping to a stressful socio-economic environment. This would result in an "arousal" at
the hypothalamic level, with an increased neuroendocrine
secretion along the sympathoadrenal and/or pituitary adrenal axes, in other words increased activity of the sympathetic nervous system and increased concentrations of
ACTH, cortisol and adrenal androgens in the circulation.
The suggestions of depressive symptoms associated with the
W/H ratio seem of particular interest here because of the
wellknown increased cortisol secretion in depression.

As already mentioned above, a part of a hypothalamic
arousal syndrome is involving the sympathetic nervous system. Symptoms of increased activity of the sympathetic
nervous system are also found in association with the W/H
ratio. These include slight hypertension, increased plasma
renin, cardiac output and heart rate, (unpublished observations) as well as increased concentrations of circulating free fatty acids (FFA).(Kissebah et al, 1985).

Corticosteroids and abdominal localization of adipose
tissue.

The next important question is then how an increased W/H
ratio might be associated with such an "arousal syndrome".
As mentioned above a defeat situation in mice and monkeys,
as well as in stressed humans is associated with an elevated neuroendocrine secretion, including ACTH, stimulating
cortisol secretion. Increased ACTH and cortisol secretion
is known to be associated with abdominally localized adipose tissue, as seen clearly in Cushing's disease. This
can also be seen after distribution of exogenous corticosteroids, such as in severe bronchial asthma. The detailed
mechanisms here are, however, not clear, and might include
both an increased mobilization of peripheral depots via an

activation of the lipolytic system of the adipocytes and an increased lipid accumulation via activation of abdominal lipoprotein lipase activity. It might be of significance that the density of corticosteroid hormone receptors seems to be higher in intraabdominal than other examined adipose tissue. (For more details of this specific area, see review by Rebuffé-Scrive in this issue).

Adrenal corticosteroids and the W/H ratio.

Can an increased activity of the ACTH-adrenal cortex axis be found in relation to an increased W/H ratio? Krotkiewski et al (1966) have already 20 years ago observed elevated urinary excretion of both 17-keto and 17-ketogenic steroids in android obese women. We have recently made a similar examination and found a week and barely significant positive correlation between the W/H ratio and urinary excretion of free cortisol in women with slight or moderate obesity. It seems likely, that if a relation between the W/H ratio and cortisol excretion is present this would be easier to find under field conditions where every-day stress is involved.

Preliminary experiments have also been performed with stress tests under laboratory conditions. These included both psychological and physiological stress with measurements of plasma concentrations of cortisol, prolactin and growth hormone. Only physical stress in the form of cold pressure test, and in the form of the discomfort of the intravenous needle stick, gave responses in the hormones. There seems to be a positive correlation between intraabdominally localized adipose tissue and plasma cortisol concentration in these tests (unpublished observations).

Vague et al,(1985) have previously shown positive correlations between the degree of android obesity and the response to ACTH stimulation of cortisol, androstenedione and testosterone. It therefore seems possible that when the system is stressed by physical stress or direct hormonal stimulation the W/H ratio is positively correlated with adrenocortical secretions. More studies are, however, needed here before definite conclusions can be arrived at.

An attempt to synthesis.

The role of hypothalamic arousal.

   At this point an attempt to synthesis will be made. It
is thus clear that the W/H ratio is associated with a number of diseases in both cross-sectional and longitudinal
studies. It also seems clear that the W/H ratio is associated with a number of observations indicating psychosocial maladjustment, and poor coping to environmental
stress. The simplest way to connect these observations
seem to be via a condition of hypothalamic arousal, which
causes an increase in both the sympatico-adrenal and the
pituitary adrenal axes.

Cortisol may then cause an abdominal localization of adipose tissue as a "stabile" symptom of such and "arousal
syndrome". Cortisol would, however, probably also have
other effects. These include a decreased insulin sensitivity of the periphery, providing an explanation to this
phenomenon with elevated W/H ratio. Whether aldosterone is
elevated as a part of the increased stimulation of the
adrenal cortical hormones is not known, but would be a
piece of valuable information in relation to hypertension.

   How does smoking fit into this picture? It may be recalled that both women and men with increased W/H ratio smoke
comparably much, while those with increased BMI smoke comparably little. Smoking seems by itself cause symptoms
similar to that of hypothalamic arousal, because both the
activity of the sympathetic nervous system, in terms of
increased heart rate and blood pressure, and urinary cortisol secretion are markedly increased after smoking in
normal subjects (Amemiya and Björntorp, unpublished). It
seems unlikely, however, that smoking is the cause to the
symptoms of chronic arousal found to be associated with
increased W/H ratio because smoking is not a risk factor
for stroke or cardiovascular disease in women (Ohlson et
al, 1985, Welin et al, 1987, Lapidus et al, 1984), and the
W/H ratio is a risk factor for cardiovascular disease
independent of smoking in men (Larsson et al, 1984). It
seems more likely that the basic psycho-social situation
of the subjects examined is the primary factor, followed
by the use of stimulants, including alcohol and smoking.

Increased activity of the central sympathetic nervous system has been considered to be a likely pathway for the pathogenesis of early essential hypertension (Julius and Esler, 1975). The correlation between a high W/H ratio and hypertension might therefore be another consequence of this "arousal syndrome".

One might ask whether other neuroendocrine secretions might be disturbed along with the sympatho-adrenal and pituitary-adrenal axes. A good candidate here would be the secretions of the follicle stimulating and the luteinizing hormones. The delicate balance between these two secretions is an important prerequisite for ovulation, progesterone secretion and menstruation. There is a disturbance in these functions associated with an increased W/H ratio (Hartz et al, 1983). It may be recalled that monkeys subjected to a defeat syndrome by stress also ovulate irregularly and produce too little progesteron (Kaplan et al, 1984). It therefore seems reasonable to assume that these disturbances also are part of a disturbed neuroendocrine secretion from the hypothalamus, now affecting the pituitary-ovarian axis, although so far no direct measurements of the function of this axis has been performed in relation to adipose tissue distribution.

This possibility is of particular potential significance for the association between the W/H ratio and endometrial carcinoma. This disease has been thought to be closely associated to an increased, uninterrupted secretion of estrogen, having a carcinogenic effect on the mucosal cells. This would be the situation if ovulation, progesterone production and menstruation are not occurring regularly to exchange the endometrial mucosa which under such conditions is exposed to estrogen during prolonged periods of time.

The role of obesity

By this theory it then seems possible to link the W/H ratio to several of the risk factors for cardiovascular disease, stroke, NIDDM and female carcinomas. The remaining question then is to try to analyse how BMI is involved. It may then be recalled that in addition to the W/H ratio BMI was positively associated to plasma triglyceride concentration hypertension, and NIDDM. It is known that the abdominal adipose tissues have a lively lipolytic activity (for details, see the review by Rebuffé-Scrive in this issue). An increase of the size of the abdominal adipose tissue such as in abdominal obesity, as indicated by an elevated W/H ratio plus elevated BMI, would then presumably result in increased concentrations of free fatty acids (FFA), as has also been described (Kissebah et al, 1985). Increased circulatin FFA might have several consequences. One would be to decrease peripheral glucose transport and decrease insulin sensitivity (Randle et al, 1963). Insulin resistance, is considered to be one of the corner-stones in the pathogenesis of NIDDM. Furthermore, increased FFA concentrations, particularly when produced from the visceral depots into the portal circulation, would increase very low density lipoprotein production by the liver resulting in increased of primarily plasma triglyceride concentration. In this way hypertriglyceridemia, insulin resistance and an increased risk for NIDDM might be thought to be causally related to the production of excess FFA.

This leaves us with the problem of hypertension and its association to both the W /H ratio and BMI. If we accept that the association to the W/H ratio is due to a hypothalamic arousal syndrome, including the central sympathetic nervous system, then the question remains how BMI is linked to elevated blood pressure. Let us again assume that an increased activity of the central nervous system is involved in the pathogenesis of early essential hypertension. It has been suggested that the sympathetic activity might be increased in obesity as a consequence of a positive caloric balance (Landsberg and Young, 1978). This then would presumably be another type of activation of the central sympathetic nervous system, involving more specifically this particular branch of the neurophysiological response and not involving the cortical parts as with the stress activation of the hypothalamic area. This of course is entirely hypothetical.

It is of considerable interest, that both the W/H ratio and BMI are associated to hypertension, but only the W/H ratio is associated with increased risk for stroke (Welin et al, 1987). These observations suggest that hypertension in the obese is less malignant if factors associated with the elevated W/H ratio are not involved. These findings and interpretations are reminiscent of previous suggestions of a relative innocense of hypertension in obesity

(Barrett-Connors and Khaw, 1985).

The role of increased androgenicity.

A finding which is related to an increased W/H ratio, and which has not been discussed, is the elevated levels of free testosterone and low sex hormone binding globuline concentrations in women (Evans et al, 1983). It is not clear how the increased free testosterone concentration is brought about. At least two alternatives seem possible. One alternative is an adrenal origin of the androgens, directly or indirectly produced by the elevated stimuli of the adrenal cortex, as shown by Vague's (1985) stimulation by ACTH. Another alternative might be an increased secretion from the ovarian follicles, a hypothetical consequence of a disturbed pituitary-ovarian axis discussed above. Whatever the mechanism it is probable that the increased androgenicity seen in women with an elevated W/H ratio is caused by this abberation in hormonal secretion. Such androgenicity is expressed by a tendency to hirsutism in these women. Furthermore, findings in women of increased muscle mass and a muscle fiber composition, similar to the characteristics of men, are probably other expressions of increased androgenicity (Krotkiewski and Björntorp, 1986). It is of particular interest that these muscle characteristics can be produced experimentally by testosterone injections in rats (Krotkiewski et al, 1980). Furthermore, such muscle tissue, containing a relative abundance of white, fast twitch fibers is relative insensitive to insulin stimulation (Hom and Goodner, 1984), and contains less insulin receptors (Boren et al, 1981). The insulin resistance found associated with a high W/H ratio in women with such muscle tissue (Krotkiewski and Björntorp, 1986) might thus be at least partly explained by this factor.

Conclusions

In this review an altempt has been made to explain the relationships between obesity factors, particularly the distribution of adipose tissue, and health prcblems. The interpretations of the current situation is based on the information available at present, and has, of course, to be partly hypothetical where information is missing. At this stage, however, it seems warranted to suggest that obesity, defined as an increase of total fat mass, and abdominal distribution of body fat, are treated as different entities. It seems very likely that these two factors have different pathogenetic background, and it seems clear that they are associated with widely different health factors. The distribution factor is more closely associated than obesity to a spectrum of indicators of poor health, from feeling of stress to serious vascular catastrophies and malignancies. Obesity seems by itself to be associated mainly with metabolic abberations such as insulin resistance and hypertriglyceridemia, as well as with hypertension. Obesity might therefore be a more benign condition than previously thought when the adipose tissue distribution factor has not been taken in consideration. As a matter of fact, certain observations indicate a particularly good health in obese subjects. It should, however, be clearly emphasized that the information on which this review is based, has mainly been obtained in populations of non-selected subjects from the population, with about 20% moderately obese, and with very few severely obese subjects. There is abundant evidence that morbid obesity is a clear health hazzard with a mortality (Burton et al, 1985) of the same order as mammary carcinoma. Why this is so is not clear, but also here it seems advicable to separate different potential factors contributing more or less strongly to the excess morbidity and mortality of this syndrome.

REFERENCES

Barrett-Connors E, Kwah KT. (1985). Is hypertension more benign when associated with obesity? Circulation 72:53-60.
Bengtsson C, Blohmé G, Hallberg L et al. (1973). The study of women in Gothenburg 1968-69 - population study. General design, purpose and sampling results. Acta Med Scand 193:311-318.
Björntorp P. (1985). Regional patterns of fat distribution. Ann.Int.Med.103:994-995.
Bonen A, Tan M.H. and Watson-Wright W.M. (1981). Insulin binding and glucose uptake in rodent skeletal muscle. .Diabetes 30:702-704.
Burton BT, Foster WR, Hirsch J and vanItallie TB. (1985). Health implications of obesity: an NIH concensus development conference. Int J Obesity 9:155-170.

Evans PJ, Hoffman R-G, Kalkhoff R.K. and Kissebah A.H. (1983). Relationship of androgenic activity to body fat topography, fat cell morphology and metabolic abberations in menopausal women. J Clin Endocr Metab 57:304-310.

Frankenhaeuser M. The symphatetic-adrenal and pituitary-adrenal response to challenge: Comparison between the sexes. (1983). In: Dembroski TM, Schmidt TH and Blümchen G eds. Biobehavioural Bases of Coronary Heart Disease, Human Psychophysiology, Karger Biobehvioral Medicine Series,2:91-105.

Hartz AJ, Rupley DC, Kalkhoff RD, and Rimm AA (1983). Relationship of obesity to diabetes:influence of obesity level and body fat distribution. Prev Med 12:351-357.

Henry JP, Stephen PM. Stress, health, and the social environment. A sociobiological approach to medicine. Springer, New York, 1977.

Hom FG and Goodner CJ. (1984). Insulin dose-response characteristics among individual muscle and adipose tissues measured in the rat in vivo with ^{3}(H)2-deoxyglucose. Diabetes 33:153-159.

Julius S and Esler M (1975). Autonomic nervous cardiovascularregulation in borderline hypertension. Amer J Cardiol 36:685-696.

Kaplan JR, Adams MR, Clarkson TB, and Koritnik DR (1984). Psychosocial influences on female protection among Cynomolgus Macaques. Atherosclerosis 53:283-295.

Kissebah AH, Evans DJ, Peiris A and Wilson CR (1985). Endocrine characteristics of regional obesities: Role of sex steroids. In: Vague et al, (eds) Metabolic Complications of Human Obesities, Excerpta Medica, Amsterdam, pp.115-130.

Kissebah AH, Vydelingum N, Murray R, Evans D, Hartz A, Kalkhoff R and Adams P. (1983). Relation of body fat distribution to metabolic complications of obesity. J Clin Endocr Metab 54:254-260.

Krotkiewski M, Butruk E and Zembrzuska Z (1966). Les fonctions cortico-surrenales dans les divers types morphologiques d'obesité. Le Diabete, 19:229-233.

Krotkiewski M and Björntorp P (1986). Muscle tissue in obesity with different distribution of adipose tissue, effects of physical training. Int J Obesity 10:331-341.

Landsberg L and Young LB. (1978). Fasting, feeding and regulation of the sympathetic nervous system. N Eng J Med 298:1295-1301.

Larsson B, Svärdsudd K, Welin L, Wilhelmsen L, Björntorp P and Tibblin G. (1984). Abdominal adipose tissue distribution, obesity and risk of cardiovascular disease and death: 13 year follow-up of participants in the study of men born in 1913. Brit Med J 288:1401-1404.

Larsson B, Seidell J, Svärdsudd K, Welin L, Tibblin G and Björntorp P (1987). Obesity, adipose tissue distribution and health in men. The Study of Men Born in 1913. Submitted for publ.

Lapidus L, Bengtsson C, Larsson B, Pennert K, Rybo E and Sjöström L. (1984). Distribution of adipose tissue and risk of cardiovascular disease and death: a 12 year follow-up of participants in the population study of women in Gothenburg, Sweden. Brit Med J 289:1257-1261.

Lapidus L, Bengtsson C, Hällström T and Björntorp P (1987). Obesity, adipose tissue distribution and health in women-results from a population study in Gothenburg, Sweden. Submitted for publication.

Mason JW. Organization of the multiple endocrine responses to avoidance in the monkey. Psychosomatic Medicine 30:774-790.

Ohlsson LO, Larsson B, Svärdsudd K, Welin L, Eriksson H, Wilhelmsen L, Björntorp P and Tibblin G. (1985). The influence of body fat distribution on the incidence of diabetes mellitus. 13.5 years follow-up of the participants in the study of men born 1913. Diabetes 34:1055-1058.

Peiris AN, Mueller RA, Struve MF, Smith GA and Kissebah AH. (1987). Relationships of androgenic activity to splanchnic insulin metabolism and peripheral glucose utilization in premenopausal women. J Clin Endocr Metab 64:162-169.

Randle PJ, Garland PB, Hales CN, and Newsholme EA. (1963). The glucose fatty acid cycle. Its role in insulin sensitivity and the metabolic disturbances of diabetes mellitus. Lancet 2:785-789.

Simopoulos A. (1985). Fat intake, obesity, and cancer of the breast and endometrium. Med Oncol Tumour Pharmacother. 2:125-135.

Tibblin G. (1967). High blood pessure in men aged 50 - A population study of men born in 1913.(1967). Acta Med Scand 178:453-458.

Vague J, Meignen JM, Negrin JF, Thomas M, Tramoni M and Jubelin J (1985). La diabete de la femme androide. Trente-cinq ans aprés. Sem Hop. Paris 61:1015-1025.

Welin L, Svärdsudd K, Wilhelmsen L, Larsson B and Tibblin
   G. (1987). Family history and other risk factors for
   stroke. The Study of Men Born in 1913. N Engl J Med, in
   print.
Wolf S and Godell H (1968). Stress and disease.
   Charles Thomas, NY 1968.

Fat Distribution During Growth and Later Health Outcomes
pages 193–201 © *1988 Alan R. Liss, Inc.*

FAT DISTRIBUTION AND RISK FOR DEATH, MYOCARDIAL INFARCTION
AND STROKE

Bo Larsson

Department of Medicine I, University of Göteborg, 413 45 Göteborg, Sweden

INTRODUCTION:

In most studies the degree of obesity is associated
with several risk factors for arteriosclerosis, but obesity
is not consistently associated with coronary heart risk
(Larsson B et al 1981). Recent epidemiologic studies have
indicated that the distribution of fat deposits may be a
better predictor of arteriosclerotic vascular disease than
is the degree of obesity. I will discuss studies on the
association between adipose tissue distribution and "hard
endpoints" like death, myocardial infarction and stroke
(Table I). Other authors will deal with the connections
between fat distribution and risk factors for cardiovascular disease like glucose intolerance, blood lipids, and
blood pressure.

The importance of a distinction between central and
peripheral type of fat distribution was stressed by Vague
already in the fifties. In clinical cross-sectional studies
he indicated that "atherosclerosis is more influenced by
the degree of masculine differentiation than by excessive
weight". (Vague J et al 1955). Not until recently any
attempt have been made to confirm his findings.

REVIEW OF LITERATURE:
U S A
      Studies of the Framingham cohort, after more than 20
years of follow-up, showed that obesity was associated to
the risk of cardiovascular disease also independent of its
association to blood pressure, serum cholesterol and blood

Table 1. Fat distribution and CHD incidence. Prospective epidemiological studies.

Study	Framingham Heart Study	Honolulu Heart program	Paris Prospective Study	Prospective Men Born in 1913	Population Study of Women
Population size	2420 F 1934 M	7692 M	7746 M	792 M	1462 F
Age at baseline (yrs)	34-68	-	42-53	54	38-60
Fat distribution measure	Subscapular skinfold	Subscapular skinfold	Sum of skinfolds Ratio upper/lower circumference	Waist/Hip circumference	Waist/Hip circumference
Follow-up duration (yrs)	22	12	6.6	13	12
Number of events	-CHD	448 CHD	128 CHD	91 CHD 33 stroke 101 death	23 MI 13 stroke 76 death
Linear dose-response evident	-	yes	yes		yes
Independent of other CHD risk factors	yes	yes	yes	no	yes

glucose (Hubert HB et al 1983). At the fourth biennial examination, involving 2420 women and 1934 men aged 34-68, some measurements of body configuration and of regional distribution of fat was included (Stokes J et al 1985). Table 2 shows the association between 22-year coronary heart disease (CHD) incidence and various indices of obesity after adjusting for age and other CHD risk factors. The standardized coefficients allow comparison of the relative importance of the risk factors. Subscapular skinfold measurement appears to be the best measure in both men and women. The relative importance of subscapular skinfold thickness with other risk factors for CHD showed that in both sexes it is one of the more important risk factors.

Table 2. The relative independent contributions of certain indices of obesity to the 22-year incidence of CHD. The Framingham heart study.

Index of obesity	Standardized regression coefficient	
	Men	Women
Subscapular skinfold	0.306	0.183
Abdominal skinfold	0.265	(0.079)
Waist circumference	0.162	(0.021)
Body mass index	0.185	0.136

Comments:
   This analysis indicates that truncal obesity, expressed as subscapular skinfold thickness, is a better predictor of coronary heart disease than degree of obesity measured as body mass index (BMI) or waist circumference.

   Since obesity indices act as risk factors for coronary heart disease also via serum cholesterol, blood pressure and blood glucose it would have been interesting to see results from age standardized simple regression analysis also.

   Recently a report from the Honolulu Heart Program (Donahue RP et al 1987) showed the relation between central

body fat distribution, determined by measurement of subscapular skinfold thickness, and the development of coronary
heart disease. A 12 year follow-up of 7692 men showed that
the risk of coronary heart disease was directly related to
subscapular skinfold thickness stronger than to BMI (Fig.1)
The independent effect of subscapular skinfold thickness
was significant after adjustment for BMI and other risk-
factors for CHD. In contrast the independent effect of BMI
was not significant after adjustment for subscapular skinfold thickness.

Comments:
    For a given level of BMI, central subcutaneous distri-
bution of fat was an independent risk factor for CHD in
men of Japanese ancestry.

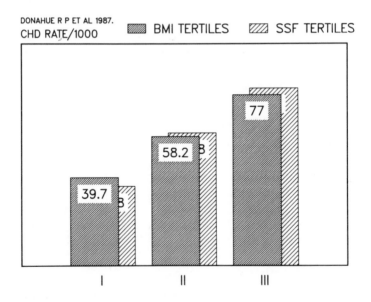

DONAHUE R P ET AL 1987.
CHD RATE/1000   ▨ BMI TERTILES   ▨ SSF TERTILES

Figure 1. Age adjusted 12-year incidence of coronary
heart disease in tertiles of subscapular skinfold thickness
(SSF) and body mass index (BMI).

France
    Relationships between adiposity measurements and the
incidence of coronary heart disease have also been analy-

sed in the Paris Prospective Study I (Ducimetiere P et al
1985). 7746 men aged 42-53 years have been followed up from
5 to 9 years and events were classified as angina pectoris,
or myocardial infarction and sudden death.

The subscapular, axiliary and subumbilikal skinfold
thickness were the most predictive variables, whereas four
skinfold measurements at the thigh were not all associated
with CHD. The two global measurements (BMI, iliac circumference) were moderately significantly associated with CHD.

The sum of subscapular, axiliary and subumbilical skinfold thickness (S_1) over the sum of 4 skinfold thickness of
the thigh (S_2) was more closely associated with CHD risk
than any individual measurement. The age adjusted annual
incidence of CHD was about doubled for those in the upper
quintile of the S_1/S_2 distribution in comparison with those
in the lower quintile. The index S_1/S_2 remained a significant predictor of CHD risk also when conventional CHD risk
factors were taken into account. The global measure of obesity (BMI) was not a significant predictor for CHD in that
multivariate analysis.

Comments:
Predominance of fat in the upper part of the body, as
indicated by ratio of skinfolds, was a better predictor of
atherosclerotic disease than the overall degree of obesity.

In a later more detailed analysis of this population
(Ducimetiere P et al 1986), using subcutaneus fat distribution from 13 skinfold thicknesses, it was shown that trunk
fat deposits was a strong CHD risk factor also after controlling for other CHD risk factors.

Sweden
Men: In 792 54 year old men followed-up for 13 years
The Study of Men Born in 1913 (Larsson B et al 1984) the
relation between baseline measurements of abdominal adipose
tissue distribution (waist to hip circumference ratio),
commonly used indices of the degree of obesity and the
incidence of stroke, ischaemic heart disease and death from
all causes was studied. Body mass index, sum of three skinfold thicknessess, waist or hip circumference were not
significant predictors of any of three endpoints used.
Waist to hip ratio was a significant predictor for stroke,
ischaemic heart disease and death from all causes, also
when BMI or sum of the three skinfolds was accounted for.

The ratio was however not a predictor when smoking, blood pressure and serum cholesterol were taken into account.

In a more detailed analysis of risk factors for stroke after 19 years follow-up of this male cohort 7.2% developed stroke (Welin L et al. To be published). Waist to hip ratio was number two after blood pressure in a list of risk factors ranked in order of etiologic fraction. Body mass index was not a significant predictor of stroke.

Comments:
This was the first prospective study that seemed to confirm Vagues old hypothesis "that atherosclerosis is even more influenced by the degree of masculine differentiation than by excessive weight" (Vague J 1956). The study also indicated that men with high waist to hip ratio but low BMI might have the highest risk for cardiovascular disease and death.

Women:
Results from a longitudinal population study of 1462 women 38-60 followed up for 12 years The Population Study of Women in Gothenburg (Lapidus L et al 1984) showed that the waist to hip circumference ratio was a significant predictor of myocardial infarction, stroke and death whereas body mass index was a significant predictor for myocardial infarction only. The risk ratio between the highest and the lowest quintile of the waist to hip circumference distribution was 2.8 for myocardial infarction, 3.8 for stroke and 2.0 for death from all causes. Among the 10% women with the lowest ratio not a single women developed myocardial infarction or stroke. The association with incidence of myocardial infarction remained in multivariate analysis and was independent of age and body mass index (Fig 2) and also independent of smoking habits, serum cholesterol, serum triglycerides and systolic blood pressure.

Comments:
In women the relation between the waist to hip circumference ratio and myocardial infarction, stroke and death was stronger than for any other anthropometric variables studied. The risk associated with increasing ratio seem to be higher for women than for men. As for men the highest risk of CHD was noted for those who were lean with a high waist to hip ratio.

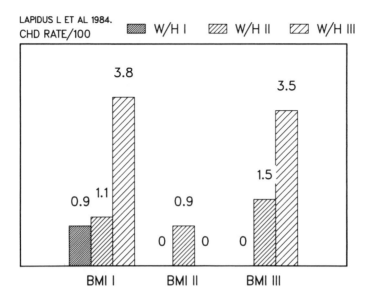

Figure 2. Age adjusted 12-year incidence of coronary heart disease in tertiles of waist to hip ratio (W/H) within each tertile of body mass index (BMI).

DISCUSSION:

   The purpose of epidemiology is to develop information on which prevention of disease may be based. The initial step is to look for risk factors for disease and the next, often difficult step, is to find out if the risk factor in question is alterable and if the ateration is benificial.

   The criteria for drawing causal inferences from observational studies as these reviewed include the strength and graded nature of the association, a clear temporal relationship with power to predict future risk, consistency between studies and biologic plausibility. Most of these criteria are met by the studies reviewed but only experimental studies can prove causality.

   Central or abdominal fat mass distribution is now identified as an important risk factor for CHD in five prospective studies from all over the world, but no intervention studies that could prove causality have been made.

Waiting for such we should go on studying the importance of genetic and environmental factors as determinants of the adipose tissue distribution. A certain adipose tissue distribution might be an indicator of a hithero unknown underlying factor that also increases the risk for vascular disease and death. It is therefore still difficult to assign the specific effect of a certain adipose tissue distribution alone.

ACKNOWLEDGEMENTS:
This study was supported by grants from the Swedish Medical Research Council (B86-27X-06276-05), the King Gustav V and Queen Victoria´s Foundation, the Medical Association of Gothenburg and the University of Gothenburg.

REFERENCES

Donahue RP, Abbot RD, Bloom E, Reed DM and Yano K (1987). Central obesity and coronary heart disease in men. Lancet 821-824.
Ducimetiere P, Richard J, Cambien F, Avous P and Jacqueson A (1985). Relationship between adiposity measurements and the incidence of coronary heart disease in a middle-aged male population - The Paris Prospective Study I. Am J Nutr.4:31-38.
Ducimetiere P, Richard J and Cambien F (1956). The pattern of subcutaneous fat distribution in middle-aged men and the risk of coronary heart disease: The Paris Prospective Study. Int J Obesity 10;229-240.
Hubert HB, Feinleib M and McNamara PM (1983). Obesity as an independent risk factor for cardiovascular disease. A 26-year follow-up of participants in the Framingham heart study. Circulation 67:768-777.
Lapidus L, Bengtsson C, Larsson B, Pennert K, Rybo E, Sjöström L (1984). Distribution of adipose tissue and risk of cardiovascular disease and death: a 12 year follow up of participants in the population study of women in Göteborg, Sweden. Br Med J 289:1261-1263.
Larsson B, Björntorp P, Tibblin G (1981). The health consequences of moderate obesity. Int J Obes. 5:91-116.
Larsson B, Svärdsudd K, Welin L, Wilhelmsen L, Björntorp P, Tibblin G (1984).Abdominal adipose tissue distribution, obesity and risk of cardiovascular disease and death. Br Med J 288:1401-1404.

Stokes J, Garrison R , Kannel WB (1985). The independent contribution of various indices of obesity to the 22-year incidence of coronary heart disease: The Framingham study. In Vague J ed. Metabolic complications of human obesity. Amsterdam: Elsevier 49-57.

Vague J (1956). The degree of masculine differentiation of obesities: A factor determining predisposition to diabetes, atherosclerosis, gout, and uric calculocus disease. Am J Nutr. 4:20-34.

Fat Distribution During Growth and Later Health Outcomes
pages 203–220 © 1988 Alan R. Liss, Inc.

MECHANISMS ASSOCIATING BODY FAT DISTRIBUTION TO GLUCOSE
INTOLERANCE AND DIABETES MELLITUS

Ahmed H. Kissebah, Alan Peiris and David J. Evans
Clinical Research Center
Medical College of Wisconsin
9200 West Wisconsin Avenue
Milwaukee, Wisconsin 53226

INTRODUCTION

Despite frequent assertions of a strong association between obesity and noninsulin-dependent diabetes mellitus, the nature of this relationship remains controversial. Descriptive and epidemiologic studies suggest a variety of factors that influence expression of diabetes in the obese population including social background, genetics and degree of overweight. The complexity of this relationship is further illustrated by the observation that the regional distribution of body fat is more closely aligned with glucose intolerance and overt diabetes than obesity per se. This relationship was recognized by Vague (1) and Feldman (2) in retrospective clinical studies. In a report from this institution (3), a continuous rise in the frequency of diabetes was observed with an increased distribution of fat to the upper body as assessed by the waist:hip girth ratio (WHR). Relative risk analysis yielded a risk factor of 3.17 for obesity and fat localization to the upper body increased this risk to 10.34. The importance of these epidemiologic associations has been confirmed in other populations (4-8). Furthermore, in a prospective study of healthy premenopausal women, WHR was an important predictor of glucose intolerance and hyperinsulinemia, and exerted an effect independent of and additive to that of obesity (9-16). The metabolic events by which regional body fat distribution influences glucose-insulin homeostasis and the exact role of obesity in these events are obscure. Our research (9-22) has shown that the fat depot is separated into 2 functionally distinct organs: an upper body depot (both intra- and extra-abdominal) which is metabolically capable of influencing the metabolic profile, and a lower body depot which exerts minimal influence upon glucose-insulin homeostasis. A sequence has also been proposed in which increasing androgenic activity (secretion and sensitivity) is considered a primary event, influencing both the pattern of body fat distribution and the metabolic aberration accompanying upper body fat predominance in the female. These studies as well as the supporting evidence from other laboratories are summarized below.

RELATIONSHIP OF BODY FAT DISTRIBUTION TO GLUCOSE TOLERANCE AND INSULIN LEVELS

To determine whether the site of body fat predominance predicts aberrations in insulin-glucose homeostasis, a cohort of premenopausal Caucasian women was evaluated. The distribution of fat between the upper and lower body was assessed from the WHR which varied from 0.64 to 1.02. Increasing WHR was accompanied by progressively increasing fasting plasma glucose and insulin, and higher insulin and glucose responses to oral glucose challenge. Partial and multiple regression analysis revealed that the effects of body fat topography are independent of and additive to those of obesity. Within obese subjects alone, percent ideal body weight (%IBW) had no predictive value, but WHR remained a significant predictor of plasma glucose and insulin concentrations.

In these studies, body fat distribution was assessed by WHR which has been found to be as effective in predicting the metabolic profile as more complicated procedures including multiple skinfold thickness, Vague's diabetogenic fat mass index, Ashwell's fat distribution score, and arm:thigh adipose ratio determined by CT scanning. Other anthropometric measures assessing the relative distribution of fat between the trunk and the thigh such as waist:thigh circumference ratio and subscapular:medial thigh skinfold ratio predicted the metabolic profile equally well. More important, however, was the highly significant correlation between the metabolic profile and the distribution of fat between the intra- and extra-abdominal sites, emphasizing the importance of the male type of fat distribution (higher intra:extra-abdominal ratio) in this association. WHR also correlated with the intra:extra-abdominal fat mass ratio.

METABOLIC SEQUENCE ASSOCIATING BODY FAT DISTRIBUTION TO THE
ABNORMALITIES IN INSULIN-GLUCOSE HOMEOSTASIS

The co-existence of hyperinsulinemia and impaired glucose tolerance in upper body segment obesity (UBSO) suggests
that diminished insulin sensitivity is the underlying abnormality. Thus, the first series of studies examined the
following questions: 1) Does the insulin resistance in UBSO
affect peripheral glucose disposal? 2) Is it expressed at
the tissue level, particularly in skeletal muscle? 3) Does
it involve a receptor and/or postreceptor defect? 4) Is it
a primary or secondary event, and what metabolic sequence is
involved?

The in vivo insulin effects on overall glucose metabolism were determined using the insulin impedance test and
the insulin euglycemic clamp procedure. WHR correlated
positively with the steady-state plasma glucose (SSPG) attained during the insulin impedance test and negatively with
the amount of glucose metabolized (M/I) during the euglycemic
clamp determined at a steady-state plasma insulin (SSPI) of
~100 uU/ml, suggesting diminishing sensitivity of insulin-
mediated glucose disposal. This relationship remained even
after adjusting for the effects of obesity per se.

Since skeletal muscle is a major utilizer of glucose,
impaired insulin sensitivity in this organ could be a major
factor in the pathogenesis of diminished glucose disposal.
As an index of insulin action in this organ, basal and
insulin-stimulated activities of glycogen synthase I (GSI)
were determined in quadriceps muscle biopsies. Insulin is
known to promote glycogen deposition by increasing %GSI in
skeletal muscle.

Obese women, separated into 3 age- and weight-matched
subgroups by increasing WHR, demonstrated a significant decline in %GSI response to submaximal insulin levels as WHR
increased. This decline correlated highly with the increase
in SSPG, suggesting that the defect in skeletal muscle insulin sensitivity contributes to the impairment in overall
glucose disposal. Insulin specific binding to circulating
monocytes was also decreased as WHR increased. The decrease
in insulin receptor number correlated with the decline in
skeletal muscle %GSI and the increase in SSPG. At supramaximal SSPI (~1000 uU/ml), a subgroup of the UBSO women
achieved normal SSPG, suggesting that the defect in their

glucose disposal resides at the receptor level. However, some UBSO women exhibited reductions in maximal glucose disposal with high SSPG even though their %GSI response was normalized, suggesting the presence of an additional post-receptor defect(s) affecting other pathways of glucose metabolism.

The significant intercorrelation between the metabolic variables measured is compatible with the complex glucose-insulin regulatory system in which a pertubation at one point evokes a multitude of secondary changes. Multiple regression pathway analysis revealed that WHR was most strongly associated with increasing plasma insulin levels.

The second series of studies thus examined the relationship of body fat distribution to splanchnic insulin metabolism and addressed the following questions. 1) Does the hyperinsulinemia of UBSO result from increased pancreatic secretion, diminished hepatic extraction of insulin, or both? 2) What is the influence of obesity level and the degree of insulin resistance? 3) What is the relationship between the abnormalities in splanchnic insulin metabolism and aberration in insulin action?

The principle for the methodology used is as follows: since insulin and its connecting peptide (c-peptide) are secreted from the pancreas equimolarly and since hepatic extraction of c-peptide, in contrast to insulin, is negligible, measurements of peripheral c-peptide turnover estimate prehepatic or pancreatic insulin production. Peripheral insulin turnover, on the other hand, estimates total body flux excluding the amount retained by the liver during the first portal passage. The difference between these 2 measurements quantifies the hepatic insulin extraction.

Compared to the nonobese, obese women have higher prehepatic insulin production and portal vein insulin levels basally and following i.v. or oral glucose stimulation. In age- and weight-matched UBSO and LBSO subjects, prehepatic insulin production and portal vein insulin levels at all time-points during oral glucose stimulation were comparably increased. Prehepatic insulin production was correlated with the degree of overweight but not WHR or peripheral insulin sensitivity, suggesting that insulin hypersecretion is primarily linked to obesity and not influenced by the distribution of body fat or the presence of insulin resistance.

Compared to the nonobese or LBSO, UBSO subjects demonstrated a significant decrease in hepatic insulin extraction both basally and during i.v. or oral glucose stimulation. Within the obese group, increasing WHR was correlated with decreasing hepatic insulin extraction fraction. Consequently, posthepatic insulin delivery was progressively increased and correlated well with the degree of peripheral hyperinsulinemia. Furthermore, the decrease in hepatic insulin extraction in the UBSO subjects was proportionate to the accompanying diminution in peripheral insulin sensitivity.

The third series of studies examined the relationship of abnormalities in insulin secretion and hepatic insulin extraction to the overall clearance of insulin and the disturbance in insulin-mediated regulation of glucose metabolism. Insulin metabolic clearance rate (MCR), glucose production, and glucose utilization were determined in groups of nonobese, LBSO or UBSO women at insulin infusion rates of 10, 20, 40, and 300 mU/min/m^2 utilizing the euglycemic clamp technique.

UBSO was associated with a decline in insulin MCR, this decline being observed at sub- and supramaximal insulin concentrations, suggesting that both receptor and nonreceptor mechanisms are involved. The defect in peripheral glucose utilization was closely aligned with the decline in insulin MCR, also being observed at sub- and supramaximal insulin levels. Insulin suppression of glucose production was impaired, but overcome by the increase in portal vein plasma insulin concentration.

Compared to the nonobese, the LBSO dose-response curve for the insulin-mediated suppression of hepatic glucose production was shifted to the right. The curve for the UBSO showed a greater rightward shift. In both the nonobese and the two obese subgroups, however, hepatic glucose production was virtually completely suppressed at an insulin infusion rate of 40 mU/min/m^2. The insulin-stimulated glucose utilization curve for the LBSO also showed a rightward shift compared to the nonobese. The curve for the UBSO subjects exhibited a greater rightward shift and a marked reduction of maximal glucose utilization rate. We conclude that obesity and body fat distribution influence glucose metabolism via independent and additive mechanisms. An increase in relative body weight is thus associated with a moderate decline in hepatic and peripheral insulin sensitivity. Upper body fat localization is characterized by a greater diminution in hepatic and peripheral insulin sensitivity, as well as a marked reduction in maximal stimulation of peripheral glucose utilization.

Not all abnormalities of glucose-insulin homeostasis in NIDDM are explained by the presence of obesity and/or upper body fat predominance. Additional defects, presumably related to genetic background which influences insulin regulation of hepatic glucose production and/or insulin secretion might thus be involved in the progression to NIDDM. The metabolic events leading to this interaction are summarized below:

DEGREE OF OVERWEIGHT	UPPER BODY FAT LOCALIZATION
↑ Insulin secretion	↓ Hepatic insulin extraction
↓ Hepatic & peripheral insulin sensitivity (receptor)	↓↓ Hepatic & peripheral insulin sensitivity (receptor)
	↓ Peripheral insulin responsivity (postreceptor)

GENETIC TRAIT
Dysrhythmicity and ↓ insulin secretion
↓ Hepatic insulin responsivity (postreceptor)

↑ = Increased
↓ = Decreased

ETIOLOGIC MECHANISMS ASSOCIATING BODY FAT DISTRIBUTION TO THE ABNORMALITIES IN INSULIN-GLUCOSE HOMEOSTASIS

At least 3 hypotheses can be proposed to explain the association of body fat distribution to the metabolic cascade described above. These 3 hypotheses represent the developmental stages of our current research.

The first hypothesis assumes that individuals with UBSO have adipocytes in the areas around the waist (subcutaneous and visceral) that are morphologically and metabolically different from those deposited in the thigh region, resulting in increased plasma FFA flux and thus overexposure of hepatic and extrahepatic tissues to FFA.

This hypothesis receives credence from the following observations:

1. Upper body adipocytes are large in volume and exhibit high rates of basal and adrenaline-stimulated lipolysis, presumably due to increased β- to α-adrenergic activities as well as diminished sensitivity to the antilipolytic action of insulin.

2. UBSO women demonstrate higher nocturnal excretions of plasma FFA, despite higher plasma insulin levels.

3. Feeding a high fat diet to rats increases portal vein plasma FFA level and hepatic TG content, correlating with a decline in hepatic insulin extraction (23).

4. Animal and human studies (24-26) suggest that FFA could inhibit insulin stimulation of peripheral glucose metabolism, and insulin suppression of hepatic glucose production.

Thus, if similar mechanisms operate in UBSO, an increase in hepatic exposure to FFA could lead to increased posthepatic insulin delivery and hyperinsulinemia. Increased FFA could also diminish hepatic and peripheral insulin sensitivity. However, no studies have yet been undertaken to demonstrate the presence of in vivo differences in splanchnic FFA flux and/or hepatic FFA channeling between UBSO and LBSO individuals. Furthermore, an understanding of the cellular and subcellular mechanisms by which FFA overexposure could influence hepatic insulin processing and catabolism is lacking. More importantly, factors favoring the preferential deposition of highly lipolytic adipocytes in visceral regions of UBSO subjects are still unexplained.

The second hypothesis assumes that body fat distribution with its adipocyte morphologic and metabolic characteristics and the abnormalities in insulin-glucose homeostasis are linked via an aberration in androgenic activity.

In healthy, premenopausal women without significant history of hirsutism, amenorrhea, or clinical evidence of endocrine disorders, we observed no significant relationship between body fat distribution and plasma level of total testosterone, androstenedione, dihydroepiandrosterone sulfate or estradiol. In contrast, there was a highly significant trend to a decrease in SHBG and increase in %FT with increasing WHR. Since in females plasma SHBG levels are determined largely by the androgen:estrogen balance, the decrease in

SHBG and the increase in %FT thus indicate a relative increase in androgenic activity.

The strong correlation between the increase in androgenic activity and WHR suggests that body fat distribution might be a manifestation of the increased body exposure to unbound androgens. The degree of androgenic activity (SHBG and %FT) correlates with the increase in abdominal but not thigh adipocyte volumes, suggesting that hypertrophy of the abdominal adipocytes in UBSO might also be a manifestation of hyperandrogeneity. UBSO women, like men, preferentially deposit fat intra-abdominally; the increase in intra:extra-abdominal fat mass ratio correlated highly with the increase in androgenic activity. Furthermore, in nonobese women, despite similar degrees of lean body mass, increasing plasma androgen levels, as in women with idiopathic hirsutism or polycystic ovarian disease, were associated with increasing WHR. Finally, Rebuffe-Scrive (27) recently reviewed the regional morphologic and biochemical characteristics of adipocytes from men and women. Her findings support the hypothesis of the intersexual regional specialization of the adipose tissue depot. Whereas the femoral-gluteal depot is primarily a storage organ dedicated to such female stresses as pregnancy and lactation, the abdominal-visceral depot is dedicated primarily to storage of easily and rapidly mobilizable energy reserves. This anatomical and functional specialization is governed by the sex hormone balance.

The growth potential of adipose tissue is contingent upon the number of cells capable of accumulating fat (preadipocytes). If sex hormones are determinants of body fat distribution, they may also affect regional recruitment and differentiation of preadipocytes. To investigate this, we developed a flow cytometric procedure utilizing a specific antibody to rat adipose tissue LPL, a putative marker for cells committed to becoming adipocytes. We utilized this procedure to quantify the differentiated and undifferentiated preadipocyte pools present in vascular adipose tissue stroma of visceral (perinephric and parametrial) and subcutaneous (abdominal and femoral) regions of female rats. We also evaluated the possible role of ovarian factors in establishing regional disparity in preadipocyte recruitment and differentiation, and the eventual transformation to mature adipocytes. Sexual maturation of the female rat was associated with significant increases in the fat cell mass and number in all regions. This increase was accompanied by

a significant decrease in the available pool of preadipocytes in all depots except the femoral. We conclude that,
in contrast to other regions, the femoral depot possesses an
infinite capacity to provide precursor cells capable of
rapid differentiation and transformation into mature adipocytes. This characteristic appears to be maintained by
ovarian factors. Interestingly, previous studies have reported that the visceral depot in male rats contains an
infinite pool of preadipocytes with enhanced capability for
replication. Our preliminary observations thus raise the
interesting question as to whether variations in regional
distribution of adipocyte precursors are sex-linked? If so,
how much of the observed disparity is related to sex hormones;
is it modified by overexposure to androgens and, if so, do
androgens exert their effects directly?

The importance of sex hormone activity in influencing
body fat distribution is supported by the following observations: 1) the onset of androgen secretion in the pubertal
male or administration of exogenous testosterone to the
hypogonadal male is accompanied by localization of fat in
the upper body (28) and a decrease in SHBG levels (29). 2)
In individuals undergoing sexual transformation, testosterone treatment in females increases cell volume in upper body
adipocytes, whereas estrogen therapy in men increases fat
cell number in the thigh (30). 3) In women with polycystic
ovary syndrome, obesity and excess plasma androgens are
frequently associated, the increase in fat deposition co-
inciding with the increase in androgen production (31).
Many of these women exhibit a predominance of upper body
fat, the male habitus. Conversely, men with lower body fat,
the typical female habitus, have increased levels of E_2 (32).
4) In experimental animals, androgens increase and estrogens
decrease the activity of adipocyte lipoprotein lipase (LPL)
and in turn adipose size (33-36). An increase in LPL is the
first abnormality to appear after administration of exogenous sex steroids and precedes changes in food intake, adipocyte volume, and body weight (33). This abnormality has
been demonstrated in animal and human models of obesity and
is not reversed by weight reduction (36,37).

In premenopausal women, the degree of androgenic activity correlated significantly with the aberrations in plasma
glucose and insulin levels. Increasing androgenic activity
also correlated with the diminution in peripheral insulin
sensitivity and the decline in hepatic insulin extraction.

These findings suggest that the association between upper body fat localization and the aberrations in hepatic insulin extraction and peripheral insulin sensitivity and the result-ant changes in the metabolic profile might be mediated by a common mechanism involving the increase in androgenic activ-ity. This contention is supported by the finding of signif-icantly impaired peripheral insulin sensitivity in nonobese hyperandrogenized hirsute women. This impairment is overcome by administration of the antiandrogen, spironolactone.

The influence of increased androgen activity on carbo-hydrate metabolism is supported by the following observa-tions: 1) diabetes is more common in males than in age- and relative weight-matched females (38). When expressed per kg of lean body weight, insulin-mediated glucose disposal mea-sured during the euglycemic clamp is 45% lower in healthy men compared to women similar in age and body weight (39). 2) Administration of testosterone derivatives to women results in impaired glucose tolerance and hyperinsulinemia (40,41). 3) Hyperandrogenism and insulin resistance are associated in women with polycystic ovary disease and acanthosis nigricans, and may regress after estrogen therapy (42-44). 4) Experimental exposure of animals to encephalo-myocarditis virus, streptozotocin or subtotal pancreatectomy results in a higher frequency of diabetes in male than female animals (45-47). 5) Estrogen administration reduces activity of rat liver gluconeogenic enzymes, alters the glu-cagon response, and promotes a decrease in plasma glucose (48,49).

Support for the influence of androgens on hepatic removal of insulin comes from the elevation of plasma insulin, but not c-peptide levels, in men compared to age- and weight-matched women (50,51). Testosterone and insulin have similar clearances with approximately 50% undergoing removal from the splanchnic circulation via hepatic activity. Androgen receptors have been demonstrated in the hepatic parenchymal cells of both rats and humans (52). Furthermore, studies in sexually mature rats demonstrate that hepatic insulin ex-traction is less in males than in age- and weight-matched females (53).

Previous studies have shown that individual body fat patterns are not altered remarkably by weight reduction (54). Increasing WHR in nonobese or ex-obese women is also correlated with an increasing risk of diabetes (3). Does variation in androgenic activity in the nonobese continue to predict body fat pattern as it does in obese individuals? We contend that this relationship continues for 2 reasons: 1) in nonhirsute obese premenopausal women, no significant change in plasma SHBG and %FT or total T was observed after short-term calorie restriction or dietary restabilization following long-term weight loss, and 2) in nonobese women with and without hirsutism, increasing plasma androgen levels were associated with proportionately increasing WHR.

The third hypothesis assumes that the association between the sex hormone balance, body fat distribution and the abnormalities in insulin-glucose homeostasis is exacerbated by a genetic and/or early developmental aberration occurring at the time of sexual dimorphism.

The reasons for suggesting this hypothesis are as follows:

1. The association between body fat distribution and abnormalities in hepatic insulin extraction or peripheral insulin sensitivity, when adjusted for the effects of SHBG and %FT, although markedly reduced, are still detectable, suggesting that the androgenic balance is not the sole determinant of these relationships.

2. Compared to men with similar degrees of lean body mass, hirsute women have greater impaired peripheral insulin sensitivity. Although the plasma androgen levels are higher in hirsute than in nonhirsute women, their level is much lower than that of men.

3. In studies of hirsute women, treatment with the antiandrogen, spironolactone, reduces androgen levels to normal and improves peripheral insulin sensitivity but does not restore insulin-glucose homeostasis completely to normal.

Why the liver would be sensitive to such small changes in androgen levels remains obscure. Could the androgen sensitivity in UBSO women be due, in part, to an aberrant sexual dimorphism? As reviewed recently, animal studies (53,55,56) have indicated the presence of higher levels of 5 α-reductase activity in the female liver capable of converting testosterone to its active metabolite, dihydrotestosterone. Sex-related differences in hepatic metabolism of sex steroids, several plasma proteins, and drugs are all well recognized. The relative abundance of hepatic androgen receptors is also sex-dependent. These sex differences in hepatic activities appear to be imprinted by prenatal and neonatal exposure to sex steroids, primarily regulated by sex hormone activity. No studies, however, have yet addressed the relationship of sexual dimorphism to hepatic insulin processing and insulin action.

Krotkiewski and Bjorntorp (57) have demonstrated that UBSO women, like men, have a high preponderance of fast twitch fibers while LBSO women resemble normal women, having a preponderance of slow twitch fibes in their quadriceps muscle. The degree of aberration of plasma insulin and glucose levels correlated well with relative abundance of fast twitch b fibers. Differences in insulin receptor number, substrate processing, and insulin sensitivity between muscle fiber types are well recognized. Whether the characteristic muscle fiber composition of UBSO is also part of an aberrant sexual dimorphism is unknown.

As reviewed in this symposium, UBSO individuals demonstrate a multitude of behavioral and psychological maladjustments to stress. They also suffer from menstrual irregularities, suggesting the co-existence of a neuroendocrine disorder. Pre- and perinatal exposure to androgens is known to influence behavior and maturation of the neuroendocrine gonadal axis (58,59). Could the neuroendocrine disorder in UBSO also be part of aberrant sexual dimorphism? If so, to what extent and by what mechanism could this disorder influence glucose-insulin homeostasis?

Finally, body fat distribution appears to be, in part, genetically determined (60) and each of the metabolic complications associated with it, including NIDDM, hyperlipidemia, hypertension, and coronary heart disease, has a major genetic component in its pathogenesis. Perinatal overexposure to androgens might also result from a genetic disorder. To what extent these associations could be influenced by genetic linkages is unknown?

The possible direct and indirect sites of interaction between androgenic activity and the abnormal metabolic profile in UBSO are summarized as follows:

MECHANISMS ASSOCIATING BODY FAT DISTRIBUTION TO
THE ABNORMALITIES IN INSULIN AND GLUCOSE HOMEOSTASIS

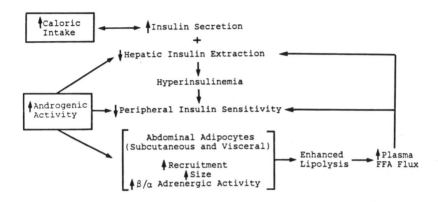

ACKNOWLEDGMENTS

This work was supported, in part, by grant #RR00058 from the National Institutes of Health General Clinical Research Centers Branch.

REFERENCES

1. Vague J (1956). The degree of masculine differentiation of obesities: a factor determining predisposition
   to diabetes, atherosclerosis, gout and uric calculus
   disease. Am J Clin Nutr 4:20.
2. Feldman R, Sender A, Siegelaub AB, Oakland MS (1969).
   Differences in diabetic and nondiabetic fat distribution patterns by skinfold measurements. Diabetes 18:478.
3. Hartz A, Rupley D, Kalkhoff R, Rimm A (1983). Relationship of obesity to diabetes: influence of obesity level
   and body fat distribution. Prev Med 12:351.
4. Larsson B (1985). Obesity and prospective risk for
   associated diseases. With special reference to the
   importance of adipose tissue distribution. In Vague J,
   Bjorntorp P, Guy-Grand B, Rebuffe-Scrive M, Vague P
   (eds): "Metabolic Complications of Human Obesities,"
   Amsterdam: Excerpta Medica, pp 21.

5. Ducimetiere P, Richard J, Cambien F, Avons P, Jacqueson A (1985). Relationships between adiposity measurements and the incidence of coronary heart disease in middle-aged male population--The Paris prospective study I. In Vague J, Bjorntorp P, Guy-Grand B, Rebuffe-Scrive M, Vague P (eds): "Metabolic Complications of Human Obesities," Amsterdam: Excerpta Medica, pp 31.
6. Stokes J III, Garrison RJ, Kannel WB (1985). The independent contributions of various indices of obesity to the 22-year incidence of coronary heart disease: The Framingham heart study. In Vague J, Bjorntorp P, Guy-Grand B, Rebuffe-Scrive M, Vague P (eds): "Metabolic Complications of Human Obesities," Amsterdam: Excerpta Medica, pp 49.
7. Haffner SM, Stern MP, Hazuda HP, Rosenthal M, Knapp JA, Malina RM (1986). Role of obesity and fat distribution in noninsulin-dependent diabetes mellitus in Mexican Americans and non-Hispanic whites. Diabetes Care 9:153.
8. Krotkiewski M, Bjorntorp P, Sjostrom L, Smith U (1983). Impact of obesity on metabolism in men and women: importance of regional adipose tissue distribution. J Clin Invest 72:1150.
9. Kissebah A, Vydelingum N, Murray R, Evans D, Hartz A, Kalkhoff RK, Adams P (1982). Relation of body fat distribution to metabolic complications of obesity. J Clin Endocrinol Metab 54:254.
10. Evans DJ, Hoffmann RG, Kalkhoff RK, Kissebah, AH (1984). Relationship of body fat topography to insulin sensitivity and metabolic profiles in premenopausal women. Metabolism 33:68.
11. Kalkhoff R, Hartz A, Rupley D, Kissebah AH (1983). Relationship of body fat topography to insulin sensitivity and metabolic profiles in premenopausal women. J Lab Clin Med 102:621.
12. Evans DJ, Hoffmann RG, Kalkhoff RK, Kissebah AH (1983). Relationship of androgenic activity to body fat topography, fat cell morphology, metabolic aberrations in premenopausal women. Clin Endocrinol Metab 57:304.
13. Evans DJ, Murray R, Kissebah AH (1984). Relationship between skeletal muscle insulin resistance, insulin-mediated glucose disposal, and insulin binding; effects of obesity and body fat topography. J Clin Invest 74:1515.

14. Kissebah AH, Evans DJ, Peiris A, Wilson CR (1985). Endocrine characteristics in regional obesities: role of sex steroids. In Vague J, Bjorntorp P, Guy-Grand B, Rebuffe-Scrive M, Vague P (eds): "Metabolic Complications of Human Obesities," Amsterdam: Excerpta Medica, pp 115.

15. Peiris A, Mueller RA, Smith GA, Struve MF, Kissebah AH (1986). Splanchnic insulin metabolism in obesity: influence of body fat distribution. J Clin Invest 78:1648.

16. Peiris AN, Mueller RA, Struve MF, Smith GA, Kissebah AH (1987). Relationship of androgenic activity to splanchnic insulin metabolism and peripheral glucose utilization in premenopausal women. J Clin Endocrinol Metab 64:162.

17. Peiris A, Hennes M, Evans DJ, Wilson CR, Lee M, Kissebah AH (1987). Relationship of anthropometric measurments of body fat distribution to the metabolic profile in premenopausal women. Acta Medica Scand (in press).

18. Peiris AN, Struve MF, Kissebah AH (1987). Relationship of body fat distribution to the metabolic clearance of insulin in premenopausal women. Int J Obesity (in press).

19. Peiris AN, Struve MF, Mueller RA, Lee M, Kissebah AH (1987). Glucose metabolism in obesity: influence of body fat distribution. J Clin Invest (submitted for publication).

20. Evans DJ (1986). Body fat distribution and metabolic complications. MD Thesis, University of Cardiff, UK.

21. Kissebah AH, James R, Krakower G, Arnaud C, Etienne J, Keller R (1985). Flow cytometric analysis of fat cell precursors: regional differences in adipose depots. Int J Obesity 9:A126.

22. Krakower GR, James RJ, Arnaud C, Etienne J, Keller RH, Kissebah AH (1987). Regional adipocyte precursors in the female rat: influence of ovarian factors. J Clin Invest (in press).

23. Stromblad G, Bjorntorp P (1986). Reduced hepatic insulin clearance in rats with dietary-induced obesity. Metabolism 35:323.

24. Randle P, Garland P, Hales C, Newsholme E (1963). The glucose-fatty acid cycle. Its role in insulin sensitivity and the metabolic disturbances of diabetes mellitus. Lancet I:785.

25. Ferrannini E, Barrett EJ, Bevilacqua S, DeFronzo RA (1983). Effect of fatty acids on glucose production and utilization in men. J Clin Invest 72:1737.

26. Bevilacqua S, Bonadonna R, Buzzigoli G, Boni C, Ciociaro D, Maccari F, Giorico MA, Ferrannini E (1987). Acute elevation of free fatty acid levels leads to hepatic insulin resistance in obese subjects. Metabolism 36:502.

27. Rebuffe-Scrive M (1987). Regional adipose tissue metabolism in men and in women during menstrual cycle, pregnancy, lactation and menopause. Int J Obesity (in press).

28. Vague J (1947). La differenciation sexuelle-facteur determinant des formes de l'obesite. Presse Med 55:339.

29. Vermeulin A, Verdonck L, Van der Straeten M, Orie N (1969). Capacity of testosterone-binding globulin in human plasma and influence of specific binding of testosterone on its metabolic clearance rate. J Clin Endocrinol Metab 29:1470.

30. Vague J, Meignen JM, Negrin JF (1984). Effects of testosterone and estrogens on deltoid and trochanter adipocytes in two cases of transsexualism. Horm Metab Res 16:380.

31. Yen SSC (1980). The polycystic ovary syndrome. Clin Endocrinol 12:177.

32. Sparrow D, Bosse R, Rowe JW (1980). The influence of age, alcohol consumption, and body build on gonadal function in men. J Clin Endocrinol Metab 51:508.

33. Steingrimsdottir L, Brasel J, Greenwood MR (1980). Hormonal modulation of adipose tissue lipoprotein lipase may alter food intake in rats. Am J Physiol 239:E162.

34. Wade GN, Gray JM (1979). Theoretical review. Gonadal effects on food intake and adiposity: a metabolic hypothesis. Physiol Behav 22:583.

35. Krotkiewski M, Kral JG, Karlsson J (1980). Effects of castration and testosterone substitution on body composition and muscle metabolism in rats. Acta Physiol Scand 109:233.

36. Gruen R, Hietanen E, Greenwood MRC (1978). Increased adipose tissue lipoprotein lipase activity during the development of the genetically obese rat (fa/fa). Metabolism 27 (Suppl 2):1955.

37. Schwartz RS, Brunzell JD (1981). Increase of adipose tissue lipoprotein lipase activity with weight loss. J Clin Invest 67:1425.

38. Garn SM (1957). Fat weight and fat placement in the female. Science 125:1091.

39. Yki-Jarvinen H (1984). Sex and insulin sensitivity. Metabolism 33:1011.
40. Landon J, Wynn V, Samols E (1963). The effect of anabolic steroids on blood sugar and plasma insulin levels in man. Metabolism 12:924.
41. Beck P (1973). Contraceptive steroids: modification of carbohydrate and lipid metabolism. Metabolism 22:841.
42. Burghen GA, Givens JR, Kitabchi AE (1980). Correlation of hyperandrogenism with hyperinsulinism in polycystic ovarian disease. J Clin Endocrinol Metab 50:113.
43. Kahn CR, Flier JS, Bar RS, Archer JA, Gordon P, Martin MM, Roth J (1976). The syndromes of insulin resistance and acanthosis nigricans. Insulin receptor disorders in man. N Engl J Med 294:739.
44. Cole C, Kitabchi AE (1978). Remission of insulin resistance with orthonovum in a patient wtih polycystic ovarian disease and acanthosis nigricans. Clin Res 26: 412A.
45. Morrow PL, Freedman A, Craighead JE (1980). Testosterone effect on experimental diabetes mellitus in encephalomyocarditis (EMC) virus infected mice. Diabetologia 18:247.
47. Paik SG, Michelis MA, Kim YT, Shin S (1982). Induction of insulin-dependent diabetes by streptozotocin: inhibition by estrogens and potentiation by androgens. Diabetes 31:724.
46. Rodriguez RR (1965). Influence of oestrogens and androgens on the production and prevention of diabetes. In Leibel BS, Wrenshall GA (eds): "On the Nature and Treatment of Diabetes," Amsterdam: Excerpta Medica, pp 288.
47. Mandour T, Kissebah A, Wynn V (1977). Mechanisms of oestrogen and progesterone effects on lipid and carbohydrate metabolism: alterations in the insulin:glucagon molar ratio and hepatic enzyme activity. Eur J Clin Invest 7:181.
48. Mandour T (1974). Effect of steroids on liver lipogenic and gluconeogenic enzymes: role of insulin and glucagon. PhD Thesis, London Univ Publ, London.
49. Krotkiewski M, Bjorntorp P, Sjostrom L, Smith U (1983). Impact of obesity on metabolism in men and women. Importance of regional adipose tissue distribution. J Clin Invest 72:1150.
50. Hale P, Wright J, Nattrass M (1985). Differences in insulin sensitivity between normal men and women. Metabolism 34:1133.

51. Roy AK, Chatterjee B (1983). Sexual dimorphism in the liver. Annu Rev Physiol 45:37.
52. Ashwell M, S Chinn, S Stalley, JS Garrow (1978). Female fat distribution--a photographic and cellularity study. Int J Obesity 2:289.
53. McCarroll AM, Buchanan KD (1973). Physiological factors influencing insulin clearance by the isolated perfused rat liver. Diabetologia 9:174.
55. Gustafsson J-A, A Mode, G Norstedt, P Eneroth, T Hokfelt (1983). Growth hormone: a regulator of the sexually differentiated steroid metabolism in rat liver. In "Developmental Pharmacology," New York: AR Liss, pp 37.
56. Bardin CW, Catterall JF (1981). Testosterone: a major determinant of extragenital sexual dimorphism. Science 211:1285.
57. Krotkiewski M, Bjorntorp P (1985). The effects of physical training in obese women and men and in women with apple- and pear-shaped obesity. In Vague J, Bjorntorp P, Guy-Grand B, Rebuffe-Scrive M, Vague P (eds): "Metabolic Complications of Human Obesities," Amsterdam: Excerpta Medica, pp 259.
58. Ehrhardt AA, Meyer-Bahlburg HFL (1981). Effects of prenatal sex hormones on gender-related behavior. Science 211:1312.
59. MacLusky NJ, Naftolin F (1981): Sexual differentiation of the central nervous system. Science 211:1294.
60. Bouchard C (1985). Inheritance of fat distribution and adipose tissue metabolism. In Vague J, Bjorntorp P, Guy-Grand B, Rebuffe-Scrive M, Vague P (eds): "Metabolic Complications of Human Obesities," Amsterdam: Excerpta Medica, pp 87.

Fat Distribution During Growth and Later Health Outcomes
pages 221–241 © 1988 Alan R. Liss, Inc.

REGIONAL ADIPOSE TISSUE DISTRIBUTION AND PLASMA LIPOPROTEINS.

Jean-Pierre Després, Angelo Tremblay and Claude Bouchard. Physical Activity Sciences Laboratory, Laval University, Ste-Foy, Quebec, Canada, G1K 7P4.

INTRODUCTION

Obesity is considered as a health hazard and represents a significant health problem in many countries including Canada as 10 to 15% of Canadians above 30 years of age have a body mass index above 30 (Fitness Canada, 1986). Although the causal link between obesity and cardiovascular disease has been debated (Larsson et al., 1981), recent longitudinal studies that have used large samples followed over long periods of time have shown that obesity is a significant and independent predictor of cardiovascular disease events (Hubert et al., 1983; Lapidus et al., 1984; Ducimetière et al., 1985). However, the association between obesity and cardiovascular disease is, at best, moderate. Björntorp (1984, 1985) has suggested that this weak association is due to the fact that a long «incubation» period is necessary to detect the obesity-associated complications. Another possibility, however, is that only a subgroup of obese subjects is at risk for the development of cardiovascular disease, thus diluting the cardiovascular risk to the whole obese population, making it very difficult to detect any relationship between obesity and cardiovascular complications. Vague et al. (1986), in a recent review of this concept, mentioned that fat mass per se has little effect on the progression of obesity toward diabetes and atherosclerosis and that a preferential deposition of fat in the upper part of the body (as seen in android obesity) was a necessary condition for the observation of the metabolic complications of obesity. Recent reports have indicated that this model should be considered seriously. Larsson et al. (1984) as well as Lapidus et al. (1984) have studied prospectively the association between obesity, adipose tissue distribution and the development of cardiovascular disease and they both reported that an excessive deposition of fat in the abdominal region was strongly associated with cardiovascular disease and mortality, and that this relationship was independent of obesity. Recent reports from the Paris prospective study (Ducimetière et al., 1986), from the Framingham cohort (Stokes et al., 1985) and from the Honolulu Heart Program (Donahue et al., 1987) also indicate that upper body fat is independently associated with coronary heart disease and related death. Therefore, it appears that the moderate association that has been reported between obesity and cardiovascular disease can be attributed, at least partly, to the fact that subjects with abdominal obesity are primarily carrying a clear increased cardiovascular disease risk, a concept that was introduced by Professor Jean Vague from the University of Marseille 30 years ago (Vague, 1956).

ADIPOSE TISSUE DISTRIBUTION AND PLASMA LIPOPROTEINS

Although recent studies have reported clear associations between body fat distribution and coronary heart disease, the mechanisms for this association remain to be established. In concordance with the results of Vague (1956) who first recognized its related metabolic disorders, many reports have shown that the localization of adipose tissue was associated with cardiovascular risk factors such as glucose intolerance and insulin resistance, diabetes, changes in plasma lipid and lipoprotein concentrations and hypertension. The present report will focus on the relation of adipose tissue distribution to plasma lipids and lipoproteins.

Disturbances in glucose homeostasis and increased susceptibility to diabetes and hypertension are not the only factors that could contribute to the association between fat distribution and cardiovascular disease. Indeed, since the early study of Albrink and Meigs (1965) showing that excess trunk fat was associated with high serum triglyceride levels, other reports have indicated that body fat distribution is associated with plasma lipid and lipoprotein levels. Allard and Goulet (1968) reported that serum triglyceride was more closely associated with the subscapular skinfold than with the anterior thigh fat depot . They also reported that subjects with an «hyperandroid» distribution of body fat had higher serum cholesterol and triglyceride levels than subjects with an «intermediate» distribution of fat (between gynoïd and android).

Additional studies that have further addressed the metabolic complications associated with changes in fat distribution have also reported associations between adipose tissue topography and serum lipids. Kissebah et al. (1982), Krothiewski et al. (1983) as well as Evans et al. (1984) have also shown that high serum triglyceride concentrations were related to abdominal obesity. Evans et al. (1984) have shown that this effect of fat distribution was independent from the level of obesity. The association between fat distribution and serum cholesterol levels has not, however, been found to be consistent. We have recently reported that a high proportion of abdominal fat was associated not only with high serum triglyceride levels but also with low concentrations of serum HDL-cholesterol (Després et al., 1985).

The hypothesis that adipose tissue distribution is involved in regulating serum lipids and lipoproteins was first suggested by the observation of obvious sex differences in the association between fatness and serum lipids (Després et al., 1985). Indeed when we compared serum cholesterol (CHOL), triglyceride (TG), HDL-CHOL and the HDL-CHOL/CHOL ratio in lean, average and overfat individuals, a different pattern was observed in men compared to women (Table 1). Indeed, when comparing the lean men to thoses with an average level of fat, there was readily a significant change in all serum lipids studied whereas in women, significant changes were only noted in the overfat group for serum CHOL, TG and for the HDL-CHOL/CHOL ratio. In addition, there was no significant effect of adiposity on serum HDL-CHOL concentration in women. These results suggest that the association between obesity and the lipoprotein-lipid profile is weaker in women than in men.

TABLE 1. Serum lipid values in lean, average and overfat men and women

| Variable | Men | | | Difference |
	Lean (I)	Average (II)	Overfat (III)	
CHOL	211.6±45.9	243.2±43.2	231.9±38.9	*IvsII *IvsIII
TG (log 10)	1.99±0.20	2.16±0.26	2.21±0.23	†IvsII †IvsIII
HDL-CHOL	50.7±12.3	43.8±10.8	40.0±11.7	†IvsII †IvsIII
HDL-CHOL/CHOL	0.25±0.07	0.19±0.06	0.19±0.05	†IvsII †IvsIII

| | Women | | | |
	Lean (I)	Average (II)	Overfat (III)	
CHOL	194.4±34.4	201.8±37.6	220.8±45.5	†IvsIII †IIvsIII
TG (log 10)	1.86±0.19	1.91±0.18	1.99±0.18	†IvsIII *IIvsIII
HDL-CHOL	59.5±14.5	61.6±16.1	58.3±16.3	NS
HDL-CHOL/CHOL	0.31±0.08	0.31±0.08	0.28±0.09	*IvsIII *IIvsIII

Values are means ± SD
* Significantly different, $p < 0.05$; † $p < 0.01$
NS: not significant.
HDL-CHOL: serum high density lipoprotein cholesterol.
Adapted from Després et al., Metabolism, 1985.

Indeed, when we measured the association between body fatness and serum lipids in both sexes, we observed trends for a weaker association in women than in men.

Table 2 shows the correlation coefficients between % body fat, fat mass, the sum of six subcutaneous skinfolds and serum lipids in men and women.

TABLE 2. Correlations between subcutaneous fat, % body fat, total fat mass and serum lipids in both sexes.

Variable	Men			
	CHOL	TG	HDL-CHOL	HDL-CHOL /CHOL
Σ 6 skinfolds	0.17*	0.30**	-0.28**	-0.35**
% body fat	0.26**	0.34**	-0.21**	-0.35**
fat mass	0.21**	0.33**	-0.24**	-0.35**
	Women			
Σ 6 skinfolds	0.20**	0.27**	-0.16*	-0.26**
% body fat	0.25**	0.26**	-0.03NS	-0.18*
fat mass	0.24**	0.24**	-0.11NS	-0.23**

* $p < 0.05$; ** $p < 0.01$
NS: not significant
Adapted from Després et al., Metabolism, 1985, and Després et al., unpublished observations.

Serum HDL-CHOL concentrations were not significantly associated with % body fat nor with fat mass in women. In addition, the relation of adiposity to serum TG and HDL-CHOL/CHOL ratio was somewhat weaker in women ($-0.18 \leq r \leq -0.26$) compared to men ($r = -0.35$). Only serum CHOL did not appear to display this sex difference.

This weaker association of serum lipids with adiposity in women than in men was also reflected by the correlations between subcutaneous skinfolds and serum lipids presented in Table 3. Firstly, in both sexes, skinfolds were positively correlated with serum TG and negatively correlated with serum HDL-CHOL and the HDL-CHOL/CHOL. The correlation between adiposity and serum CHOL was no longer significant when the effect of age on serum CHOL was controlled by covariance analysis (results not shown). Indeed, as it is well-known that serum CHOL levels are closely associated with age, it is important to control for its effect when studying the association between adiposity and serum cholesterol. Control for age, however, failed to eliminate the association between adiposity and serum TG and HDL-CHOL (results not shown).

TABLE 3. Correlations between various skinfold measurements and serum lipids

Skinfolds	Men			
	CHOL	TG	HDL-CHOL	HDL-CHOL /CHOL
Triceps	0.11	0.19†	-0.21†	-0.26†
Biceps	0.13₊	0.25†	-0.24†	-0.29†
Subscapular	0.20†	0.33†	-0.32†	-0.40†
Suprailiac	0.07₊	0.12₊	-0.15*	-0.18†
Abdomen	0.22†	0.36†	-0.27†	-0.38†
Calf	0.04₊	0.15*	-0.19†	-0.18†
Trunk/Ext	0.20†	0.20†	-0.14*	-0.26†
Subs + Abdo	0.22†	0.37†	-0.31†	-0.41†
Biceps + Calf	0.08₊	0.20†	-0.23†	-0.24†
Subs + Abdo / Bic + Calf	0.23†	0.22†	-0.15*	-0.29†

	Women			
	CHOL	TG	HDL-CHOL	HDL-CHOL /CHOL
Triceps	0.21†	0.21†	-0.15*	-0.26†
Biceps	0.20†	0.20†	-0.14*	-0.23†
Subscapular	0.14*	0.22†	-0.17†	-0.23†
Suprailiac	0.14*	0.24†	-0.16*	-0.21†
Abdomen	0.20†	0.27†	-0.14*	-0.25†
Calf	0.16*	0.19†	-0.05	-0.14*
Trunk/Ext	0.03₊	0.15*	-0.09	-0.11₊
Subs + Abdo	0.18†	0.26†	-0.16*	-0.25†
Biceps + Calf	0.19†	0.22†	-0.09	-0.20†
Subs + Abdo / Bic + Calf	0.03	0.13	-0.10	-0.12

* $p < 0.05$; † $p < 0.01$
Adapted from Després et al., Metabolism, 1985, and from Després et al., unpublished observations.

Secondly, skinfolds that displayed the highest associations with serum TG and HDL-CHOL were the subscapular and the abdominal skinfolds. Various combinaisons and ratios were computed but they did not display higher associations with serum lipids than these two skinfolds taken indidually. In women, correlations tended to be lower and regional differences in the associations between skinfolds and serum TG and HDL-CHOL were less obvious. This situation might be attributed to the fact that our sample consisted of non-obese, healthy women. As higher levels of body fat have to be present in women to observe metabolic disturbances compared to men (Schwane and Cundiff, 1979; Krotkiewski et al., 1983; Després et al., 1985), our sample may not be appropriate to evaluate the effect of fat distribution in women. We can only point out that, in a sample of non-obese healthy women, the effect of subcutaneous fat distribution on plasma lipoprotein levels was not evident. In obese women, Kissebah et al. (1985) reported an association between the waist-to-hip circumferences ratio and fasting HDL-CHOL concentration that was independent from the level of obesity. In a large sample of Mexican Americans, Haffner et al. (1987) reported that the waist-to-hip ratio was an independent predictor of HDL-CHOL levels in women. Therefore, it appears that fat distribution is also associated with plasma lipoprotein metabolism in women.

Our results, however, indicated an effect of adipose tissue localization on plasma lipoprotein-lipid levels in men. As the amount of abdominal fat increases with the level of obesity and as there is a good correlation between the absolute amount of abdominal fat and obesity in men, it was important to determine whether abdominal fat has an effect on serum lipids and HDL-CHOL that is independent from total adiposity. We recently studied this phenomenon in a sample of 429 adult men (Després et al., in press). As previously reported, we observed significant associations between total adiposity (BMI) and serum lipids, and significant correlations between the proportion of subcutaneous trunk fat, the abdominal skinfold, and serum lipids (0.01 > p < 0.001). Analyses of variance were computed to evaluate the respective contributions of subcutaneous fat distribution and of total adiposity (as estimated by the BMI) on the variance of serum lipids. Table 4 indicates that both variables had significant effects on serum TG ($p < 0.001$), HDL-CHOL ($p < 0.05$) and HDL-CHOL/CHOL ($p < 0.001$).

TABLE 4. Analysis of variance for the effects of subcutaneous fat distribution (as measured by the trunk/extremity skinfolds ratio) and of the body mass index on serum triglycerides, HDL-CHOL and HDL-CHOL/CHOL.

		BMI tertiles			
Triglycerides		I	II	III	
T/E ratio	I	94.0	125.3	129.0	F=7.9
tertiles	II	127.6	138.3	200.8	p<0.001
	III	108.0	178.3	166.1	
		F = 13.6, p < 0.001			
		I	II	III	
HDL-CHOL					
T/E ratio	I	52.0	48.9	45.6	F=4.6
tertiles	II	48.7	45.1	43.8	p<0.01
	III	46.4	45.6	44.0	
		F = 3.0, p < 0.05			
		I	II	III	
HDL-CHOL/CHOL					
T/E ratio	I	0.28	0.23	0.22	F=14.1
tertiles	II	0.22	0.21	0.19	p<0.001
	III	0.23	0.21	0.20	
		F = 11.5, p < 0.001			

Values are in mg/dl
Adapted from Després et al., Int. J. Obesity, in press.

However, when the respective effects of abdominal fat (as measured by the abdominal skinfold) and total adiposity (BMI) on serum lipids were evaluated, analysis of variance indicated that the variance in serum TG and HDL-CHOL was solely explained by variations in abdominal fat and not by total adiposity (Table 5). Only the HDL-CHOL/CHOL variance was significantly explained by both the amount of abdominal fat and total adiposity.

TABLE 5. Analysis of variance for the effects of abdominal fat (as measured by the abdominal skinfold)
and of the body mass index on serum triglycerides, HDL-CHOL and HDL-CHOL/CHOL.

		BMI tertiles			
Triglycerides		I	II	III	
Abdominal	I	93.8	151.1	134.1	F=1.9
skinfold	II	157.1	135.7	138.5	NS
tertiles	III	152.9	168.3	186.8	
		F = 4.8, p < 0.01			
		I	II	III	
HDL-CHOL					
Abdominal	I	50.4	46.5	47.4	F=2.3
skinfold	II	50.5	48.6	48.4	NS
tertiles	III	47.9	42.4	42.4	
		F = 3.5, p < 0.05			
		I	II	III	
HDL-CHOL/CHOL					
Abdominal	I	0.27	0.22	0.21	F=5.0
skinfold	II	0.23	0.23	0.21	p<0.01
tertiles	III	0.22	0.19	0.19	
		F = 5.0, p < 0.01			

Values are in mg/dl; NS = not significant
Adapted from Després et al., Int. J. Obesity, in press.

It therefore appeared that, in this study, the
association between obesity and serum lipids and HDL-CHOL
was primarily explained by the amount of abdominal fat.
Partial correlation coefficients with control over the
effect of total adiposity on serum lipids eliminated the
association between skinfolds and serum TG and HDL-CHOL
with the exception of the subscapular and abdominal
skinfolds (Table 6), emphasizing their independent
contribution to the serum HDL-CHOL variance.

These results indicate that the absolute amount of
abdominal fat is more important than the relative
distribution of subcutaneous fat in the association
between adipose localization and serum HDL-CHOL. It must
be noted, however, that the trunk/extremity skinfolds

TABLE 6. Partial correlations between subcutaneous skinfolds and serum lipids and lipoproteins after control for the effect of the BMI on the dependent variables.

Skinfolds	CHOL	TG	HDL-CHOL	HDL-CHOL/CHOL
Triceps	-0.03	-0.06	-0.06	-0.03
Biceps	-0.01	-0.00	-0.06	-0.04
Subscapular	0.04	0.09	-0.16**	-0.15**
Suprailiac	-0.06	-0.03	0.00	0.05
Abdomen	0.09	0.20***	-0.13*	-0.16**
Calf	-0.07	-0.05	-0.03	0.03

* p <0.01; ** p < 0.005; *** p < 0.0001

ratio describes only the distribution of subcutaneous fat. As omental fat has been suggested as important in the etiology of the metabolic complications of obesity (Björntorp, 1984; Kissebah et al., 1985; Sparrow et al., 1986; Fujioka et al., 1987), further work will be needed to elucidate its association with plasma lipoprotein levels. A recent study by Fujioka et al. (1987) reported trends for higher TG and lower HDL-CHOL levels in male subjects with an increased proportion of deep fat compared to subjects with a high proportion of subcutaneous fat. Differences were, however, not significant, this lack of effect being probably caused by the samll sample size. They reported, however, significant correlations between the ratio of deep to subcutaneous fat and serum CHOL and TG concentrations (Fujioka et al., 1987) suggesting that, indeed, the proportion of omental fat might be an important variable in the association between fat topography and plasma lipoprotein levels. Further work in this area will be required to further understand the association between deep adipose tissue and plasma lipoproteins.

Nonetheless, an additional question remains to be answered. As there is a well-known negative relationship between serum TG and HDL-CHOL levels, we had to test the possibility that the low HDL-CHOL levels observed in abdominal obesity are attributed to the effect of fat topography on serum TG levels, as high serum TG concentrations are observed in abdominal obesity. In our sample, we observed significant negative correlations between serum TG and HDL-CHOL ($r = -0.33$, $p < 0.0001$) and HDL-CHOL/CHOL ($r = -0.54$, $p < 0.0001$). As fat distribution affects serum TG and HDL-CHOL in opposite directions, it was justified to test the possibility that some of the effects of excess abdominal fat on serum HDL-CHOL could be mediated by the increased TG levels associated with altered body fat distribution. We, therefore, removed the effect of TG on serum HDL-CHOL by covariance analysis and we studied the independent association between the BMI, the trunk/extremity skinfold ratio, the abdominal skinfold and serum HDL-CHOL (Table 7). After control for serum TG levels, the trunk/extremity skinfolds ratio was no longer correlated with serum HDL-CHOL but the amount of abdominal fat was still significantly correlated with serum HDL-CHOL ($r = -0.16$, $p < 0.01$). These results indicate that there is a significant association between the absolute amount of subcutaneous abdominal fat and serumm HDL-CHOL that is independent from obesity and serum TG levels.

TABLE 7. Relationships between the relative distribution of subcutaneous fat (trunk/extremity skinfolds ratio), the amount of abdominal fat (abdominal skinfold), the body mass index and serum HDL-CHOL and HDL-CHOL/CHOL after adjustment by covariance analysis for the effect of serum triglycerides.

Variable	BMI	Abdominal skinfold	T/E ratio
HDL-CHOL (corrected for TG)	-0.16**	-0.16**	-0.06[NS]
HDL-CHOL/CHOL (corrected for TG)	-0.27***	-0.24***	-0.13*

* $p < 0.01$; ** $p < 0.005$; *** $p < 0.001$;
NS: not significant
Adapted from Després et al., Int. J. Obesity, in press.

MECHANISMS

The mechanisms for this independent abdominal fat-plasma HDL-CHOL association remain to be established. It has been documented that plasma high density lipoproteins can interact specifically and saturably with human fat cells (Fong et al., 1985) and that regional variation exists in the fat cell-HDL metabolism (Salter et al., 1987; Després et al., 1987). Indeed, it has been shown in purified adipocyte plasma membrane preparations (Salter et al., 1987) and in collagenase isolated fat cells (Després et al., 1987) that large subcutaneous abdominal adipocytes possess more HDL binding sites than small omental cells. In addition, a positive correlation between abdominal fat cell size and the level of adipocyte HDL-binding has been reported (Després et al., 1987). This increased fat cell: HDL interaction observed in abdominal obesity could be an additional mechanism by which abdominal fat is associated with plasma HDL-CHOL concentration. Indeed, Salter et al. (1987) have reported significant negative correlations between the levels of subcutaneous and omental fat cells HDL binding and plasma HDL-CHOL concentration. Whether this association represents a cause-effect relationship remains to be determined but it gives support to the notion that abdominal fat cells play a role in the regulation of plasma HDL-CHOL levels.

In addition to this hypothetical mechanism, a role for insulin as a mediator of the effects of body fat distribution on plasma lipoproteins has been suggested. Numerous reports have shown that subjects with excess upper body fat have high fasting and post-glucose insulin levels (Kissebah et al., 1982; Krotkiewski et al., 1983; Evans et al., 1984). In a recent experiment in which we subjected young men to a 3-week overfeeding period, we observed that changes in fasting insulin and in the insulin response to oral glucose induced by overfeeding were significantly correlated with changes in serum triglycerides (Després et al., 1987), emphasizing the association between the insulin metabolism and VLDL secretion by the liver (Olefsky et al., 1974; Kissebah et al., 1976). Following overfeeding, we also reported that the greater was the increase in serum TG, the greater was the reduction in serum HDL-CHOL (Després et al., 1987), suggesting that an increase in VLDL secretion and high TG levels associated with high insulin levels could have consequences on the concentration or composition of other lipoprotein fractions (Schonfeld et al., 1976; Deckelbaum et al., 1984). We have also obtained additional evidence that insulin could be involved in the association between adipose tissue distribution and plasma lipoprotein metabolism when we subjected 12 young men to a 22 day aerobic exercise training program that induced a daily caloric deficit of 1000 kcal (Poehlman et al., 1986; Tremblay et al., 1987). At the end of this program, subjects had lost weight and their plasma insulin response to an oral glucose challenge was markedly reduced, a well-documented effect of exercise-training. Changes in plasma lipoprotein and insulin levels were, however, totally dissociated from changes in total adiposity (Després et al., submitted) but significantly correlated with changes in the proportion of trunk fat. Subjects that displayed the greatest reduction in trunk fat showed the most substantial reduction in plasma insulin levels and in some lipoproteins. In addition, significant correlations were observed between changes in the insulin reponse to glucose and changes in plasma lipoproteins suggesting synchronized changes in fat distribution, insulin metabolism and plasma lipoproteins. Therefore, it appears that the effect of fat distribution on plasma lipoproteins is partly linked to the effect of adipose tissue localization on insulin metabolism, an association that was extensively reviewed by Dr. Kissebah during this meeting.

From the results presented and from the literature available on the possible mechanisms by which adipose tissue distribution is associated to cardiovascular risk factors (Björntorp, 1984, 1985; Kissebah et al., 1985; Stern and Haffner, 1986), a preliminary model for the association between excess abdominal fat and reduced plasma HDL-CHOL levels is presented (Figure 1).

Firstly, an increased relative proportion of abdominal fat is associated with the enlargement of abdominal fat cells (omental or subcutaneous) compared to femoral fat cells. The very lively lipolysis of these large abdominal cells would release more free fatty acids (FFA) in the portal circulation than in a situation where

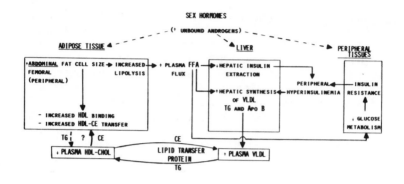

FIGURE 1. Preliminary model for the association between excess abdominal fat and reduced plasma HDL-cholesterol levels.

fat is stored peripherally. This condition, associated with increased levels of unbound androgens, has been proposed to play a role in the reduced hepatic extraction of insulin (Kissebah et al., 1985), contributing to produce peripheral hyperinsulinemia. These high plasma FFA levels also reduce the peripheral glucose metabolism, leading to an insulin resistant state. Hyperinsulinemia and high FFA levels would also induce an increased hepatic synthesis of VLDL, TG and Apo B. The presence of high TG (VLDL) in the plasma would then alter the composition of the other lipoprotein fractions, including HDL, contributing to reduce the cholesterol content of the HDL fraction. The roles of plasma lipoprotein lipase (LPL) and of hepatic lipase (HL) are not presented in this model as their associations with body fat distribution are not known. The role of LPL, a key enzyme in lipoprotein metabolism, will have to be investigated as a slow catabolism of VLDL, which has been reported in obese and/or hyperinsulinemic subjects (Lewis et al., 1972;

Wilson et al., 1978; Brunzell et al., 1979), would be associated with a decreased production of HDL as a good proportion of HDL particles comes from the action of LPL on triglyceride-rich lipoproteins (Eisenberg, 1984). In addition, the association between hepatic lipase and fat distribution is not known although Kissebah et al. (1985) have suggested that this enzyme may be involved in the body fat localization-plasma lipoproteins association.

In addition to these mechanisms, as human fat cells have the ability to interact specifically with high density lipoproteins (Fong et al., 1985), it is possible that the increased mass of abdominal adipose tissue could play a role in the metabolism of plasma HDL and that the abdominal adipose cells-HDL metabolism could be an additional factor for the association between fat distribution and plasma lipoproteins. As HDL is involved in cholesterol ester delivery to numerous organs (Andersen and Dietschy, 1978; Strauss et al., 1982), and that a disproportionate uptake of HDL-cholesterol compared to HDL-apoproteins has been documented in a variety of tissues (Glass et al., 1983; Leitersdorf et al., 1984), the interaction of HDL with enlarged abdominal fat cells could lead to the depletion of HDL-cholesterol esters, a phenomenon that could explain the negative association between abdominal obesity and plasma HDL-CHOL levels.

SUMMARY AND CONCLUSIONS

The literature is generally in agreement in showing that the distribution of adipose tissue is associated with plasma lipoprotein levels, especially with TG-containing lipoproteins (VLDL) and with the proportion of serum cholesterol transported by high density lipoproteins. We have reported that the absolute amount of subcutaneous abdominal fat is critical in the association between obesity and serum TG and HDL-CHOL concentrations. The effect of abdominal fat on serum TG levels is important but it is not the sole mediator of the fat distribution-plasma HDL-CHOL association and insulin is involved in the relation of abdominal obesity to serum TG levels. However, only a portion of the effect of abdominal fat on serum HDL-CHOL is mediated by the effect of fat distribution on serum TG as there is a significant residual association between the amount of abdominal fat and HDL-CHOL concentration after control for serum TG levels.

Although there is evidence that body fat distribution is associated with plasma lipoprotein levels, further work is needed to better understand the mechanisms of this association and studies on large samples of subjects with simultaneous measurements of the full plasma lipoprotein and apoprotein profiles, of the key enzymes involved in lipoprotein metabolism (LPL and HL) along with extensive measures of fat topography (axial tomography) and with controls over sex hormones and insulin metabolism are needed. Meanwhile, although the mechanisms are not completely understood, the independent effect of adipose tissue distribution on plasma HDL-CHOL levels is an additional factor that contributes to explain the increased cardiovascular disease risk observed in abdominal obesity (Larsson et al., 1984; Lapidus et al., 1984; Stokes et al., 1985; Ducimetière et al., 1986; Donahue et al., 1987).

REFERENCES

Albrink MJ, Meigs JW (1965) The relationship betwen serum triglycerides and skinfold thickness in obese subjects. Ann NY Acad Sci 131: 673-683.

Allard C, Goulet C (1968) Serum lipids: An epidemiological study of an active Montreal population. Can Med Ass J 98: 627-637.

Andersen JM, Dietschy JM (1978) Relative importance of high and low density lipoproteins in the regulation of cholesterol synthesis in adrenal gland, ovary and testis from the rat. J Biol Chem 253: 9024-9032.

Björntorp P (1984) Hazards in subgroups of human obesity. Eur J Clin Invest 14: 239-241.

Björntorp P (1985) Obesity and the risk of cardiovascular disease. Ann Clin Res 17: 3-9.

Brunzell JD, Porte D Jr, Bierman EL (1979) Abnormal lipoprotein-lipase-mediated plasma triglyceride removal in untreated diabetes mellitus associated with hypertriglyceridemia. Metabolism 28: 901-907.

Deckelbaum RJ, Granot E, Oschry Y, Rose L, Eisenberg S (1984) Plasma triglyceride determines structure-composition in low and high density lipoproteins. Arteriosclerosis 4: 225-231.

Després JP, Allard C, Tremblay A, Talbot J, Bouchard C (1985) Evidence for a regional component of body fatness in the association with serum lipids in men and women. Metabolism 34: 967-973.

Després JP, Poehlman ET, Tremblay A, Lupien PJ, Moorjani S, Nadeau A, Pérusse L, Bouchard C (1987) Genotype-influenced changes in serum HDL cholesterol after short-term overfeeding in man: association with plasma insulin and triglyceride levels. Metabolism 36: 363-368.

Després JP, Fong BS, Julien P, Jimenez J, Angel A (1987) Regional variation in HDL metabolism in human fat cells: effect of cell size. Am J Physiol (Endocrinol Metabol) 252: E654-E659.

Després JP, Tremblay A, Pérusse L, Leblanc C, Bouchard C (in press) Abdominal adipose tissue and serum HDL-cholesterol: association independent from obesity and serum triglyceride concentration. Int J Obesity

Després JP, Moorjani S, Tremblay A, Poehlman ET, Lupien PJ, Nadeau A, Bouchard C (submitted) Heredity and changes in plasma lipids and lipoproteins following short-term exercise-training in man: association with changes in adipose tissue distribution and plasma insulin.

Donahue RP, Abbott RD, Bloom E, Reed DM, Yano K (1987) Central obesity and coronary heart disease in men. Lancet April: 822-824.

Ducimetière P, Richard J, Cambien F (1986) The pattern of subcutaneous fat distribution in middle-aged men and the risk of coronary heart disease: The Paris Prospective Study. Int J Obesity 10: 229-240.

Eisenberg S (1984) High density lipoprotein metabolism. J Lipid Res 25: 1017-1058.

Evans DJ, Hoffmann RG, Kalkhoff RK, Kissebah AH (1984) Relationship of body fat topography to insulin sensitivity and metabolic profiles in premenopausal women. Metabolism 33: 68-75.

Fitness Canada (1986) Ottawa, Government of Canada.

Fong BS, Rodrigues PO, Salter AM, Yip BP, Després JP, Gregg R, Angel A (1985) Characterization of high density lipoprotein binding to human adipocyte plasma membranes. J Clin Invest 75: 1804-1812.

Fujioka S, Matsuzawa Y, Tokunaga K, Tarui S (1987) Contribution of intra-abdominal fat accumulation to the impairment of glucose and lipid metabolism in human obesity. Metabolism 36: 54-59.

Glass C, Pittman R, Weinstein DB, Steinberg D (1983) Dissociation of tissue uptake of cholesterol ester from that of apoprotein A-I of rat plasma high density lipoprotein: selective delivery of cholesterol ester to liver, adrenal, and gonad. Proc Natl Acad Sci USA 80: 5435-5439.

Haffner SM, Stern MP, Hazuda HP, Pugh J, Patterson JK (1987) Do upper-body and centralized adiposity measure different aspects of regional body-fat distribution? Relationship to non-insulin-dependent diabetes mellitus, lipids, and lipoproteins. Diabetes 36: 43-51.

Hubert HB, Feinleb M, McNamara PM, Castelli WP (1983) Obesity as an independent risk factor for cardiovascular disease: A 26-year follow-up of participants in the Framingham Heart Study. Circulation 67: 968-977.

Kissebah AH, Alfarsi S, Adams PW, Wynn V (1976) Role of insulin resistance in adipose tissue and liver in the pathogenesis of endogenous hypertriglyceridemia in man. Diabetologia 12: 563-571.

Kissebah AH, Vydelingum N, Murray R, Evans DJ, Hartz AJ, Kalkhoff RK, Adams PW (1982) Relation of body fat distribution to metabolic complications of obesity. J Clin Endocrinol Metab 54: 254-260.

Kissebah AH, Evans DJ, Peiris A, Wilson CR (1985) Endocrine characteristics in regional obesities: role of sex steroids. In: Metabolic complications of human obesities. Vague J et al, eds, Amsterdam: Elsevier Science Publishers, pp 115-130.

Krotkiewski M, Björntorp P, Sjöström L, Smith U (1983) Impact of obesity on metabolism in men and women. Importance of regional adipose tissue distribution. J Clin Invest 72: 1150-1162.

Lapidus L, Bengtsson C, Larsson B, Pennert K, Rybo E, Sjöström L (1984) Distribution of adipose tissue and risk of cardiovascular disease and death: a 12 year follow-up of participants in the population study of women in Gothenburg, Sweden. Br Med J 289: 1261-1263.

Larsson B, Björntorp P, Tibblin G (1981) The health consequences of moderate obesity. Int J Obesity 5: 97-116.

Larsson B, Svärdsudd K, Welin L, Wilhelmsen L, Björntorp P, Tibblin G (1984) Abdominal adipose tissue distribution, obesity, and risk of cardiovascular disease and death: 13 year follow-up of participants in the study of men born in 1913. Br Med J 288: 1401-1404.

Leitersdorf E, Stein O, Eisenberg S, Stein Y (1984) Uptake of rat plasma HDL subfractions labeled with (^{3}H) cholesteryl linoleyl ether or with ^{125}I by cultured rat hepatocytes and adrenal cells. Biochim Biophys Acta 796: 72-82.

Lewis B, Marcini M, Mattock M, Chait A, Frazier TR (1972) Plasma triglycerides and fatty acid metabolism in Diabetes Mellitus. Eur J Clin Invest 2: 445-453.

Olefsky JM, Farquhar JW, Reaven GM (1984) Reappraisal of the role of insulin in hypertriglyceridemia. Am J Med 57: 551-560.

Poehlman ET, Tremblay A, Nadeau A, Dussault J, Thériault G, Bouchard C (1986) Heredity and changes in hormones and metabolic rates with short-term training. Am J Physiol (Endocrinol Metab) 250: E711-E717.

Salter AM, Fong BS, Jimenez J, Rotstein L, Angel A (1987) Regional variation in high-density lipoprotein binding to human adipocyte plasma membranes of massively obese subjects. Eur J Clin Invest 17: 16-22.

Schonfeld G, Weidman SW, Witztum JL, Bowen RM (1976) Alterations in levels and interrelations of plasma apolipoproteins induced by diet. Metabolism 25: 261-275.

Schwane JA, Cundiff DE (1979) Relationships among cardiorespiratory fitness, regular physical activity, and plasma lipids in young adults. Metabolism 28: 771-776.

Sparrow D, Borkan GA, Gerzof SG, Wisniewski C, Silbert CK (1986) Relationship of fat distribution to glucose tolerance. Results of computed tomography in male participants of the normative aging study. Diabetes 35: 411-415.

Stern MP, Haffner SM (1986) Body fat distribution and hyperinsulinemia as risk factors for diabetes and cardiovascular disease. Arteriosclerosis 6: 123-130.

Stokes J III, Garrison RJ, Kannel WB (1985) The independent contributions of various indices of obesity to the 22-year incidence of coronary heart disease: The Framingham heart study. In: Metabolic complications of human obesities. Vague J et al, eds, Amsterdam: Elsevier Science Publishers, pp 49-57.

Strauss JF III, McGregor JC, Gwynne JT (1982) Uptake of high density lipoproteins by rat ovaries in vivo and dispersed ovarian cells in vitro. Direct correlation of high density lipoprotein uptake with steroidogenic activity. J Steroid Biochem 16: 525-531.

Tremblay A, Poehlman E, Nadeau A, Pérusse L, Bouchard C (1987) Is the response of plasma glucose and insulin to short-term exercise-training genetically determined? Horm Metab Res 19: 65-67.

Vague J (1956) The degree of masculine differenciation of obesities: a factor determining predisposition to diabetes, atherosclerosis, gout, and uric calculous disease. Am J Clin Nutr 4: 20-34.

Vague J, Vague P, Meignen JM, Jubelin J, Tramoni M (1986) Obésités androïde et gynoïde: Passé et présent. Méd Nutr 11: 11-22.

Wilson DE, Glad BW, Working PK, Adler ME (1978) Post-heparin plasma lipase activities in obesity: Failure to increase with adipose organ enlargement. Metabolism 27: 1084-1094.

Fat Distribution During Growth and Later Health Outcomes
pages 243–261 © *1988 Alan R. Liss, Inc.*

FAT DISTRIBUTION AND BLOOD PRESSURES

R. M. Siervogel and Richard N. Baumgartner

Division of Human Biology, Department of Pediatrics,
Wright State University School of Medicine, 1005 Xenia
Avenue, Yellow Springs, Ohio 45387-1695

INTRODUCTION

Body size and fatness show particularly strong positive associations with blood pressure levels in both children and adults (Bøe et al. 1957; Stamler et al. 1975a, b, 1978; Siervogel et al. 1980, 1982). Elevated blood pressure alone is an important risk factor for coronary heart disease and there are strong positive associations of obesity with hyperlipidemia, hypertension, and glucose intolerance (Kannel and Dawber 1973; Weinsier et al. 1976; Kannel and Gordon 1980). Furthermore these conditions are risk factors for coronary heart disease and non-insulin dependent diabetes (Kannel 1976, 1985; Tyroler et al. 1975). Recent studies indicate that adipose tissue distribution may be a risk factor for hypertension also (Stallones et al. 1982; Kalkhoff et al. 1983; Blair et al. 1984; Weinsier et al. 1985; White et al. 1986; Shear et al. 1987).

Vague (1956) was among the first to draw attention to the importance of the anatomical distribution of adipose tissue in relation to disease risk. He was concerned particularly with what he called "android obesity", since a central, or upper-body fat distribution was characteristic mostly of men. Android obesity appeared to be strongly associated with metabolic-endocrine disorders especially when it occurred in women, but little attention was paid to this issue until recently.

Some early studies suggested associations between adipose tissue distribution and serum levels of triglycerides in men (Albrink and Meigs 1964), and cholesterol in men and in women (Montoye et al. 1966). Other studies have indicated strong associations with glucose intolerance, hyperinsulinemia, and hyperlipidemia in obese men and women (Kissebah et al. 1982; Kalkhoff et al. 1983; Krotkiewski et al. 1983; Evans et al. 1984; Foster et al. 1987). Epidemiological research has confirmed these associations (Szathmary and Holt 1983; Contaldo et al. 1986; Haffner et al. 1986a; Reichley et al. 1987; Baumgartner et al. 1987), and demonstrated associations between adipose tissue distribution and non-insulin dependent diabetes, heart disease, and stroke (Feldman et al. 1969; Hartz et al. 1984; Mueller et al. 1984; Ohlson et al. 1985; Haffner et al. 1986b; Larsson et al. 1984; Lapidus et al. 1984; Ducimetière et al. 1986). Nevertheless, clinical and epidemiologic investigations have been less consistent regarding associations between adipose tissue distribution and blood pressure.

THEORETICAL AND METHODOLOGICAL CONCERNS

Several theoretical and methodological issues confuse research on the associations of adipose tissue distribution with risk factors for disease.

Theoretical Issues

Although a model is being developed which may explain the association between excess abdominal adipose tissue (a centripetal adipose tissue distribution) and hyperlipidemia and hyperinsulinism, some key aspects of this model remain obscure (Stern and Haffner 1986). The lack of a plausible mechanism for an association with blood pressure is one weakness.

Clinical and population studies have shed some light on the natural history of centripetal fat distribution and on its associations with glucose and lipid metabolism. A centripetal distribution of adipose tissue is a characteristic of males which develops in adolescence, regardless of ethnicity (Mueller 1982; Baumgartner et al. 1986), and increases with aging (Borkan et al. 1982, 1985; Mueller et al. 1986). Centripetal fat deposition is controlled to some extent by levels of sex hormones, and recent clinical studies have reported significant correlations between the waist/hip circumference index of fat patterning and serum levels of free-testosterone and hormone-binding globulin in each sex (Stefanick et al. 1987; Evans et al. 1983). There is considerable evidence that sex hormones play a role in the regulation of lipid metabolism (Stefanick et al. 1987).

Abdominal adipocytes are more labile metabolically than gluteal and femoral adipocytes (Östman et al. 1979; Lafontan et al. 1979; Bolinder et al. 1983), and abdominal obesity may be associated with a greater flow of free-fatty acids to the liver through the portal circulation (Smith 1985). Abdominal obesity is primarily hypertrophic, whereas lower body obesity is mostly hyperplastic (Kissebah et al. 1982; Krotkiewski et al. 1983). Hypertrophic adipocytes are insulin resistant, but insulin resistance in adipose tissue can account for only a fraction of total body resistance (Stern and Haffner 1986). There is decreased insulin responsiveness in the skeletal muscle of obese women with upper body fat patterns (Evans et al. 1984).

In summary, it has been hypothesized that excess androgens may produce centripetal fat distribution, as well as reduce hepatic extraction of insulin, leading to an increase in serum levels of insulin (Evans et al. 1983, 1984). Obesity with a centripetal distribution results in increased insulin resistance in adipose tissue and in increased free fatty acids, which may enhance insulin resistance in muscle and alter lipid metabolism in the liver (Björntorp 1984; Stern and Haffner 1986). Associations of centripetal adipose tissue distribution and hyperinsulinemia, insulin resistance, and hyperlipidemia are explained by this model. An association with hypertension might be due to a secondary effect of hyperinsulinemia on sodium retention in the kidney, or to increased activity of the sympathetic nervous system (Björntorp 1984).

Methodological Issues

Despite progress in the development of a theoretical model explaining associations between adipose tissue distribution and risk factors for disease, several methodological difficulties impede research on this topic. A major problem is the definition and anthropometric measurement of adipose tissue distribution. Considerable effort has been devoted to this problem by some scientists (Skerlj et al. 1953; Edwards et al. 1951; Garn 1955; Shephard et al. 1969; Badora 1975; Ashwell et al. 1978; Mueller and Reid 1979; Bailey et al. 1982; Norgan and Ferro-Luzzi 1986; Baumgartner et al. 1986), most of which has been inadequately considered by clinicians and epidemiologists, with a few exceptions (Ducimetière et al. 1986; Reichley et al. 1987).

Adipose tissue distribution has been indexed by a variety of methods. Most of these indices are considered to reflect contrasts between the upper and lower body distribution of adipose tissue or between the trunk and the extremities. Examples of some indices that have been used include: ratios of circumferences (waist/hip circumference ratio, arm to thigh circumference); ratios of estimated areas (adipose tissue and muscle areas in the upper arm and in the thigh); ratios of pairs of skinfold thicknesses (subscapular to triceps skinfold thicknesses), simple differences between skinfolds at different sites (e.g., between skinfolds on the trunk and those on the thigh, or between standardized values for the lateral chest and medial calf skinfold thicknesses); skinfold at one site statistically controlled for effects of skinfold thickness at another site; and more complex combinations of skinfolds (e.g. principal component scores). Many of these indices are, for convenience, referred to by the same name; for example, "centripetal fat pattern index", although some are considered to index an upper-lower body adipose tissue distribution. Surprisingly, one recent study used a single skinfold (subscapular) as an index of "central obesity" (Donahue et al. 1987).

The quantification of centripetal adipose tissue distribution poses multiple problems which may confuse investigations of its associations with risk factors for diseases. Skinfold thicknesses are direct measurements of skin and of adipose tissue, but they can only measure variation in the distribution of subcutaneous adipose tissues. If standardized methods are employed, circumferences can be measured with less error than skinfold thicknesses, especially in the obese (Bray et al. 1978), but the differences are small (Mueller and Malina 1987).

Several studies using circumferences to define centripetal fat distribution have not used standardized methods, but have relied on self-reported measurements (Hartz et al. 1984), or have failed to report how the circumferences were measured (Lanska et al. 1985; Evans et al. 1983). In other studies, "hip circumference" has been measured at the level of the iliac crest, rather than at the maximum extension of the buttocks or at the maximum lateral extensions of the greater trochanters (Larsson et al. 1984; Ohlson et al. 1985). Hip circumference measured at the level of the iliac crest is virtually the same as abdominal circumference measured at the level of the umbilicus, and the ratio of these two measurements will be highly sensitive to measurement errors. "Waist/hip ratios", in general, have narrow ranges of variation (e.g., coefficients of variation less than 10%) and may be more sensitive to measurement errors than ratios based on skinfold thicknesses. Carefully controlled comparisons have not been made between centripetal fat pattern indices based on skinfold thicknesses with those based on circumferences for relative sensitivity and specificity in discriminating subjects with diabetes, hypertension, or hyperlipidemia.

Studies using area measurements of adipose tissue from computer assisted tomography cross-sectional images have suggested that intra-abdominal adipose tissue is increased in non-insulin dependent diabetes (Shuman et al. 1986; Sparrow et al. 1986). It is not clear if a centripetal distribution of subcutaneous adipose tissue is associated with increased intra-abdominal adipose tissue. Indices based on circumferences, such as the waist/hip ratio (Kalkhoff et al. 1983) or waist/thigh ratio (Ashwell et al. 1985), measure variation in intra-abdominal as well as subcutaneous adipose tissue, but also include variation in muscle and bone (Baumgartner et al. 1987b). Some studies suggest that increased skeletal and muscle mass may be associated with increased blood pressures (Weinsier et al. 1985), insulin resistance (Evans et al. 1984), and elevated plasma lipids (Krotkiewski and Björntorp 1986). If true, associations of these risk factors with weight/stature^2 (W/S^2) and with indices of adipose tissue distribution may confound centripetal obesity with increased muscularity and fat-free mass.

ASSOCIATIONS OF VARIOUS MEASURES OF ADIPOSE TISSUE DISTRIBUTION AND RISK FACTORS

Adipose tissue distribution was first reported to have important associations with plasma lipids and lipoproteins. The thickness of the costal skinfold, controlling for the thickness of the forearm skinfold was shown to have a significant positive association with the level of serum triglycerides in men (Albrink and Meigs 1964). Serum levels of cholesterol also were found to be more highly associated with subscapular skinfold thicknesses than with triceps skinfold thicknesses in men and in women (Montoye et al.1966).

Centripetal adipose tissue distribution, indexed by the waist/hip circumference ratio, has been reported to be associated significantly, independent of age and W/S^2, with mortality from stroke and from ischemic heart disease in prospective studies of men and women (Larsson et al. 1984; Lapidus et al. 1984). Centripetal fat pattern, defined by the difference between the thicknesses of skinfolds on the trunk and those on the thigh, was shown to be a potent predictor of angina pectoris and myocardial infarction in a 6.6 year follow-up of men in the Paris Prospective Study (Ducimetière et al. 1983). An index derived from the combination of principal components based on skinfolds that involved overall adiposity and a trunk-thigh contrast showed a positive relationship with systolic blood pressure, total cholesterol and triglycerides and was the best predictor of coronary heart disease in the same study (Ducimetière et al. 1986).

The "brachio-femoral adipomuscular ratio" is a complex index of fat and muscle distribution, defined by the ratios of adipose tissue and muscle areas in the upper arm and in the thigh (Vague 1956). When adipose tissue distribution is defined by this ratio, plasma levels of triglycerides were significantly higher in women with upper body segment obesity than in age- and weight-matched women with lower body segment obesity (Kissebah et al. 1982). In a later study of 110 obese women in whom adipose tissue distribution was defined by the waist/hip circumference ratio, Kalkhoff et al. (1983) did not find a significant difference in plasma triglyceride levels between the means of the quartile with the lowest waist/hip circumference ratio and those in the highest quartile (upper body segment obesity), although there was a tendency for those in the upper group to have higher levels.

The ratio of the subscapular to triceps skinfold thicknesses showed significant positive associations with plasma levels of triglycerides in both Anglo and Mexican-American men and women, after controlling for W/S^2 and for age in the San Antonio Heart Study (Haffner et al. 1986c). This indicates that a subcutaneous centripetal adipose tissue distribution is related to level of triglycerides; however, the proportions of variance in triglycerides explained by this index were small (1 to 2 percent). In the same study, plasma levels of HDL cholesterol had weak, negative associations with centripetal adipose tissue distribution, after controlling for estrogen use in women, and alcohol consumption in men, but only a small proportion of the overall variation was explained (1 to 3 percent).

ASSOCIATIONS BETWEEN ADIPOSE TISSUE DISTRIBUTION AND LEVEL OF BLOOD PRESSURE

Although adipose tissue distribution has been studied extensively with regard to glucose and lipid metabolism, comparatively few studies have analyzed associations between adipose tissue distribution and blood pressures. In 6243 adolescent (12-17 years) boys and girls sampled in the U.S. Health Examination Survey, Stallones et al. (1982) did not find a significant association between blood pressures and the difference between standardized values for the lateral chest and medial calf skinfold thicknesses after adjustment for age and weight. Nevertheless, this index had a significant positive association with systolic blood pressure, after adjustment for age and an index of fatness, but prior to an adjustment for weight. Relationships between blood pressures and indices of total body fatness or fat pattern may be less important in adolescents than in adults.

A recent analysis based on 3784 subjects ages 5 to 24 years enrolled in the Bogalusa Heart Study, indicated a significant association between systolic blood pressure and the subscapular skinfold thickness after controlling for age, sex, race, and triceps skinfold thickness; however, the percentages of variation explained in systolic blood pressures were small ($< 3.5\%$) and associations were particularly weak for ages 13-17 years (Shear et al. 1987). Similarly, significant associations of systolic and diastolic blood pressures with subscapular skinfold thickness controlling for sex, race and age in 5506 adults from the First Health and Nutrition Examination Survey have been reported, but without corrections for overall level of adiposity (Blair et al. 1984). The subscapular skinfold thickness was reported to a have stronger positive correlations with blood pressures in white and in black men than the the triceps skinfold thickness (Blair et al. 1984).

Centripetal fat distribution, defined by the ratio of the subscapular and triceps skinfold thicknesses, was not correlated significantly with mean arterial pressure in 399 obese patients of a weight control clinic; although upper body fatness, defined by the ratio of arm to thigh circumferences, was reported to have a significant correlation with mean arterial pressure, after adjustment for lean body mass, age and an index of body build in the same study (Weinsier et al. 1985).

Three studies have reported associations between blood pressures and the waist/hip circumference ratio as an index of fat patterning. Kalkhoff et al. (1983) studied 110 white premenopausal women (mean age 39.5 years) who were 50% or more above ideal body weight, but otherwise healthy. They found that women with an upper body fat distribution tended to have higher blood pressures, poorer carbohydrate tolerance and more insulin resistance than did women with a lower body fat distribution. Systolic and diastolic blood pressures were significantly correlated with the waist to hip circumference ratio, even after adjusting for age and overall obesity using the weight to height ratio. In a sample of 20,325 women, Hartz et al. (1984) estimated the relative risk of hypertension, adjusted for age and relative weight, to be 1.74 for upper body segment obesity compared to lower body segment obesity. The waist/hip circumference ratio was reported to have small, but significant, positive correlations, adjusted for age and weight/stature, with both systolic ($r = 0.26$) and diastolic ($r = 0.29$) blood pressures in women (Kalkhoff et al. 1983). In a cross-sectional study of 10,405 adult participants in the Canada Fitness Survey, White and associates (1986) found significant associations between the prevalence of hypertension and the waist/hip circumference ratio , as well as the subscapular skinfold thickness. The risk of hypertension, however, was related more strongly to age and to W/S^2 than to either th waist/hip ratio or subscapular skinfold thickness.

In a study of dehydroepiandrosterone sulfate (DHEAS) variation in black adolescents and its relationship to blood pressure levels and body fat, Katz et al. (1986) reported that girls, but not boys, with high levels of DHEAS had higher blood pressure levels than those with lower DHEAS levels, even after adjusting for W/S^2. In addition, they found a positive association between DHEAS levels and centripetal adipose tissue distribution defined as higher values of and index of the ratio of subscapular to subscapular plus triceps skinfold thicknesses. The study sample consisted of 384 children ranging in age from 12 to 16 years.

STUDIES AT THE DIVISION OF HUMAN BIOLOGY

We have been involved in two recent studies examining the relationships between the distribution of adipose tissue and level of blood pressure, lipids and lipoproteins, or glucose levels (Baumgartner et al. 1987a; Baumgartner and Siervogel 1987). The first involves data from participants in the Fels Longitudinal Growth Study and the second, data from participants in a cross-sectional genetic study of hypertension and associated variables (Siervogel et al. 1980). Study design and the type and diversity of the variables measured in the two studies differ and thus each was used to address slightly different questions.

Fels Longitudinal Growth Study

The data used for the Fels analysis were selected from serial data on body composition, including body density from hydrostatic weighing and levels of fasting blood lipids and lipoproteins from participants in the Fels Longitudinal Study. The analysis was based on cross-sectional data from 152 men and 151 women, 18 to 57 years of age (Mean ± s.d. = 33.5 ± 9.4 years). This subsample includes all adult participants measured at the first examination in the serial study of body composition who had appropriate data.

To date, the Fels data have been used to answer at the question: "How much variation in blood pressure (and separately, lipids/lipoproteins) can be explained by a simple index of fat distribution after age, and general level of fatness have been taken into account?" The logarithm of the ratio of the subscapular to lateral calf skinfold thicknesses as an index (TES) of trunk-extremity skinfold contrasts in adipose tissue distribution. The rationale for using such a simple index of fat patterning was fourfold: 1) we wanted an index that was simple and could be widely applied in epidemiological studies, 2) the simpler the index, the larger the sample size available, because more individuals had complete data, 3) the specific index used was most highly correlated ($r = 0.7$ to 0.8) with a multivariate index derived from principal components analysis of seven skinfolds (subscapular, triceps, suprailiac, biceps, lateral calf, anterior chest, and mid-axillary) in a subsample with complete data and 4) this simple index has been suggested by others to be more sensitive than indices contrasting the trunk with the arm (Mueller and Stallones 1981). TES scores greater than zero indicate a centripetal fat pattern, and scores less than zero indicate a peripheral one.

Baumgartner et al. (1987a) found that subscapular skinfold thicknesses were relatively larger than the calf skinfold thicknesses in the men, but not in the women. Whereas 85 per cent of the men had centripetal adipose tissue distributions (scores > zero) only about 40 per cent of the women had this pattern. TES was correlated significantly with plasma lipids and lipoprotein cholesterols and blood pressures in the men, with the pattern and directions of the correlations the same as for per cent body fat. In the women, TES had significant positive correlations with plasma triglycerides and diastolic blood pressure, and was negatively correlated with HDL cholesterol.

Age and age^2 accounted for between 17 and 30 per cent of the variance in plasma lipids, lipoprotein cholesterols, and blood pressures in the men. Per cent body fat accounted for between 2 and 7.5 per cent of the remaining variance in these variables. Systolic and diastolic blood pressures explained about 5.6 per cent of the variance remaining in plasma triglycerides, after controlling for age, age^2 and per cent body fat. TES was not related independently and significantly to systolic or diastolic blood pressure in men nor was it significantly associated with total plasma cholesterol, HDL or LDL cholesterol, or plasma triglycerides in the men after controlling for age, age^2, per cent body fat, and systolic and diastolic blood pressures through multiple regression.

In the women, TES had a small, but significant positive association with plasma triglycerides ($R^2 = 0.045$, $p < 0.01$), and a significant negative association with plasma HDL-cholesterol ($R^2 = 0.066$, $p < 0.0005$) after effects due to age, age^2, per cent body fat and systolic and diastolic blood pressures had been removed. Age and age^2 explained about 8 per cent of the variance in plasma levels of HDL cholesterols, and per cent body fat accounted for about 9 per cent of the remaining variance.

TES was associated significantly ($R^2 = 0.038$, $p < 0.05$) with diastolic blood pressure in the women, after controlling for age, age^2, per cent body fat, and plasma lipids and lipoprotein cholesterols. Age and age^2 explained about 18 per cent of the variance in diastolic blood pressure in the women, and per cent body fat explained about 3.5 per cent of the variance remaining after adjustment for age. Thus, the adipose tissue distribution was associated with diastolic blood pressure as strongly as total "fatness" in the women. Age and age^2 accounted for about 11 per cent of the variance in systolic blood pressure in the women, and per cent body fat and plasma levels of total cholesterol accounted for 6.6 per cent and 5.4 per cent, respectively, of the residual variance.

Familial Hypertension Study

In the analyses using the familial hypertension data set the question was somewhat different; that is: After controlling for age, what variables are the best predictors of blood pressure (or lipids, or glucose level). The cross-sectional data used for these analyses were taken from records for the first visit of white participants in this study (Siervogel et al. 1980). Data for participants with diagnoses of non-insulin dependent diabetes, gout, hyperthyroidism, Cushing syndrome, gall bladder disease or cirrhosis were deleted, since these may be associated with altered adipose tissue distribution, as were data for six women who were either pregnant or lactating at the time of data collection. The final data set included variables measured in 470 healthy participants from four large kindreds, each kindred ascertained from one adult male with diastolic blood pressure greater than 95 mmHg. There were 79 boys and 73 girls from 8 to 18 years of age, and 146 men and 172 women aged 18 to 88 years.

The data set included measurements of systolic, 4th and 5th phase diastolic blood pressures, fasting plasma cholesterol, triglycerides, HDL and LDL cholesterols, fasting glucose, and 1 and 2 hr serum glucose levels from a standard glucose tolerance test. Since the distributions of the plasma lipids were significantly skewed, these variables were log-transformed for most analyses. Anthropometric variables included weight, stature, upper arm circumference, and triceps, subscapular and suprailiac skinfold thicknesses. Socioeconomic variables were years of eduction and income. Behavioral variables included current smoking of cigarettes, pipes or cigars, current use of oral contraceptives or estrogen replacement in women, and current use of cardiovascular medications, diuretics, lipid-lowering drugs, insulin, or steroids. Ages at menarche and at menopause were included for women, as well as for hysterectomy or ovarectomy.

W/S^2 was computed as an index of relative adiposity. Upper arm muscle area (UAMA) was computed as an index of relative muscularity from upper arm circumference (UAC) and triceps skinfold thickness (T) by the formula: $(UAC-\pi(T/10))^2/4\pi$. An index of adipose tissue distribution was obtained by principal components analysis (Reichley et al. 1987). The loadings for the component considered to reflect fat patterning were -0.73 for the triceps skinfold thickness, 0.12 for the subscapular skinfold thickness, and 0.67 for the suprailiac skinfold thickness. The component accounted for 57 per cent of the total variance in fat patterning as measured by these skinfolds. A standardized index (PCTE = principal components trunk-extremity index), reflecting contrasts in trunk-extremity adipose tissue distribution was computed from transformations of the loadings for the component.

Two analytic approaches were taken towards analysis of the associations between blood pressures, lipids and glucose values and body composition, behavioral and socioeconomic variables. In the first analytic approach, separate stepwise multiple regressions were made for blood pressures, plasma lipids and serum glucose values on W/S^2, PCTE, UAMA and their interactions for each sex and age group. Education, income and smoking were included as independent variables in regressions for adults, and oral contraceptive use, hormone use, hysterectomy/ovarectomy and menopausal status were included in regressions for women. Age and age^2 were forced into each regression prior to the stepwise entry of the other independent variables.

Level of adiposity, as indexed by W/S^2, was associated significantly with systolic and diastolic blood pressures in adults and children of both sexes, and with levels of plasma lipids and serum glucose in adults. In the adults, smoking also was related to plasma levels of lipids, and UAMA was related to blood pressures in the women and in the children. Adipose tissue distribution, as measured by the PCTE, was not found to be associated significantly, after adjustment for age and W/S^2, with blood pressures, plasma lipids, or glucose tolerance in children or adults of either sex. The interaction of PCTE with UAMA was significantly associated with 4th phase diastolic blood pressure in women, and the interaction of PCTE with UAMA and W/S2 was significantly associated with 5th phase diastolic blood pressure in the boys and with 1 hour glucose levels in the women.

In the second analytic approach, subjects were first categorized on the basis of the joint relationships among blood pressures, plasma lipids, and serum glucose values, and then the associations of the categories with body composition, behavioral and socioeconomic variables were analyzed. Cluster analyses were made of blood pressures, plasma lipids, and serum glucose values for each sex. The cluster analyses defined groups of participants with distinct profiles for these variables. These groups were then regressed on the body composition, behavioral and socioeconomic variables using least-squares discriminant analysis.

Groups of men and of women were defined that had higher than average blood pressures, plasma cholesterol, triglycerides, and LDL cholesterol, lower than average HDL cholesterol, and higher than average serum glucose levels (fasting, 1 and 2 hour). Groups for each sex also were distinguished in which plasma lipids or glucose values were higher than average. Membership in these "high risk" groups was shown to be associated with age and W/S2 in the men, and with age, W/S2, the interaction of age and W/S2, and with smoking in women. The PCTE index of adipose tissue distribution did not discriminate significantly among these groups.

CONCLUSIONS

Although the results of previous studies are not directly comparable to ours due to differences in design and the types of measurements used, the magnitudes of the reported associations between adipose tissue distribution and risk factors generally have been small, particularly with regard to blood pressures (Stallones et al. 1982; Blair et al. 1984; Weinsier et al. 1985; White et al. 1986; Shear et al. 1987). The results of our work indicate that strong associations exist between blood pressures, levels of plasma lipids and of serum glucose and adiposity for each sex that are independent of age, but associations with adipose tissue distribution, if present, are weak (Baumgartner et al. 1987a; Baumgartner and Siervogel 1987).

Perhaps one of the more important developments that could facilitate progress in the understanding of adipose tissue distribution in relation to risk factors is improved measurement of this distribution. Well-defined standard anthropometric methods should be used. In addition, workers should avoid using the same name for a variety of different indices and should publish an adequate description of the methods used to derive specific indices. Too frequently, indices derived in different ways or by using anthropometric variables measured in a non standard fashion, are compared as if they were the same. This may occur because these different indices have used the same name, such as "centripetal fat pattern index".

ACKNOWLEDGEMENTS

This work was supported by Grant HDAM-12252 from the National Institutes of Health, Bethesda, MD.

REFERENCES

Albrink MJ, Meigs JW (1964) Interrelationship between skinfold thickness, serum lipids and blood sugar in normal men. Am J Clin Nutr 15:255-61.

Ashwell M, Chinn S, Stalley S, Garrow JS (1978) Female fat distribution--a photographic and cellularity study. Int J Obesity 2:289-302.

Ashwell M, Cole TJ, Dixon AJ (1985) Obesity: new insight into the anthropometric classification of fat distribution shown by computed tomography. Br Med J 290:1692-4.

Badora G (1975) The distribution of subcutaneous fat tissue in young women and men. Stud Phys Anthrop 1:91-108.

Bailey SM, Garn SM, Katch VL, Guire KE (1982) Taxonomic identification of human fat patterns. Am J Phys Anthrop 59:361-6.

Baumgartner RN, Roche AF, Guo S, Lohman T, Boileau RA, Slaughter MH (1986) Adipose tissue distribution: The stability of principal components by sex, ethnicity and maturation stage. Hum Biol 58:719-35.

Baumgartner RN, Roche AF, Chumlea WC, Siervogel RM, Glueck CJ (1987a) Fatness and fat patterns: Associations with plasma lipids and blood pressures in adults 18 to 57 years of age. Am J Epidem (in press).

Baumgartner RN, Heymsfield SB, Roche AF, Bernadino M (1987b) Quantification of abdominal composition by computed tomography. Am J Clin Nutr (under review).

Baumgartner RN, Siervogel RM (1987) Associations of blood pressures, lipids and glucose with indices of adiposity and adipose tissue distribution. (under review).

Björntorp P (1984) Adipose tissue in obesity (Willendorf Lecture). In: Recent Advances in Obesity Research IV - Proceedings of the 4th International Congress on Obesity. J. Hirsch and T. VanItallie (eds) J. Libbey: London, pp. 163-70.

Blair J, Habicht J-P, Sims EAH, Sylwester D, Abraham S (1984) Evidence for an increased risk for hypertension with centrally located body fat and the effect of race and sex on this risk. Am J Epidemiol 119:526-40.

Bøe J, Humerfelt S, Wedervag F (1957) The blood pressure in a population: Blood pressure readings and height and weight determinations in the adult population of the city of Bergen. Acta Med Scand 157(suppl 321):1-336.

Bolinder J, Kager L, Östman J, Arner P (1983) Differences at the receptor and postreceptor levels between human omental and subcutaneous adipose tissue in the action of insulin on lipolysis. Diabetes 32:117-23.

Borkan GA, Gerzof SG, Robbins AH, Hults DE, Silbert CK, Silbert JE (1982) Assessment of abdominal fat content by computed tomography. Am J Clin Nutr 36:172-7.

Borkan GA, Hults DE, Gerzof SG, Robbins AH (1985) Comparison of body composition in middle-aged and elderly males using computed tomography. Am J Phys Anthrop 66:289-95.

Bray GA, Greenway FL, Molitch ME, Dahms WT, Atkinson RL, Hamilton K (1978) Use of anthropometric measures to assess weight loss. Am J Clin Nutr 31:769-73.

Contaldo F, Giuseppe DB, Salvatore P, Trevisan M, Farinaro E, Mancini M (1986) Body fat distribution and cardiovascular risk in middle-aged people in Southern Italy. Atherosclerosis 61:169-72.

Donahue RP, Abbott RD, Bloom E, Reed DM, Yano K (1987) Central obesity and coronary heart disease in men. The Lancet 1:821-4.

Ducimetière P, Richard J, Cambien F (1986) The pattern of subcutaneous fat distribution in middle-aged men and the risk of coronary heart disease: The Paris Prospective Study. Int J Obesity 10:229-40.

Ducimetière P, Avons P, Cambien F, Richard JL (1983) Corpulence history and fat distribution in CHD etiology. Euro Heart J 4(suppl):8.

Edwards DA (1951) Differences in the distribution of subcutaneous fat with sex and maturity. Clin Sci 10:305-15.

Evans DJ, Hoffmann RG, Kalkhoff RK, Kissebah AH (1983) Relationship of androgenic activity to body fat topography, fat cell morphology, and metabolic aberrations in premenopausal women. J Clin Endocrin Metab 57:304-10.

Evans DJ, Murray R, Kissebah AH (1984) Relationship between skeletal muscle insulin resistance, insulin-mediated glucose disposal, and insulin binding. Effects of obesity and body fat topography. J Clin Invest 74:1515-25.

Feldman R, Sender AJ, Siegelaub AB (1969) Difference in diabetic and nondiabetic fat distribution patterns by skinfold measurements. Diabetes 18:478-86.

Foster CJ, Weinsier RL, Birch R, Norris DJ, Bernstein RS, Wang J, Pierson RN, Van Itallie TB (1987) Obesity and serum lipids: an evaluation of the relative contribution of body fat and fat distribution to lipid levels. Int J Obesity 11:151-61.

Garn SM (1955) Relative fat patterning: an individual characteristic. Hum Biol 27:75-89.

Haffner SM, Stern MP, Hazuda HP, Pugh J, Patterson JK, Malina R (1986a) Upper body and centralized adiposity in Mexican Americans and Non-Hispanic Whites: relationship to body mass index and other behavioral and demographic variables. Int J Obesity 10:493-502.

Haffner SM, Stern MP, Hazuda HP, Rosenthal M, Knapp JA, Malina RM (1986b) Role of obesity and fat distribution in non-insulin-dependent diabetes mellitus in Mexican Americans and Non-Hispanic Whites. Diabetes Care 9:153-61.

Haffner SM, Stern MP, Hazuda HP, Rosenthal M, Knapp JA (1986c) The role of behavioral variables and fat patterning in explaining ethnic differences in serum lipids and lipoproteins. Am J Epidemiol 123:830-40.

Hartz AJ, Rupley DC, Rimm AC (1984) The association of girth measurements with disease in 32,856 women. Am J Epidemiol 119:71-80.

Kalkhoff RK, Hartz AH, Rupley D, Kissebah AH, Kelber S (1983) Relationship of body fat distribution to blood pressure, carbohydrate tolerance, and plasma lipids in healthy obese women. J Lab Clin Med 102:621-7.

Kannel WB, Gordon T (1980) Physiological and medical concomitants of obesity: The Framingham Study. In: Bray GA ed. Obesity in America. Washington, D.C.: Department of Health, Education and Welfare, (DHEW publication no. (NIH)80-359), pp. 125-63.

Kannel WB (1985) Lipids, diabetes, and coronary heart disease: insights from the Framingham Study. Am Heart J 110:1100-6.

Kannel WB (1976) Coronary risk factors: I. Recent highlights form Framingham Study. Aust NZ J Med 6:373-86.

Kannel WB, Dawber TF (1973) Hypertensive cardiovascular disease: the Framingham Study. In: Hypertension: Mechanisms and Management, edited by Onesti G, Kim KE. New York: Grune and Stratton, pp. 93-110.

Katz SH, Hediger ML, Zemel BS, Parks JS (1986) Blood pressure, body fat, and dehydroepiandrosterone sulfate variation in adolescence. Hypertension 8:277-84.

Kissebah AH, Vydelingum N, Murray R, Evans DJ, Hartz AJ, Kalkhoff RK, Adams PW (1982) Relation of body fat distribution to metabolic complications of obesity. J Clin Endocrin and Metab 54:254-60.

Krotkiewski M, Björntorp P, Sjöström L, Smith U (1983) Impact of obesity on metabolism in men and women. J Clin Invest 72:1150-62.

Krotkiewski M, Björntorp P (1986) Muscle tissue in obesity with different distribution of adipose tissue effects of physical training. Int J Obesity 10:331-41.

Lafontan M, Dang-Tran L, Berlan M (1979) Alpha-adrenergic antilipolytic effect of adrenaline in human fat cells of the thigh: comparison with adrenaline responsiveness of different fat deposits. Euro J Clin Invest 9:261-6.

Lanska DJ, Lanska MJ, Hartz A, Kalkhoff RK, Rupley D, Rimm AA (1985) A prospective study of body fat distribution and weight loss. Int J Obesity 9:241-46.

Lapidus L, Bengtsson C, Larsson B, Pennert K, Rybo E, Sjöström L (1984) Distribution of adipose tissue and risk of cardiovascular disease and death: a 12 year follow up of participants in the population study of women in Gothenberg, Sweden. Br Med J 289:1257-61.

Larsson B, Svärdsudd K, Welin L, Wilhelmsen L, Björntorp P, Tibblin G (1984) Abdominal adipose tissue distribution, obesity, and risk of cardiovascular disease and death: 13 year follow up of participants in the study of men born in 1913. Br Med J 288:1401-4.

Montoye HJ, Epstein FH, Kjelsberg MO (1966) Relationship between serum cholesterol and body fatness: an epidemiologic study. Am J Clin Nutr 18:397-406.

Mueller WH (1982) The changes with age of the anatomical distribution of fat. Soc Sci and Med 16:191-6.

Mueller WH, Stallones L (1981) Anatomical distribution of subcutaneous fat: skinfold site choice and construction of indices. Hum Biol 53:321-35.

Mueller WH, Joos SK, Hanis CL, Zavaleta AN, Eichner J, Schull WJ (1984) The diabetes alert study: growth, fatness and fat patterning, adolescence through adulthood in Mexican Americans. Am J Phys Anthrop 64:389-99.

Mueller WH, Deutsch MI, Malina RM, Bailey DA, Mirwald RL (1986) Subcutaneous fat topography: age changes and relationship in cardiovascular fitness in Canadians. Hum Biol 58:955-73.

Mueller WH, Reid RM (1979) A multivariate analysis of fatness and relative fat patterning. Am J Phys Anthrop 50:199-208.

Mueller WH, Malina RM (1987) Relative reliability of circumferences and skinfolds as measures of body fat distribution. Am J Phys Anthrop 72:437-439.

Norgan NG, Ferro-Luzzi A (1986) Simple indices of subcutaneous fat patterning. Ecol Food Nutr 18:117-23.

Ohlson L-O, Larsson B, Svärdsudd K, Welin L, Eriksson H, Wilhelmsen L, Björntorp P, Tibblin G (1985) The influence of body fat distribution on the incidence of diabetes mellitus: 13.5 years of follow-up of the participants in the study of men born in 1913. Diabetes 34:1055-8.

Östman J, Arner P, Engfeldt P, Kager L (1979) Regional differences in the control of lipolysis in human adipose tissue. Metabolism 28:1198-1205.

Reichley KB, Mueller WH, Hanis CL, Joos SK, Tulloch BR, Barton S, Schull WJ (1987) Centralized obesity and cardiovascular disease risk in Mexican Americans. Am J Epidemiol 125:373-86.

Shear CL, Freedman DS, Burke GL, Harsha DW, Berenson GS (1987) Body fat patterning and blood pressure in children and young adults: The Bogalusa Heart Study. Hypertension 9:236-244.

Shephard RJ, Jones G, Ishii K, Kaneko M, Olbrecht AJ (1969) Factors affecting body density and thickness of subcutaneous fat. Data on 518 Canadian city dwellers. Am J Clin Nutr 22:1175-89.

Shuman WP, Newell Morris LL, Leonetti DL, Wahl PW, Moceri VM, Moss AA, Fujimoto WY (1986) Abnormal body fat distribution detected by computed tomography in diabetic men. Invest Radiol 21:483-8.

Siervogel RM, Frey MAB, Kezdi P, Roche AF, Stanley E (1980) Blood pressure, electrolytes and body size: Their relationships in young relatives of men with essential hypertension. Hypertension 2:I-83-92.

Siervogel RM, Roche AF, Chumlea WC, Morris JG, Webb P, Knittle JL (1982) Blood pressure, body composition, and fat tissue cellularity in adults. Hypertension 4:382-6.

Skerlj B, Brozek J, Hunt, Jr. EE (1953) Subcutaneous fat and age changes in body build and body form in women. Am J Phys Anthrop 11:577-600.

Smith U (1985) Regional differences in adipocyte metabolism and possible consequences *in vivo*. Int J Obesity 9:145-8.

Sparrow D, Borkan GA, Gerzof SG, Wisniewski C, Silbert CK (1986) Relationship of fat distribution to glucose tolerance. Results of computed tomography in male participants of the normative aging study. Diabetes 35:411-5.

Stallones L, Mueller WH, Christensen BH (1982) Blood pressure, fatness, and fat patterning among USA adolescents from two ethnic groups. Hypertension 4:483-6.

Stamler J, Stamler R, Rhomberg P, Dyer A, Berkson D, Reedus W, Wannamaker J (1975a) Multivariate analysis of the relationship of six variables to blood pressure: Findings from Chicago community surveys, 1965-1971. J Chronic Dis 28:499-525.

Stamler J, Rhomberg P, Schoenberger JA, Shekelle R, Dyer A, Shekelle S, Stamler R, Wannamaker J (1975b) Multivariate analysis of the relationship of seven variables to blood pressure. J Chronic Dis 28:527-48.

Stamler R, Stamler J, Riedlinger WF, Algera G, Roberts R (1978) Weight and blood pressure: Findings in hypertension screening of 1 million Americans. JAMA 240:1607-10.

Stefanick ML, Williams PT, Krauss RM, Terry RB, Vranizan KM, Wood PD (1987) Relationships of plasma estradiol, testosterone, and sex hormone-binding globulin with lipoproteins, apolipoproteins, and high density lipoprotein subfractions in men. J Clin Endocrin Metab 64:723-30.

Stern MP, Haffner SM (1986) Body fat distribution and hyperinsulinemia as risk factors for diabetes and cardiovascular disease. Arteriosclerosis 6:123-30.

Szathmary E, Holt N (1983) Hyperglycemia in Dogrib Indians of the Northwest Territories, Canada: Association with age and a centripetal distribution of body fat. Hum Biol 55:493-515.

Tyroler HA, Heyden S, Hames CG (1975) Weight and hypertension: Evans County studies of blacks and whites. In: Epidemiology and Control of Hypertension, edited by Paul O. Miami: Symposia Specialist, pp. 177-204.

Vague J (1956) The degree of masculine differentiation of obesities: a factor determining predisposition to diabetes, atherosclerosis, gout, and uric calculus disease. Am J Clin Nutr 4:20-34.

Weinsier RL, Fuchs RJ, Kay TD, Triebwasser JH, Lancaster MC (1976) Body fat: its relationship to coronary heart disease, blood pressure, lipids and other risk factors measured in a large male population. Am J Med 61:815-24.

Weinsier RL, Norris DJ, Birch R, Bernstein RS, Wang J, Yang M-U, Pierson, Jr. RN, Van Itallie TB (1985) The relative contribution of body fat and fat pattern to blood pressure level. Hypertension 7:578-85.

White FMM, Pereira LH, Garner JB (1986) Associations of body mass index and waist/hip ratio with hypertension. CMAJ 135:313-320.

Fat Distribution During Growth and Later Health Outcomes
pages 263–284 © 1988 Alan R. Liss, Inc.

Androgens, Obesity and Body Fat Patterns

SOLOMON H. KATZ
KROGMAN GROWTH CENTER, U. OF PA.
DEPARTMENT OF PSYCHIATRY
EINSTEIN NORTHERN HOSPITAL
4019 IRVING ST.
PHILADELPHIA, PA. 19104-6003

INTRODUCTION

Since Vague (1956) initially described a masculinized fat pattern associated with diabetes, atherosclerosis, and gout, a number of studies were conducted that confirmed the epidemiological significance of this phenomenon. In general, these studies have suggested that when obesity is accompanied by a relative increase in trunk body fat as opposed to the extremity body fat, there is a significant increase in adipose cell hypertrophy as opposed to adipose cell hyperplasia, which is associated with the increased risk of a number of metabolic abnormalities. Trunk body fat is commonly defined by increases or decreases of skinfold thickness ratios of subscapular to triceps, or waist to hip ratios, respectively (see Haffner et al. 1987 for comparisons of their significance and independence). These abnormalities include hyperinsulinemia (Kissebah et al. 1982; Krotkewski et al. 1983), hypertriglyceridemia (DesPres et al. 1985), lower HDL-cholesterol (Glueck et al. 1980), increased CHD and hypertension (Stokes et al. 1985; Lapidus et al. 1984; Larsson et al. 1984), increased post-hepatic insulin levels (Peiris and Kissebah 1986a). A number of other risk factors are also associated with developmental events such as earlier onset of menarche (Frisancho and Flegal, 1982), which is in turn associated with the risk of postmenopausal breast cancer (Sherman et al. 1981) and increased blood pressure in adolescence (Katz et al. 1986).

METABOLIC MECHANISMS ASSOCIATED WITH CHRONIC PATHOLOGY

In addition to identifying these metabolic risk factors, over the last few years there have also been a number of substantial advances in determining the mechanisms that may underly the pathologies associated with the android fat pattern. Of the various chronic pathologies associated with this android pattern of obesity, one of the best studied is the metabolic characteristics of non-insulin dependent diabetes mellitus (NIDDM). In general, both basal levels of insulin, and the response of insulin to glucose challenge, are significantly elevated in individuals with android obesity versus those with the gynoid distribution (lower body) (Kissebah et al. 1982; Krotkiewski et al. 1983).

In a further study of the correlates of central or centripetal body fat, Kissebah's group (Peiris et al. 1987) demonstrated significant associations among normal premenopausal women between upper body fat (Waist/Hip ratio) and decreased glucose tolerance, increased insulin resistance, hyperinsulinemia, decreased hepatic insulin extraction, and diminished peripheral insulin sensitivity in muscle and fat. Moreover, these statistically significant associations were independent and additive to those with generalized obesity.

Several hypotheses have been forwarded to account for the apparent diminished sensitivity to the effects of insulin in promoting glucose uptake and utilization in adipose and skeletal muscle tissue (Olefsky 1976). One possible factor is hypertrophy of adipocytes and the concomitant decreased numbers of receptors, in contrast to hyperplasia of the adipocytes which is associated with the gynoid type of obesity (Salans et al. 1968; Sjostrom 1972). Other factors involve down regulation, or a decrease in insulin receptors associated with increases in circulating insulin (Olefsky 1976; Freidenberg et al. 1987), abnormalities of glucose transport ascribed to post-receptor defects, the effects of increased circulating free fatty acids (FFA) on diminished glucose uptake by both skeletal and heart muscle (Stern and Haffner 1986), and decreased hepatic insulin extraction (Kissebah et al. 1985).

Although one or more of the mechanisms proposed above may account for the increase in post-hepatic insulin levels, Kissebah et al. (1985) found an association between shifts in androgenic to estrogenic activity and the degree of impairment in insulin-mediated glucose disposal as well as an elevation in plasma insulin concentrations (Peiris et al. 1987). While the latter hypothesis is not unequivocally confirmed, a variety of evidence tends to support the role of excess androgens in accounting for a substantial portion of the pathological changes in the hepatic metabolism of glucose and insulin. Kissebah et al. (1985) and Evans et al. (1984) proposed that androgen excess directly produces decreased hepatic extraction of insulin and the accumulation of upper body fat in normal, healthy, premenopausal women. In this population, there was a significant negative association between increasing W/H ratios and decreasing plasma sex hormone binding globulin (SHBG), and an increase in percent free testosterone (T). This effect was not associated with increased thigh fat, and was independent of the degree of obesity, which itself was significantly associated with both SHBG and percent free T. Moreover, SHBG appeared to be a more sensitive marker than percent free T as an indicator of the change in balance of androgens to estrogen.

Other disorders associated with higher T production, such as oligomenorrhea, hirsutism, and primary cystic ovary disease, all exhibit the same lowering of SHBG (Enriori et al. 1986). Since other steroids such as androstenediol, 17-beta-OH steroids, and dihydrotestosterone are also bound by SHBG (Peiris et al. 1987), they, too, may contribute an important increase in androgenicity, which may account for the weak correlation between percent free T and W/H ratio. Overall, a decrease in SHBG would influence T considerably more than estradiol, and clearly lead to a shift in the androgen balance which could account for the decreased peripheral fat. Whether this condition directly leads to the development of a redistribution of body fat in adulthood, or is the product of a long-term pattern expressed earlier, is not well understood. Thus, data on the expression of this fat pattern at earlier periods in the life cycle of both sexes prior to the onset of sexual maturity may shed important new insights on the development of this pattern.

ANDROGENS IN CHILDHOOD AND ADOLESCENCE

Although there are only a limited number of studies on prepubertal fat patterning, Frischano and Flegal (1982) have confirmed that increased subscapular to triceps skinfold ratios (CFR) are significantly associated with advanced skeletal age in both sexes and with earlier menarche in girls. If androgens are involved in influencing CFR, the only major source of androgenic variation prior to the onset of puberty is the adrenal androgens, and Pintor et al. (1984) and Genazzani et al. (1978) have linked raised DHEA-S levels to increased prepubertal obesity.

Before sexual maturity, the adrenals undergo adrenarche, or maturation of the androgen secreting capacity of the adrenals. During adrenarche, the zona reticularis of the adrenal gland differentiates to secrete DHEA-S and DHEA. The timing of maturation is species-specific, and occurs at four years in the chimpanzee and at approximately six to seven years in the human, along with a mid growth spurt (Forest et al. 1982). Moreover, adrenarche only occurs in the human and chimpanzee, making it a unique and most likely recently evolved endocrine phenomenon among the higher primates (Cutler and Loriaux 1980; Katz et al. 1983; Zemel and Katz 1986).

Adrenal androgen levels have been associated with obesity in prepubertal children (Genezanni et al. 1978) and with increased BMI and skinfold thicknesses in preadolescent males (Katz et al. 1985) and in adolescent females (Katz et al. 1986; Hediger and Katz 1986). Moreover, Katz et al. (1986) reported that CFR was associated in females with increased DHEA-S levels. Further analyses of these data on females (Hediger and Katz 1986) demonstrated that DHEA-S or DHEA interacting with BMI (Quetelet's index) were the best predictors in stepwise regression analyses also involving chronological age and BMI alone, in skeletally mature and skeletally advanced females, respectively. However, the best predictor of the CFR of skeletally immature females was BMI, and not DHEA-S levels. Since DHEA-S does not reach a peak until after skeletal maturity, these data suggest that the increasing capacity to secrete DHEA-S becomes important in establishing the pattern of CFR.

ANDROGEN CORRELATES OF BODY FAT PATTERNS IN PHILADELPHIA BLACK ADOLESCENTS

Data from Katz et al. (1986) were recomputed and plotted as histograms to demostrate these important interactions in humans. Figure 1 shows the chronological age specific plots for DHEA-S levels for both sexes. There were 212 and 172 black males and females respectively aged 12-16. Although there are no reported sex differences, females in this large sample did show differences that were particularly apparent at age 14; however, these differences were not apparent at the later ages. Figure 2 shows the female mean +/- standard error of the mean skinfold data broken into age standardized groupings of DHEA-S for the low <15%, the "normal" middle 15-85%, and the high >85% for triceps and subscapular skinfolds in order to compare the trends at the upper and lower portions of the distribution. Overall, there is a trend toward relatively greater triceps than subscapular skinfolds at the lower levels of DHEA-S, and an increase in subscapular over triceps at the upper (>85%) end of the distribution. Although the overall trend is statistically significant for the associations between subscapular skinfold thickness (SFT) and DHEA-S groupings ($p<.02$), the ANCOVA procedure only demonstrated a borderline effect for the overall model for triceps SFT. (Unadjusted skinfolds for age were both significantly associated with DHEA-S levels, shown in Figure 3). However, computing the CFR (subscapular/subscapular and triceps) yielded a substantial increase (post hoc testing $p<.01$) for the upper DHEA-S groups, as opposed to the mid and lower groups, suggesting that elevated DHEA-S above the 85% in this population had an important association with CFR. We also reported that this effect of DHEA-S was associated with a significant rise in seated systologic and diastolic phase IV blood pressure, independent of increased BMI.

In males there are two sources of androgens which were measured. Accordingly, the data were analysed by two-way ANOVAS using age adjusted tertiles (tertiles were used to maintain sufficient sample size in the cross-tabulated groups) of DHEA-S and pre-, trans-, and post-gonadal testosterone (T) of <100ug/dl, 100-280 ug/dl, and >280 ug/dl levels, respectively (see Katz et al. 1985). Figure 4

DHEAS AND TESTOSTERONE BY SKELETAL AGE IN ADOLESCENT MALES

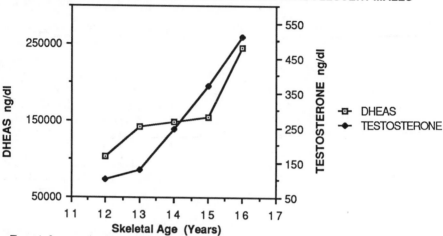

Figure 1: Cross sectional means of serum hormones (adapted from Zemel and Katz, 1986).
(note the use of the same units of measure -ng/dl)

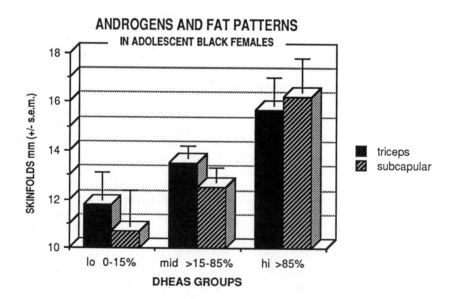

FIGURE 2

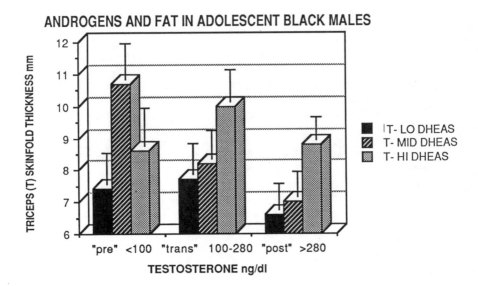

FIGURE 3

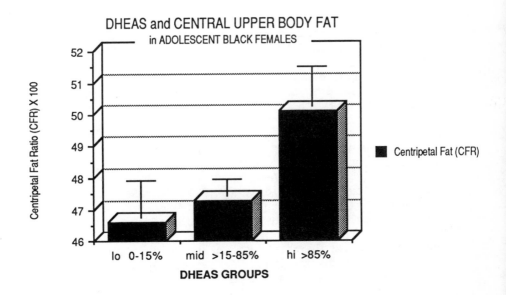

FIGURE 4

presents data on the triceps skinfold with means and standard error of the mean bars for each of the three T groups. Overall, there is a decrease in triceps SFT with increasing T, but this decrease was not statistically significant. On the other hand, there is a strong and statistically significant effect of DHEA-S on triceps which is most apparent at the trans and post groupings of T. Subscapular data are presented in Figure 5. These data indicate a substantial and statistically significant association (p<.05) of DHEA-S with subscapular skinfolds, but not with T. However, the effect of DHEA-S on the variation is much clearer in the trans and post gonadarchial groupings of the T levels. Figure 6 presents data on the CFR for males. It is strikingly different from the previous individual skinfold data in that the effects of T are highly significant (p<.001) and DHEA-S is not associated with the CFR variation. It is evident that the increasing influence of T on CFR in the male is highly dependent on T and independent of DHEA-S. This result is in sharp contrast to the very similar range of CFR which accounted for the percentage groupings of DHEA-S levels in females (Figure 3).

In order to analyze this phenomenon further a post hoc analysis of the means of each skinfold by DHEA-S tertile and T groups was undertaken. Data from this analysis are presented in Figure 7 as percentage change in each skinfold across T groups. Also, each type of skinfold was paired by tertile of DHEA-S in order to provide for the comparison of the individual SFT changes that underlie the sources of the highly significant CFR and T association. First, there is a striking decrease in overall fat in the "mid" DHEA-S groups with increasing levels of T. The other striking variation between triceps and subscapular skinfolds occurs at the upper tertile of the DHEA-S grouping. There is a consistent and statistically significnat (p<.01) increase in subscapular skinfolds with increasing DHEA-S tertiles and T maturation groupings. Thus, the principle source of variation is the overall decline in triceps and increase in subscapular skinfold thickness in the male, especially in the high DHEA-S group. Since the latter may underlie the emergence of an important cardiovascular disease risk factor (Stokes et al. 1985), these changes are marked with a star on Figure 7.

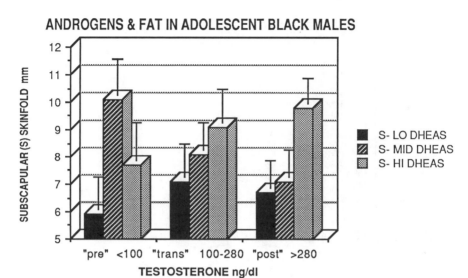

FIGURE 5

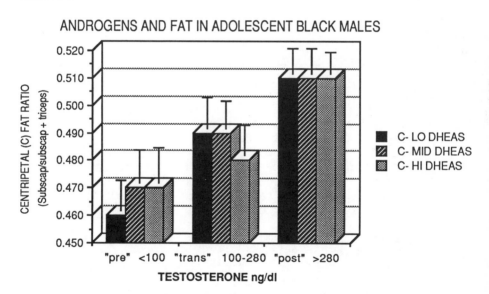

FIGURE 6

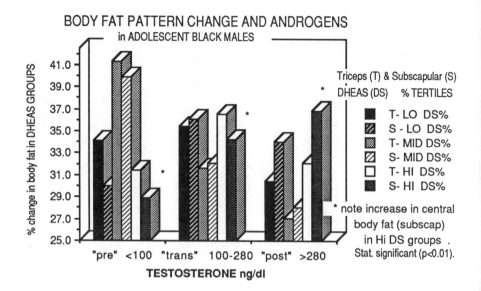

FIGURE 7

These data suggest that in males central (subscapular) fat is difficult to mobilize. In contrast, with normal maturation there is a rapid increase in the mobilization of fat from the triceps region. However, the DHEA-S group most likely to have the greatest increase in subscapular body fat is the upper tertile. Since it is known that overall increased DHEA-S is associated with increased body fat, it is the elevated fat group which is the one at greatest risk for elevated DHEA-S levels during gonadal maturation. This phenomenon appears to translate into increased CFR and increased risk of hypertension (Katz et al. 1986).

Data from both sexes taken together suggest a very important role for androgens in shaping body fat. Both adrenal and testicular androgens play a significant role in males and adrenal androgens play a highly significant role in females. These data confirm that the tendency to CFR becomes established long before the kind of pathology such as NIDDM is established in adults. However, there are changes in childhood and adolescence which may add an important risk to future pathology. These include significantly increased blood pressure, which appears to track at significantly raised levels into adulthood, thereby prognosticating the future developments of borderline hypertension (Katz et al. 1986a).

These adrenal and gonadal hormone variations are also associated with other important circumpubertal events. Katz et al. (1985) reported that increased skeletal age in males was associated with increased DHEA-S levels independent of T levels and before trans-pubertal levels of T were attained. Since raised DHEA-S is associated with increased body fat in both sexes and is associated with advanced skeletal age in males, they reasoned that the secular trend toward earlier onset of puberty was mediated through the chronic endocrine effects of raised adrenal androgens, which become aromatized in the hypothalamus and ultimately trigger an earlier onset of puberty. This hypothesis fits well with the established literature on body fat and maturation (Scott and Johnston 1982) and an increased CFR associated with advanced skeletal age and early sexual maturity in females (Frischano and Flegal 1982). Also, it suggests an additional source of important risk factors concerning the established relations between early menarche and breast cancer, and later associations of breast cancer with increased sensitivity to adrenal androgens (Kirschner et al. 1982; Bulbrook et al. 1971).

The mechanisms which underlie these substantial physiological changes remain to be determined. However, adrenal androgens require consideration along with testosterone (T) and androstenedione (A) in interpreting the endocrine basis of fat patterning. The fact that CFR and the individual skinfolds which comprise the ratios are so highly sensitive to androgens in a normal black early adolescent population clearly removes the accumulation of central body fat from the pathological context in which it has been largely evaluated in adults. These and other related data (Frisancho and Flegal 1982) strongly support a long period of development of this body fat pattern, and may help to explain how central body fat in adults is such a strong independent marker of pathology, even under conditions of relatively high measurement error and imprecise definitions (Bray et al. 1978; Mueller 1985).

ANDROGENS, OBESITY, AND FAT METABOLISM

The mechanism of the action of androgens is undoubt-
edly complex. Androgens can come from either the gonads or
adrenals, and the proportion of androgens from the testes
in males is enormous compared to that from the ovaries in
females. This difference may help to explain the substantial variation in chronic disease patterns between the
sexes. However, in either sex androgen levels may not become pathological until they are associated with long term
obesity and with other related epigenetic risk factors
which are only expressed under chronic conditions of
pathological obesity.

ADRENAL ANDROGEN METABOLISM

DHEA and DHEA-S may play an important direct role in
the regulation of body fat in both sexes. DHEA and several
of its metabolites inhibit G6PDase activity which control
the NADPH levels necessary for the synthesis of body fat,
and in the adrenal, DHEA is an important limiting factor in
cholesterol production and in steroidogenesis (Schwartz et
al. 1981; Cleary et al. 1986). Among the obese, DHEA
becomes bound to fat in enormous quantities (Feher and
Halmy 1975a). It is converted to 16Beta-OH DHEA in the
liver and is excreted in the urine in the obese (Yamaji et
al. 1980). DHEA is normally excreted in the urine; however,
in the obese, with elevated blood pressure and NIDDM, its
excretion rate is reported to fall to undetectable levels
(Sonka et al. 1965) and it is excreted entirely as urinary
16 Beta-OH DHEA (Nowaczynski et al 1977).

Conditions of gout and increased levels of serum uric
acid, along with obesity (Vague 1956) and lowered urinary
DHEA levels, have also been reported by Sonka and Gregorova
(1964). They proposed that raised purine metabolism was
associated with the absence of DHEA inhibition of G6PDase
activity. Schwartz et al. (1981) have proposed that the
anti-cancer and obesity effects of oral DHEA administration
may also operate via this inhibition of G6PDase activity.
Likewise, Cleary et al. (1986) have reported a potent anti-
obesity effect of oral administration of DHEA to Zucker
rats. Moreover, Coleman et al. (1984) have reported that
the obesity, chronic hyperglycemia, severe insulin resis-

tance, and pancreatic beta cell necrosis in the db/db mouse are completely reversible with oral administration of DHEAS and/or its metabolite, etiocholanolone. Since DHEA-sulfate can be interconverted to DHEA via the X-linked enzyme steroid sulphatase (found in skin and other body tissues), and DHEA-S has the highest plasma concentration of any steroid in the body and provides an enormous reservoir of DHEA, its role in the etiology and therapy in NIDDM and the related aspects of CVD needs further exploration.

DHEA also has other reported effects which may link it to central body fat accumulation. Sharma et al. (1963) have reported that DHEA decreases adrenal 11-Beta-hydroxylase activity, resulting in a lowered conversion and raised concentration of deoxycorticosterone (DOC) and deoxycortisol and a high level of ACTH secretion. This condition is nearly a phenocopy of the autosomal inherited and non-HLA linked 11-beta-hydroxylase deficiency which produces a hypertensive form of congenital adrenal hyperplasia in children. The latter is associated with increased ACTH, highly elevated DHEA and DHEA-S, and increased urinary excretion of 17-ketosteroids (see Katz et al. 1986; Oberfield et al. 1982). Since raised ACTH produces Cushings disease, it is possible that in addition to the blood pressure raising effects of DOC mineralocorticoid activity, there may also be a loss of body fat and muscle in selective areas, giving rise to a Cushings-like body fat distribution, which may be similar to the effects of long term therapy with glucocorticoids (Horber et al. 1986).

Another pathway for the effects of DHEA-S and T involves their aromatization, or the conversion of androgens to estrogen products (Figure 8). There are a number of reports demonstrating, in obese women, increased aromatization of androgens (MacDonald et al. 1978; Edman and MacDonald 1978). High levels of aromatase activity are found in the stromal tissue fibroblasts which provide the supporting structures to adipose tissue. Also, high aromatase activity is found in the hypothalamus and limbic system, liver, hairoots, muscle, and kidney (Forney et al. 1981; Scweikert et al. 1975; Cleland et al. 1983). Once aromatase activity is increased, it does not appear to decline after weight loss (Siiteri et al. 1976). Moreover, androstenedione (A) and T are aromatized to the estrogen products estrone and estradiol, respectively, which are fat soluble and are fat sequesterable (Edman et al. 1978).

Estradiol can also be interconverted to estrone via the action of hydroxysteroid dehydrogenase (HSD). In females, endometrial tissue HSD activity is enhanced by progesterone (Tseng and Gurpide 1979) and is reported to be significantly inhibited by DHEA and DHEA-S levels in breast and other tissues (Bonney et al. 1983). Other studies of postmenopausal women have demonstrated that plasma levels of DHEA-S are correlated inversely with the conversion of estradiol to estrone, but are not significantly associated with progesterone levels, presumably because the latter are too low in postmenopausal women to influence HSD activity (James et al. 1986). Overall, these data suggest that obesity is associated with an increased aromatization of androstenedione (A) to estrone (E1) which can be up to 2-5 times greater in obese versus normal females. Thus, fat both produces endocrine changes and is altered by the changes it produces, particularly in terms of the long term shaping of body fat distribution. Under these conditions, CFR is likely to be a long term marker for a particular type of metabolic adjustment (Whitworth and Meeks 1985).

In addition to the possible mechanisms for the adrenal androgens discussed above for females, another mechanism may account for the series of events involving both DHEA-S and T in males. A significant portion of the estradiol (E2) formed in the steroid metabolism of T is metabolized further via 2-hydroxylation to the catechol estrogen, 2-hydroxyestrone (CE) (Schneider et al. 1983), which has little or no estrogenic activity (Parvizi and Ellendorf 1980). However, CE is a specific inhibitor of catechol-O-methyltransferase (COMT) (Ball et al. 1972) and may directly interfere with the dopamine receptors involved with the mobilization of fat. Thus, the rapid increase in T in adolescent males could result in raised E1 which is then metabolized in part to CE. Small increases in CE could interfere with liver, plasma, and kidney COMT, and hence lower the metabolism of catecholamines, resulting in prolonged sympathetic increased lipoprotein lipase activity.

Also, an increase in catecholamine activity could be preferentially more effective on peripheral adipocytes than on the central ones, since the adipocytes of central body fat in the obese are stretched out and have fewer beta adrenergic receptors than do peripheral sites (Evans et al.

1983). Thus, increased levels of free T, produced by a
decrease in SHBG, which is stimulated in part by the
effects of raised adrenal androstenedione on the liver, and
in the presence of elevated levels of DHEA-S, result in
altered production of E2, E3 and increased CE levels. The
latter result in decreased liver COMT activity and increased FFA. Also, increased levels of FFA block the sensitivity of skeletal and cardiac muscle to the effects of
insulin, resulting in higher levels of insulin production
and ultimately in NIDDM. The raised levels of insulin also
enhance sympathetic activity, with increases in catecholamine levels which could further exacerbate the androgen
driven release of FFA (Landsberg and Young 1985; Rowe et
al. 1981). This mechanism (summarized on Figure 8) could
account, in Figure 7, for the rise in subscapular body fat
observed in those adolescent males with adult serum T
levels and elevated DHEA-S levels.

Additionally, raised insulin is reported to diminish
sodium excretion by the stimulation of renal sodium reabsorption (DeFronzo 1981; Kolanowski 1981), and result in
raised pressure naturesis and elevated blood pressure. The
raised sympathetic stimulation by insulin could also result
in an additional rise in blood pressure due to a further
inhibition of kidney COMT activity. Thus, the hyperinsulinemia associated with obesity suggests two factors that may
account for the association of raised blood pressure with
increases in central body fat obesity (Landsberg 1986) and
DHEA-S (Katz et al 1986). The net effects of the raised
DHEA-S and the rise in T during adolescence are raised
insulin, elevated blood pressure, and elevated body fat.

In summary, the presence of obesity results in a rise
in serum DHEA-S and DHEA concentration, presumably by stimulation via ACTH and/or some other pituitary hormonal
response to fat such as increased prolactin secretion. DHEA
may physiologically inhibit G6PDase activity, which is involved in the synthesis of fat and cholesterol and is especially important in adrenal steroidogenesis. Also, DHEA
inhibits 11-Beta hydroxylase activity, that could result in
an increase in DOC and in deoxycortisol, and be involved in
the shaping of body fat patterns. Finally, a model (Figure
8) which would link both elevated, obesity associated, serum DHEA-S levels with normal adult male levels of T and/or
increased levels of ovarian T in obese women involves excess CE formation. In adolescence (with normal thyroid

function), the rapidly rising levels of T (in part due to decreased production of liver SHBG) along with the high levels of serum DHEA-S associated with obesity, inhibit HSD activity and regulate the conversion of E2 to E1 and supply large additional quantities of A for aromatization to E1 which is then metabolized in part to CE. Since CE inhibits COMT activity, it may prolong sympathetic stimulation of fat mobilization and in turn block the hepatic uptake of insulin, possibly producing post-hepatic hyperinsulinemia, which may produce a further rise in sympathetic activity. However, only those adipocytes with adequate numbers of receptors per cell have a sufficient response to this fat mobilization. Adipocytes found in the central portion of the body that are stretched out from previous fat gain, and have too few receptors per cell surface to be stimulated, lack this response. The net effect is a gradual shaping of body fat through selective mobilization of fat, which is also altered by androgen mediated increases in muscularity, and becomes a cumulative marker for a long series of endocrine adjustments that ultimately result in the chronic diseases first described by Vague in 1956.

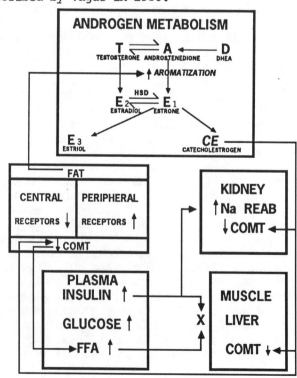

FIGURE 8:
Androgens and
Fat Metabolism
in Males

REFERENCES

Ball P, Knuppen R, Haupt M, Breuer H (1972). Interactions between estrogens and catecholamines. III. Studies on the methylation of catecholestrogens, catechol amines and other catechols by the catechol-O-methyltransferase of human liver. J Clin Endocrin 34:736–746

Bonney RC, Reed MJ, James VHT (1983). Inhibition of 17–beta– hydroxysteroid dehydrogenase activity in human endometrium by adrenal androgens. J Ster Biochem 18:59–64

Bray GA, Greenway FL, Molitch ME, Dahms WT, Atkinson RL, Hamilton K (1978). Use of anthropometric measures to assess weight loss. Am J Clin Nutr 31:769–773.

Bulbrook R, Hayward J, Spicer C (1971). Relation between urinary androgen and corticoid excretion and subsequent breast cancer. Lancet 395–397.

Cleary MP, Shepard A, Jenks B (1984). Effect of dehydroepiandrosterone on growth in lean and obese zucker rats. J Nutr 114:1242–1251.

Cleary MP, Zisk, JF (1986). Anti-obesity effect of two different levels of dehydroepiandrosterone in lean and obese middle–aged female zucker rats. Int J Obes 10:193–204

Cleland WH, Mendelson CR, Simpson ER (1983). Aromatase activity of membrane fractions of human adipose tissue stromal cells and adipocytes. Endocrin 113:2155–2160

Coleman D (1985). Antiobesity effects of etiocholanolones in diabetes (db), viable yellow (Avy), and normal mice. Endocrin 117:2279–2283

Coleman DL, Leiterp EH, Applezweig N (1984). Therapeutic effects of dehydroepiandrosterone metabolites in diabetes mutant mice (C57BL/KsJ–db/db). Endocrin 115:239–243.

Cutler GB, Loriaux DL (1980). Adrenarche and its relationship to the onset of puberty. Fed Proc 38:2384–2390.

DeFronzo RA (1981). Insulin and renal sodium handling: clinical implications. Int J Obes (Suppl 1) 5:93–104

Despres JP, Allard C, Tremblay A, Talbot J, Bouchard C (1985).Evidence for a regional component of body fatness in the association with serum lipids in men and women. Metabolism 34:967–973

Dunkel L, Sorva R, Voutilainen R (1985). Low levels of sex hormone binding globulin in obese children. J Ped 107:95–97

Edman CD, Aiman EJ, Porter JC, MacDonald PC (1978). Identification of the estrogen product of extraglandular aromatization of plasma androstenedione. Am J Obstet Gynecol 130:439–447

Edman CD, MacDonald PC (1978). Effect of obesity on conversion of plasma androstenedione to estrone in ovulatory and anovulatory young women. Am J Obstet Gynecol 130:456-461

Enriori CL, Orsini W, del Carmen Cremona M, Etkin AE, Cardillo LR, Reforzo-Membrives J (1986). Decrease of circulating level of SHBG in postmenopausal obese women as a risk factor in breast cancer: reversible effect of weight loss. Gyn Onc 23:77-86

Evans DJ, Hoffman RG, Kalkhoff RK, Kissebah AH (1983). Relationship of androgenic activity to body fat topography, fat cell morphology, and metabolic aberrations in premenopausal women. J Clin End Metab 57:304-310

Evans DJ, Hoffman RG, Kalkhoff RK, Kissebah AH (1984). Relationship of body fat topography to insulin sensitivity and metabolic profiles in premenopausal women. Metab Clin Exp 33:68-75

Feher T, Halmy L (1975a). The production and fate of adrenal DHEA in normal and overweight subjects. Hormone Res 6:303-304.

Feher T, Halmy L (1975b). Dehydroepiandrosterone and dehydroepiandrosterone sulfate dynamics in obesity. Can J Biochem 53:215-222

Forest MG, DePeretti E, David M, Sempe M (1982) L'andrenarche joue-t-elle vraiment un role determinant dans le developpement pubertaire? Ann d'Endorin (Paris) 43:465-495.

Forney JP, Milewich L, Chen GT, Garlock JL, Schwarz BE, Edman CD, MacDonald PC (1981). Aromatization of androstenedione to estrone by human adipose tissue in vitro. Correlation with adipose tissue mass, age, and endometrial neoplasia. J Clin Endocrin Metab 53:192

Freidenberg GR, Henry RR, Klein HH, Reichart DR, Olefsky JM (1987). Decreased kinase activity of insulin receptors from adipocytes of non-insulin-dependent diabetic subjects. J. Clin Invest. 79:240-250

Frisancho AR, Flegel PN (1982). Advanced maturation associated with centripetal fat pattern. Hum Biol 54:717-727.

Genazzani AR, Pintor C, Corda R (1978). Plasma levels of gonadotropins, prolactin, thyroxine, and adrenal and gonadal steroids in obese prepubertal girls. J Clin Endocrin Metab 47:974-979.

Glueck CJ, Taylor HL, Jacobs D, Morrison JA, Beaglehole R, Williams OD (1980). Plasma high-density lipoprotein cholesterol: association with measurements of body mass. Am Heart Assoc Monograph Number 73, Supple 4:62-69

Haffner SM, Stern MP, Hazuda HP, Pugh J, Patterson JK
(1987). Do upper-body and centralized adiposity measure
different aspects of regional body-fat distribution?
Diabetes 36:43-51

Hediger ML, Katz, SH (1986). Fat patterning, overweight,
and adrenal androgen interactions in black adolescent
females. Human Biol 58:585-600

Horber FF, Zurcher RM, Herren H, Crivelli MA, Robotti G,
Frey FJ (1986). Altered body fat distribution in patients
with glucocorticoid treatment and in patients on long-
term dialysis. Am J Clin Nutr 43:758-769.

James VHT, Reed MJ, Beranek PA, Bonney RC, Samuel DL,
Newton CJ, Franks S, Ghilchik MW (1986). Androgen and
estrogen metabolism in breast cancer patients. Ann NY
Acad Sci 464:117-125

Katz SH, Hediger ML, Schall JI, Valleroy LA (1983). Growth
and blood pressure. In Kotchen TA, Kotchen JM (eds):
"Clinical Approaches to High Blood Pressure in the
Young," Boston: John Wright/PSG, Inc, pp. 91-131.

Katz SH, Hediger ML, Zemel BS, Parks JS (1985). Adrenal
androgens, body fat and advanced skeletal age in puberty:
new evidence for the relations of adrenarche and
gonadarche in males. Human Biol 57:401-413

Katz SH, Hediger ML, Zemel BS, Parks JS (1986). Blood
pressure, body fat, and dehydroepiandrosterone sulfate
variation in adolescence. Hypertension 8:277-284.

Kirschner MA, Schneider G, Ertel NH, Worton E (1982).
Obesity, androgens, estrogens, and cancer risk. Cancer
Res 42:(Suppl) 3281s-3285s.

Kissebah AH, Evans DJ, Peiris A, Wilson CR (1985).
Endocrine characteristics in regional obesities: role of
sex steroids. In "Proceedings of the International
Symposium on the Metabolic Complications of Obesities,"
Amsterdam: Elsevier Science Publishers, pp 115-130

Kissebah A, Vydelingum N, Murray R, Evans DJ, Hartz AJ,
Kalkhoff RK, Adams PW (1982). Relation of body fat
distribution to metabolic complications of obesity. J
Clin Endocrin Metab 54:254-260

Kolanowski J (1981). Influence of insulin and glucagon on
sodium balance in obese subjects during fasting and
refeeding. Int J Obes (Suppl 1) 5:105-114

Krotkiewski M, Bjorntorp P, Sjostrom L, Smith U (1983).
Impact of obesity on metabolism in men and women.
Importance of regional adipose tissue distribution. J
Clin Invest 72:1150-1162

Landsberg L (1986). Diet, obesity and hypertension: an

hypothesis involving insulin, the sympathetic nervous system, and adaptive thermogenesis. Quar J Med 61:1081-1090

Landsberg L, Young JB (1985). Insulin-mediated glucose metabolism in the relationship between dietary intake and sympathetic nervous system activity. Int J Obes 9:(Suppl 2) 63-68.

Lapidus L, Bengtsson C, Larsson B, Pennert K, Rybo E, Sjostrom L (1984). Distribution of adipose tissue and risk of cardiovascular disease and death: a 12-year follow up of participants in the population study of women in Gothenburg, Sweden. Br Med J 289:1257- 1261

Larsson B, Svardsudd K, Welin L, Wilhelmsen L, Bjorntorp P, Tibblin G (1984). Abdominal adipose tissue distribution, obesity and risk of cardiovascular disease and death: a 13-year follow up of participants in the study of men born in 1913. Br Med J 288:1401-1404

MacDonald PC, Edman CD, Hemsell DL, Porter JC, Siiteri PK (1978). Effect of obesity on conversion of plasma androstenedione to estrone in postmenopausal women with and without endometrial cancer. Am J Obstet Gynecol 130:448-455

Mueller WH (1985). The biology of human fat patterning. In Norgan NG (ed): "Human Body Composition and Fat Distribution," London: Report of a European Community Workshop, pp 159-174

Nowaczynski W, Messerli FH, Kuchel O, Guthrie Jr GP, Genest J (1977). Origin of urinary 16B-hydroxydehyroepiandrosterone in essential hypertension. J Clin Endocrin Metab 44:629-638.

Oberfield SE, Levine LS, New MI (1982). Childhood hypertension due to adrenocortical disorders. Pediatr Ann 11:623-628.

Olefsky JM (1976b). The insulin receptor: its role in insulin resistance of obesity and diabetes. Diabetes 25:1154-1162

Parvizi N, Ellendorf F (1980). Recent views on endocrine effects of catecholestrogens. J Steroid Biochem 12:331-335

Peiris AN, Mueller RA, Smith GA, Struve MF, Kissebah AH (1986). Splanchnic insulin metabolism in obesity: influence of body fat distribution. J Clin Invest 78:1648-1657

Peiris AN, Mueller RA, Struve MF, Smith GA, Kissebah AH (1987). Relationship of androgenic activity to splanchnic insulin metabolism and peripheral glucose utilization in premenopausal women. J Clin Endocrin Metab 64:162–169

Pintor C, Loche S, Faedda A, Fanni V, Nuchi AM, Corda R (1984). Adrenal androgens in obese boys before and after weight loss. Human Metab Res 16:544–548.

Rowe JW, Young JB, Minaker KL, Stevens AL, Pallotta J, Landsberg L (1981). Effect of insulin and glucose infusions on sympathetic nervous system activity in normal man. Diabetes 30:219–225.)

Salans L, Knittle J, Hirsch J (1968). The role of adipose cell size and adipose tissue insulin sensitivity in the carbohydrate intolerance of human obesity. J Clin Invest 47:153–165

Schneider J, Bradlow HL, Strain G, Levin J, Anderson K, Fishman J (1983). Effects of obesity on estradiol metabolism: decreased formation of nonuterotropic metabolites. J Clin Endocrin Metab 56:973–978

Schwartz AG, Hard GC, Pashko LL, Abou-Gharbia M, Swern D (1981). Dehydroepiandrosterone: an anti-obesity and anti-carcinogenic agent. Nutr Cancer 3:46–53.

Schweikert HU, Milewich L, Wilson JD (1975). Aromatization of androstenedione by isolated human hairs. J Clin Endocrin Metab 40:413–417

Scott EC, Johnston FE (1982). Critical fat, menarche, and the maintenance of menstrual cycles: a critical review. J Adol Health Care 2:249–260.

Sharma DC, Forchielli E, Dorfman RI (1963). Inhibition of enzymatic steroid 11-B-hydroxylation by androgens. J Biol Chem 238:572–575.

Sherman B, Wallace R, Bean J, Schlabaugh L (1981). Relationship of body weight to menarcheal and menopausal age: implications for breast cancer risk. J Clin Endocrin Metab 52:488–493

Siiteri PK, Williams JE, Takaki NK (1976). Steroid abnormalities in endometrial and breast carcinoma: a unifying hypothesis. J Steroid Biochem 7:897–903

Sjostrom L (1972). Adult human adipose tissue cellularity and metabolism. Acta Med Scand (Suppl) 544:1–52

Sonka J, Gregorova I, Skamenova B (1965) Contribution a la physiopathogenie de l'obesite. I la Dehydroepiandro-sterone. Rev Franc Endocrin Clin 6:203–212.

Stern MP, Haffner SM (1986). Body fat distribution and hyperinsulinemia as risk factors for diabetes and cardiovascular disease. Arterio 6:123–130

Stokes J, Garrison RJ, Kannel WB (1986). The independent contributions of various indices of obesity to the 22-year incidence of coronary heart disease: the

Framingham Heart Study
Proc Int Symp Metab Complic Human Obes
Tseng L, Gurpide E (1979). Stimulation of various
17-beta- hydrosteroid and 20-alpha-hydroxysteroid
dehydrogenase activities by progestins in human
endometrium. Endocrin 104:1745–1748
Vague J (1956). The degree of masculine differentiation
of obesities: a factor determining predisposition to
diabetes atherosclerosis, gout, and uric calculous
disease. Am J Clin Nutr 4:20–34
Whitworth NS, Meeks GR (1985). Hormone Metabolism: body
weight and extraglandular production. Clin Obs Gyn
28:580–587
Yamaji T, Ishibashi M, Katayama S, Kinori S (1980). Serum
16B-hydroxydhydroepiandrosterone sulfate in man. J Clin
Endocrin Metab 50:955–960.
Zemel BS, Katz SH (1986). The contribution of adrenal and
gonadal androgens to the growth in height of adolescent
males. Am J Phys Anthro 71:459–466.

Fat Distribution During Growth and Later Health Outcomes
pages 285–295 © 1988 Alan R. Liss, Inc.

FAT DISTRIBUTION AND METABOLISM IN ANIMAL STUDIES

M.R.C. Greenwood, Ruth Kava, David B. West
and Roland Savard
Department of Biology, Vassar College,
Poughkeepsie, NY, 12601 (M.R.C.G. and R.K.),
Eastern Virginia Medical School, Norfolk, VA
(D.B.W.), and The University of Montreal,
Montreal, Quebec (R.S.)

INTRODUCTION

Adipose tissues differ in their metabolic and
morphological characteristics, and their hormonal
sensitivity. While all adipose tissue depots share a
common characteristic of storing triglyceride and providing
it as an energy substrate when needed, some of the
different fat depots have evolved unique characteristics.
In humans, numerous investigators have recently shown that
adipose tissue accumulation in certain regions, even in the
absence of significant adiposity, is associated with
increased morbidity and mortality (Krotkiewski, et al.,
1983; Kissebah, et al., 1982). While research in humans has
helped us to understand the importance of regional adipose
distribution, the problems inherent in sampling the various
adipose depots in humans make it difficult to understand
completely the roles played by different regional adipose
depots. Thus it is important to use animal models, and to
understand the regional regulation of adipose tissue
metabolism and morphology in these animal models, so that
appropriate and clear hypotheses may be tested with the
limited amounts of human tissue that become available.

REGIONAL ADIPOSE TISSUE CONSIDERATIONS IN PREGNANCY

In rodents and other mammals adipose tissue accumulates
during the course of a normal pregnancy. In women, this
accumulation amounts to approximately 3.5 kilograms and in
the rat approximately 7 to 17 grams (Pipe, et al., 1979;
Moore and Brasel, 1984; Lederman and Rosso, 1980). It has

been shown in the rat that lipid accumulates preferentially
in the subcutaneous depots during pregnancy and may be
mobilized preferentially from this site during lactation
(Moore, et al., 1984; Savard, et al., 1986). In general,
the increase in adipose tissue depot size in these studies
was accompanied by changes in adipose tissue cell size with
no change in adipose tissue cell number (Table 1).

TABLE 1. Changes in Adipose Depot Size and Cellularity in
Pregnant Rats at Day 20 of Gestation

	Percent of Nonpregnant Controls		
Adipose Depot:	Depot Weight	Cell Number	Cell Size
Subscapular	132%[*]	106%	133%[*]
Retroperitoneal	126%[*]	111%	125%
Parametrial	113%	97%	116%

There were 6 pregnant and 6 control rats.
[*] Indicates significantly different from
nonpregnant control (p<.05, t-test).
Data from work of Steingrimsdottir,
et al., 1980b.

The mechanism whereby adipose tissue triglyceride
accumulates in specific depots during pregnancy may be
through the action of lipoprotein lipase (LPL). This
enzyme increases its activity in specific adipose tissue
depots during pregnancy and as shown above this is
accompanied by accumulation of intracellular triglyceride.
Lipolysis in adipose tissue remains relatively unaffected
by pregnancy (Savard,., 1986). In addition, measurements
of adipose tissue blood flow have indicated that while
white adipose tissues received somewhat increased blood
flow at the end of pregnancy in the rat, blood flow to
brown adipose tissue was reduced (Kava, et al., 1986).
This reduction of blood flow to brown adipose tissue is
associated with decreased thermogenesis which is also found
during pregnancy (Tatelman, et al., 1985).

These findings suggest that, in the course of a normal pregnancy, adipose tissue metabolism is adjusted such that lipoprotein lipase activity increases and triglyceride deposition occurs in a depot-specific fashion. Food efficiency increases and this is probably aided by decreased brown adipose tissue thermogenesis. During lactation, the metabolic status is very different and adipose tissue lipoprotein lipase is significantly suppressed (Steingrimsdottir, et al., 1980a). As a result, ingested nutrients are directed to the mammary tissue for synthesis of milk and away from adipose tissue and adipose tissue lipid stores are reduced by this "gate-keeping" mechanism (Greenwood, et al., 1987).

We have hypothesized that lipid accumulation in specific depots during pregnancy is regulated by the altered hormonal status of pregnancy and could be resistant to other competing physiological stresses. To test this hypothesis, an experiment was designed in which the competing needs of lipid accumulation during pregnancy and lipid mobilization during endurance exercise were examined (Savard, et al., 1986). In this experiment, female rats were trained to swim for three hours each day. After conditioning, they were mated and then continued to swim three hours each day throughout the pregnancy. Control groups included sedentary pregnant rats and sedentary non-pregnant rats. Adipose tissue LPL, lipolytic activity and morphology were measured at day 0, day 10 and day 21 of gestation. During the course of pregnancy, both the exercising and sedentary pregnant rats gained weight at equivalent rates. The comparable rate of weight gain by the exercising rats was not due to an increase of food intake; exercising and sedentary rats consumed the same amount of food during pregnancy. Both groups displayed the well-known increment in food efficiency associated with the onset of pregnancy. Considering the energy output associated with their daily exercise regimen, the swimming pregnant animals were additionally efficient at energy utilization.

The competing stresses of exercise and pregnancy resulted in regionally specific adipose tissue responses. In the pregnant sedentary rats, parametrial adipose tissue depot weight increased as would be expected in a normal pregnancy. This increased depot mass was associated with an increase in fat cell size and increased adipose tissue lipoprotein lipase activity. In the exercising pregnant rats, parametrial adipose tissue depot weight gain was suppressed during the pregnancy, as were increments of fat cell size and lipoprotein lipase activity. Lipolysis in this depot was unaffected by either pregnancy or exercise. In contrast, in the inguinal depot, a subcutaneous depot thought to be associated with lactational stores, the response of this depot remained essentially the same in exercising and sedentary pregnant rats. That is, inguinal depot weight increased, as did LPL activity and fat cell size, despite the competing metabolic stimulus of exercise in pregnancy. Thus, during pregnancy, even in the presence of a significant lipolytic stimulus, specific adipose tissue depots may preserve accumulated lipid and maintain the nutritional stores to support a pregnancy and subsequent lactation. In this experiment both sedentary and exercised rats produced normal numbers of pups of normal weight and normal body composition (Savard, et al., 1986).

ALTERED NUTRITIONAL STATES AND REGIONAL ADIPOSE TISSUE METABOLISM

Pregnancy is not the only condition in which regionally specific adipose tissue effects may be noted. For some time, it has been of concern whether lipid is mobilized from specific adipose depots during dieting or fasting and, when repleted, returned to these same or other depots. A recently completed experiment in our laboratory suggests that subcutaneous adipose tissue in the rat is mobilized more readily than are the intraabdominal fat depots during food restriction. In a preliminary study, one group of adult male rats was fed *ad libitum* a high fat diet and then dieted and refed three times. After the final diet, rats were examined at 0, 5 and 35 days of refeeding. At these three times, rats were sacrificed and five adipose tissue depots were dissected; the dorsal subcutaneous, inguinal, retroperitoneal, epididymal and the mesenteric depots. Clear regional specificity in the pattern of fat mobilization occurred. Most of the fat lost during food restriction was mobilized from the two subcutaneous depots and the retroperitoneal depot while the epididymal and mesenteric depot were relatively preserved (Figure 1). There was no significant recovery of depot mass during the first five days of refeeding. A partial metabolic explanation for this regionally specific mobilization of triglyceride is that LPL activity was significantly lower in the inguinal compared with the epididymal depot during the restriction of food intake, while lipolysis was comparable in these two depots. This suggests that the net flux of fatty acid out of adipose tissue would be greatest in the inguinal depot (West, et al., 1987). Thus, during food restriction lipid is preferentially mobilized from subcutaneous fat depots and the lipid stores in the epididymal depot are especially protected from mobilization. During refeeding, lipid was restored to the subcutaneous depots.

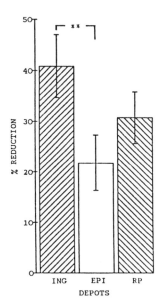

FIGURE 1. Percent reduction of depot lipid in inguinal (ING), epididymal (EPI) and retroperitoneal (RP) depots. These data were calculated by comparing depot lipid content in rats not refed after the period of food restriction (n=10) with animals refed for 35 days (n=9). ** indicate a significant difference between depots (p<.05, ANOVA and post hoc t-test). Data from the work of West, et al., 1987.

REGIONAL ADIPOSE TISSUE BLOOD FLOW AND OBESITY

In addition to significant differences in adipose tissue metabolism associated with the regional distribution of fat, there are correlated changes in adipose tissue blood flow. Regional differences in adipose tissue blood flow have been noted in several species. Recently the differences in adipose tissue blood flow have been described in spontaneously obese and genetically obese rat models (Crandall, et al., 1984; West, et al., 1987). Since obesity is known to produce significant effects on the cardiovascular system in both humans and animals, changes of adipose tissue blood flow may be important for our understanding of the altered metabolism and cardiovascular physiology in the obese.

Therefore, a study was completed measuring blood flow to adipose tissue and other organs using the labeled microsphere technique in the Zucker rat model of obesity and in lean controls (West, et al., 1987). In this experiment, known homozygous lean (FaFa) and obese (fafa) rats were used. After 12 to 16 hours of food deprivation, all rats were gavaged with a test meal consisting of their normal chow in an amount that approximated a normal meal for these rats, and blood flow was measured by the technique of Flaim and Zelis (1982). After injection of the microspheres, the heart, kidney, liver, testis, and epididymus were removed and the radioactivity was quantitated. Five adipose tissue depots; the dorsal subcutaneous, mesenteric, retroperitoneal, epididymal and inguinal fat pads also were removed, weighed, and radioactivity quantitated for the calculation of blood flow.

Blood flow expressed per cell, per unit of surface area, or per gram of tissue was decreased in all depots from obese rats. The only regionally specific effect was an increased mesenteric blood flow relative to the other depots. This was observed in both lean and obese rats. The overall reduction in adipose tissue blood flow in obese rats may be correlated with and contribute to a reduced lipolytic activity in obese adipose tissue, which predisposes obese adipose tissue to the uptake and storage rather than mobilization of lipids (West, et al., 1987).

SEXUAL DIMORPHISM IN ADIPOSITY AND GLUCOSE TOLERANCE USING THE WISTAR *fatty* RAT

The accumulation of excess adiposity in the abdominal or truncal region, a pattern characteristic of male obesity, has been associated with significant morbidity with increased risk for the development of a diabetic or glucose intolerant condition (Krotkiewski, et al., 1983; Kissebah, et al., 1982). Recently, a new animal model, the diabetic Wistar *fatty* (fafa) rat, has been described by our laboratory and others (Ikeda, et al., 1981; Kava, et al., submitted). In this strain, the genetically obese males, but not the obese females, become hyperglycemic. The diabetes in the males is diet-responsive and can be provoked early by the feeding of a high sucrose, but not a high fat, diet (Kava, et al., 1987). Although female *fatty* rats become obese, they do not develop the diabetes. This is illustrated in Table 2.

TABLE 2. Fed Plasma Glucose Levels of Wistar *fatty* Rats Fed 68% Sucrose Diet

Fed Plasma Glucose
(mg/dl)

| Group: | Age in Weeks | | | |
	5	10	18	22
Obese Males (n=7)	161 ± 6	$190 \pm 17^{*}$	$296 \pm 44^{*}$	$380 \pm 66^{*}$
Lean Males (n=7)	157 ± 4	149 ± 2	131 ± 3	128 ± 3
Obese Females (n=10	148 ± 3	167 ± 7	147 ± 4	142 ± 7
Lean Females (n=10)	139 ± 3	159 ± 7	155 ± 4	131 ± 3

Data are presented as means $\pm$ SEM.
* Indicates significantly greater than other groups ($p<.01$, ANOVA). Data from submitted manuscript by Kava, et al., 1987.

Four groups of animals, obese and lean males and females were fed a high sucrose diet from 5 to 23 weeks of age. Only the obese *fatty* male developed frank hyperglycemia after several weeks of feeding on this diet. In addition, when these animals were given a glucose tolerance test, the ability of the Wistar *fatty* male rat to increase plasma insulin levels in response to an oral glucose tolerance test was impaired. These results indicate that the obese Wistar *fatty* rat exhibits sexually dimorphic hyperglycemia by 10 weeks of age when fed a high sucrose diet.

It is not clear how gonadal steroids influence the expression of hyperglycemia in this animal model. The different gonadal hormones may influence adipose tissue regional growth and metabolism differently in the two sexes, leading to a variable susceptibility to dietary effects on adiposity and metabolism. In our preliminary studies, we have examined this question. The obese male Wistar *fatty* rats have more fat as a percentage of carcass weight and are more hypercellular than the obese females (Kava, et al., 1987). There were no other adipose tissue cellular or metabolic characteristics correlated with the sex-difference in glucose homeostasis. However, there was a significant difference in fat distribution with males having a greater proportion of fat in the superficial areas than the females (Table 3). Therefore, it is possible that alterations in

---

TABLE 3. Distribution of Adipose tissue in Wistar *fatty* Rats

Group:	Ratio of Superficial to Intraabdominal Fat[*]
Obese Males (n=7)	1.10 ± 0.06^{a}
Lean Males (n=7)	0.49 ± 0.01^{b}
Obese Females (n=10)	0.76 ± 0.06^{c}
Lean Females (n=10)	0.44 ± 0.01^{b}

Data are presented as means $\pm$ SEM.
[*] Ratio calculated as the sum of inguinal and dorsal subcutaneous depot weight divided by the sum of retroperitoneal, mesenteric and gonadal depot weights. Values with different superscripted letters are significantly different (p<.01,ANOVA). From Kava, et al., 1987.

---

the location of excess adipose tissue accumulation, perhaps due to variable control by gonadal steroids, may influence the sexual dimorphism seen in the expression of NIDDM in this new rat model, the Wistar *fatty* rat.

SUMMARY

It is apparent from examination of these several animal models that specific regional adipose tissue differences in metabolism do occur in the rat. Adipose tissue regional effects are prominent in pregnancy; they may be demonstrated during exercise, dieting and obesity, and in some cases, they may be associated with the expression of diabetes mellitus. Our understanding of the complex pathologies associated with alterations in adiposity will require greater understanding of the role that each specific adipose tissue depot plays in the homeostasis of the organism. If the regionally specific modulation of adipose tissue metabolism plays a significant role in the expression of incipient pathologies, then our understanding of the control of regional adipose tissue metabolism should lead to coherent and rational approaches to treatments.

ACKNOWLEDGEMENTS

The authors gratefully acknowledge the technical assistance of Joyce East-Palmer, Barbara Hyman, Beth Skovan and James Brown. Manuscript preparation was kindly provided by Rosette Uniacke and Bonnie Milne. Some of the work reported was supported by NIH grants HD12637 and AM26687.

Current address for Dr. West:

David B. West, Ph.D.
Department of Physiology
Eastern Virginia Medical School
Box 1980
Norfolk, VA 23501

Current address for Dr. Savard

Professor Roland Savard
University of Montreal
Department of Physical Education
CP 6128, Succursale A
Montreal, Quebec
H 3C3 J7 Canada

REFERENCES

Crandall DL, Goldstein BM, Huggins F, Cervoni P (1984). Adipocyte blood flow: influence of age, anatomic location, and dietary manipulation. Am J Physiol 247:R46-R51.

Flaim S, Zelis R (1982). Effects of diltiazen on total cardiac output distribution in conscious rats. J Pharmacol Exp Ther 222:359-366.

Greenwood MRC, Savard R, West DB, Kava R (1987). Energy metabolism and nutrient 'gating' in pregnancy and lactation. In Berry E, Blondheim SH, Eliahou HE, Shafrir E (eds): "Recent Advances in Obesity Research: V," London: John Libbey and Co., pp 258-263.

Ikeda H, Shino A, Matsuo T, Iwatsuka H, Suzuoki Z (1981). A new genetically obese-hyperglycemic rat (Wistar Fatty). Diabetes 30:1045-1050.

Kava R, West DB, Lukasik VA, Greenwood MRC (submitted for publication). Sexual dimorphism of hyperglycemia and glucose tolerance in the Wistar fatty rat.

Kava R, West DB, Lukasik VA, Greenwood MRC (1987). Adipose Tissue distribution and the sexual dimorphism of NIDDM in the Wistar fatty rat. Fed Proc 46:881.

Kava R, West DB, Lukasik V, Prinz WA, Greenwood MRC (1986). Pregnancy alters blood flow to brown and white adipose tissue in the lean Zucker rat. Fed Proc 45:601.

Kissebah AH, Vydelingum N, Murray R, Evans DJ, Hartz AJ, Kalkhoff RK, Adams PW (1982). Relation of body fat distribution to metabolic complications of obesity. J Clin Endocrinol Metab 54:254-260.

Krotkiewski M, Bjorntorp P, Sjostrom L, Smith U (1983). Impact of obesity on metabolism in men and women. J Clin Invest 72:1150-1162.

Lederman SA, Rosso P (1980). Effects of food restriction on fetal and placental growth and maternal body composition. Growth 44:77-88.

Moore BJ, Brasel JA (1984). One cycle of reproduction consisting of pregnancy, lactation or no lactation, and recovery: effects on carcass composition in ad libitum-fed and food-restricted rats. J Nutr 114:1548-1559.

Moore BJ, Olsen JL, Marks F, Brasel JA (1984). The effects of high fat feeding during one cycle of reproduction consisting of pregnancy, lactation and recovery on body composition and fat pad cellularity in the rat. J Nutr 114:1566-1573.

Pipe NGJ, Smith T, Halliday D, Edmonds CJ, Williams C, Coltart TM (1979). Changes in fat, fat-free mass and body water in human normal pregnancy. Brit J Obstet Gynaecol 86:929-940.

Savard R, Palmer JE, Greenwood MRC (1986). Effects of exercise training on regional adipose tissue metabolism in pregnant rats. Am J Physiol R837-R844.

Steingrimsdottir L, Brasel JA, Greenwood MRC (1980a). Diet, pregnancy and lactation: effects on adipose tissue, lipoprotein lipase and fat cell size. Metabolism 29:837-841.

Steingrimsdottir L, Greenwood MRC, Brasel JA (1980b). Effect of pregnancy, lactation and a high-fat diet on adipose tissue in Osborne-Mendel rats. J Nutr 110:600-609, 1980.

Tatelman, HM, Steinberg L, Winick M (1985). Whole body oxygen consumption and brown adipose tissue guanosine diphosphate (GDP) binding during pregnancy. Fed Proc 44:1161.

West DB, Brown JE, Brownell K, Greenwood MRC (1987). Regional differences in mobilization and replenishment of fat sotres in repeatedly dieted rats. Fed Proc 46:880.

West DB, Prinz WA, Francendese AA, Greenwood MRC (1987). Adipocyte blood flow is decreased in obese Zucker rats. Am J Physiol: In Press.

Fat Distribution During Growth and Later Health Outcomes
pages 297–312 © 1988 Alan R. Liss, Inc.

ALTERATION IN BODY FAT AND FAT DISTRIBUTION WITH EXERCISE

Angelo Tremblay, Jean-Pierre Després and
Claude Bouchard

Physical Activity Sciences Laboratory, Laval
University, Ste-Foy, Quebec, Canada, G1K 7P4

The energy cost of prolonged exercise of moderate
intensity can increase substantially daily energy needs.
Moreover, experimental evidence shows that a postexercise
increment in metabolic rate may also contribute to an
increment in daily energy expenditure (Tremblay et al.,
1985a, 1986; Bahr et al. 1987). If these metabolic
effects of exercise are not compensated by changes in
energy intake or in other components of energy expenditure, a training program could induce a substantial
energy deficit. Thus, exercise-training has theoreti-
cally the potential to alter considerably the adiposity
of obese individuals and could also be valuable to modify
central fat deposition.

The present chapter will be focused on the effect
of exercise-training on body fatness and fat distribution. The possibility of the existence of a sex difference in the response to exercise will also be discussed.
Finally, this chapter will be closed with an analysis of
the relationship between training-induced changes in body
fat and fat distribution and those in plasma glucose and
insulin.

EFFECT OF EXERCISE-TRAINING ON BODY WEIGHT AND FAT

Numerous training programs recommended to obese
individuals comprise aerobic exercise performed two to
five times a week during 20 to 45 min/session. Recently,
we assessed the total energy cost of this type of program

in young non obese male and female adults (Tremblay et al., 1984a). These subjects exercised on cycleergometer during 20 weeks, four times increasing to five times a week, 40 to 45 min/session, at an intensity starting at 60 and increasing to 85 percent of the heart rate reserve. Occasionally, this prescription was replaced by an intermittent exercise session. Using the heart rate method (Maxfield, 1971), we estimated that the total energy cost of exercise corresponded to 31705 and 19920 kcal for males and females, respectively. When the energy cost of sedentary activities was subtracted from this total, the training program resulted in a net total expenditure of 26007 and 15572 kcal, respectively. This represented a surplus of 185 and 110 kcal/day when expressed on a per day basis. Thus, it is clear that under such conditions, training must be maintained during a very long period of time to achieve substantial weight losses.

TABLE 1
Influence of exercise-training alone on weight loss in relation to the duration of the program in obese individuals

REFERENCE	SUBJECTS	ACTIVITY	APPROXIMATE DURATION min/week	weeks	WEIGHT LOSS min/programme	
Gwinup (1975)	Obese women	Walking	720[a]	78[a]	56,160	10.0
Krotkiewski et al. (1979)	Obese women	Jogging, dancing light gymnastics	165	24	3960	-1.2
Krotkiewski et al. (1983A)	Obese women	Jogging, dancing light gymnastics	165	12	1980	-1.8
Leon et al. (1979)	Obese men	Treadmill walking	450	16	7200	5.7
Mackeen et al. (1983)	Obese women	Jogging	80	12	960	2.1
Moody et al. (1972)	Obese women	Jogging		29	1800[b]	1.2
Woo et al. (1982)	Obese women	Walking	777	8	6320	6.8

a) Calculated from the indivudal curve of each subject.
b) Assuming that a mile was run at speed of 6 miles/hour.

These observations are concordant with the effects of exercise-training that have been generally reported in obese individuals. Indeed, as shown in table 1, minor changes in body weight were noted following programs in which duration of exercise was comparable to that described above. On the other hand, moderate weight losses (5 to 10 kg) were achieved following programs comprising a large quantity of exercise. Along these lines, it is also pertinent to indicate that five ex-obese runners recently tested in our laboratory lost 39.5 kg body weight using exercise as the main mode of treatment of their obesity (Tremblay et al. 1984b). At that time, they were running 95 km/week and they were experiencing no difficulty in maintaining a low percent body fat of 14.3%. This suggests that a long term exercise-training program comprising a large amount of exercise can result in considerable weight and fat losses. However, such a program requires substantial motivation, perseverance and availability.

EFFECT OF EXERCISE-TRAINING ON FAT DISTRIBUTION

Despite the early recognition of the role of abdominal fat deposition as a determinant of diabetes, atherosclerosis and other metabolic diseases (Vague, 1947, 1956), few attention has been given to the effect of exercise-training on fat distribution. For instance, among the three studies presented in table 1 in which moderate weight losses were observed, data pertaining to fat distribution have only been collected in the study of Leon et al. (1979). In this study, training induced a reduction in subcutaneous fat (-26.7%) comparable to that in body fat mass (-25.3%). Moreover, subcutaneous trunk fat was not preferentially reduced in comparison to subcutaneous extremity fat.

In a recent study (Després et al., 1985), we investigated the effect of a 20 week aerobic training program in 13 sedentary male subjects. As expected, a significant reduction in body fat mass and sum of skinfolds were observed following training. Trunk skinfolds were more altered than extremity skinfolds, with reductions of 22 and 12.5%, respectively. Furthermore, training did not seem to deplete preferentially subcutaneous fat.

More recently, we studied the influence of exercise-training on fat distribution using an experimental protocol inducing more pronounced changes in body fat mass. Five male overweight individuals (mean BMI = 28.8 kg/m^2) were subjected to a 100 day protocol comprising cycleergometer during 82 days. Exercise was performed twice a day for a total daily duration of 116 min, at a mean intensity of 58% $\dot{V}O_2$ max. The duration of exercise was calculated to induce a caloric deficit of 1000 kcal/day. Energy intake was maintained at the pre-training level throughout the study. This protocol resulted in body weight and fat losses corresponding to 8.6 and 6.8 kg, respectively. As shown in table 2, trunk skinfolds were slightly more reduced than extremity skinfolds in response to training. This table also indicates that the relative decrease in fat mass was more pronounced than that in subcutaneous fat. Finally, this table reveals a large interindividual variation in the response of subjects to training. Interestingly, this variation in response was particularly heterogeneous for the two indicators of fat distribution, i.e. the ratio of trunk/extremity skinfolds and that of the sum of skin-folds/fat mass.

Further evidence of the potential of exercise-training to alter central body fat is reflected by characteristics of the ex-obese runners who were tested in our laboratory (Tremblay et al., 1984b). Indeed, their mean suprailiac fat cell diameter was smaller than that of their controls (57.5 vs 86.4 um, p < 0.05) to whom they were paired for percent body fat.

In summary, all the studies discussed above indicate that exercise-training can reduce central subcutaneous fat. However, further studies are needed to establish whether this effect represents a preferential depletion in comparison to subcutaneous extremity fat and central deep fat.

SEX DIFFERENCES IN THE RESPONSE TO EXERCISE-TRAINING

Numerous studies in animals have consistently demonstrated that females increase their energy intake more than males in response to training, this resulting in an attenuation of the weight reducing effect of

TABLE 2

EFFECT OF A 100-DAY TRAINING PROGRAM ON
SUBCUTANEOUS FAT, FAT MASS AND FAT DISTRIBUTION

VARIABLE (UNIT)	BEFORE TRAINING	AFTER TRAINING	RANGE IN RESPONSE (%)[A]	MEAN DIFFERENCE (%)[A]	STATISTICAL SIGNIFICANCE
Σ7 SKINFOLDS (MM)	103.3 ± 33.6	72.9 ± 23.2	(-39.0; -15.7)	-29.4	$P < 0.01$
FAT MASS (KG)	17.0 ± 4.8	10.4 ± 3.7	(-57.3; -17.4)	-38.8	$P < 0.01$
Σ TRUNK SKINFOLDS (MM)[B]	62.9 ± 25.3	43.2 ± 18.7	(-45.1; -17.1)	-31.3	$P < 0.05$
Σ EXTREMITY SKINFOLDS (MM)[C]	40.4 ± 11.3	29.7 ± 5.2	(-36.5; -14.3)	-26.5	$P < 0.05$
Σ TRUNK SKINFOLDS / Σ EXTREMITY	1.56 ± 0.54	1.43 ± 0.41	(-27.0; 31.0)	- 8.3	NS
Σ7 SKINFOLDS / FAT MASS	6.78 ± 1.67	8.27 ± 2.53	(2.1; 67.5)	22.0	NS

VALUES ARE MEANS ± SD

[B] SUM OF SUBSCAPULAR, ABDOMEN AND SUPRAILIAC SKINFOLDS

[C] SUM OF BICEPS, TRICEPS, CALF AND THIGH SKINFOLDS

[A] $\dfrac{\text{AFTER} - \text{BEFORE}}{\text{BEFORE}} \times 100$

exercise (Oscai et al. 1973; Nance et al. 1977; Applegate et al. 1982). In humans, we also noted a reduced sensitivity to lose fat in females following aerobic exercise-training (Després et al. 1984a, Tremblay et al., 1984a).

To ascertain this concept, we recently studied the effect of a high intensity training program in young male and female adults. Thus, fourteen subjects (7 men, 7 women) participated to a 15 week cycleeregometer training program consisting of continous and intermittent exercise sessions. As presented in table 3, training produced a significant increment in $\dot{V}O_2$ max in both sexes. However, sex differences were noted in body fat changes. In men, significant decreases in percent body fat (p < 0.05), sum of seven skinfolds (p < 0.01) and suprailiac fat cell diameter (p < 0.05) were observed whereas these variables were not significantly modified in women. In addition, significant differences in subcutaneous fat loss were noted, with men losing more fat in the trunk than in the extremities whereas such a preferential fat depletion was not observed in women (table 4).

In an attempt to further characterize this sex dimorphism in the loss of fat, we recently investigated the effect of exercise on spontaneous energy intake in both sexes. Briefly, five males and five females non obese subjects were submitted to a 60 min cycleergometer exercise performed at 68% $\dot{V}O_2$ max. During the five hours following this exercise, subjects were kept in the laboratory and had free access to food. All food ingested was carefully monitored and energy intake was then derived from food tables. A second session without exercise was performed as a control situation and the order of the sessions was randomly assigned to subjects. Following exercise, the energy intake of males was similar to that noted in their control situation whereas a slight increase was observed in females. Furthermore, when subtracting the energy cost of exercise from the postexercise energy intake, males ingested 2376 kj/5 hours over the cost of exercise whereas the corresponding value in females was 4146 kj (p = 0.06). This suggests that the short-term postexercise caloric compensation in females could be higher than that seen in males.

TABLE 3

EFFECTS OF A 15 WK HIGH INTENSITY TRAINING PROGRAM ON MAXIMAL AEROBIC POWER AND PERCENT BODY FAT IN 7 MALE AND 7 FEMALE SUBJECTS

Variable (unit)	Men (n=7)			Women (n=7)		
	Before training	After training	(% change)	Before training	After training	(% change)
Weight (kg)	63.8 ± 9.0	63.9 ± 9.3	(0%)NS	50.9 ± 4.1	51.4 ± 4.9	(+1%)NS
Body mass index (kg/m^2)	21.3 ± 1.8	21.4 ± 1.2	(0%)NS	20.4 ± 1.7	20.6 ± 1.9	(+1%)NS
Percent body fat (%)	13.9 ± 4.8	11.2 ± 3.6	(-19%)*	24.1 ± 4.5	23.7 ± 5.2	(-2%)NS
Fat mass (kg)	9.0 ± 3.9	7.2 ± 2.6	(-20%)NS	12.4 ± 3.2	12.4 ± 3.7	(0%)NS
Fat free mass (kg)	54.8 ± 6.9	56.7 ± 8.1	(+3%)**	38.5 ± 2.2	39.1 ± 2.4	(+2%)NS
Sum of 7 skinfolds (mm)	63.3 ± 17.7	49.5 ± 10.9	(-22%)**	98.7 ± 27.3	89.1 ± 21.5	(-10%)NS
Fat cell diameter (µm)	84.4 ± 9.6	74.0 ± 11.3	(-17%)*	86.6 ± 9.0	89.0 ± 9.1	(+3%)NS
VO_2max (l/min)	2.93 ± 0.56	3.42 ± 0.61	(+17%)**	1.86 ± 0.31	2.34 ± 0.19	(+26%)
VO_2max (ml/kg/min)	45.3 ± 5.1	53.2 ± 3.9	(+17%)**	36.4 ± 6.0	46.1 ± 6.4	(+27%)**

VALUES ARE MEANS ± SD: THE EFFECT OF TRAINING WAS ASSESSED BY ANALYSIS OF VARIANCE. * P < 0.05, ** P < 0.01. NS: NON SIGNIFICANT. VO_2MAX: MAXIMAL AEROBIC POWER.

TABLE 4

EFFECTS OF A 15 WK HIGH INTENSITY TRAINING PROGRAM ON BODY FAT DISTRIBUTION IN 7 MEN AND 7 WOMEN.

VARIABLE (UNIT)	MEN (N=7)			WOMEN (N=7)		
	BEFORE TRAINING	AFTER TRAINING	(% CHANGE)	BEFORE TRAINING	AFTER TRAINING	(% CHANGE)
EXTREMITY SKINFOLDS (MM)	26.9 ± 8.4	22.9 ± 5.7	(-15%)*	57.3 ± 17.8	50.0 ± 13.1	(-11%)NS
TRUNK SKINFOLDS (MM)	36.4 ± 9.5	26.6 ± 5.5	(-27%)**	41.5 ± 10.5	38.2 ± 9.4	(-8%)NS
EXTREMITY/TRUNK	0.73 ± 0.05	0.86 ± 0.09	(+18%)**	1.38 ± 0.21	1.34 ± 0.20	(-3%)NS
SUM OF SKINFOLDS/ FAT MASS	7.29 ± 1.56	7.51 ± 2.79	(+3%)NS	8.02 ± 1.03	7.33 ± 0.79	(-9%)*

VALUES ARE MEANS ± SD: THE EFFECT OF TRAINING WAS ASSESSED BY ANALYSIS OF VARIANCE. * $P < 0.05$. ** $P < 0.01$. NS: NON SIGNIFICANT. EXTREMITY SKINFOLDS: SUM OF TRICEPS, BICEPS, THIGH AND CALF SKINFOLDS; TRUNK SKINFOLDS: SUM OF SUBSCAPULAR, ABDOMEN AND SUPRAILIAC SKINFOLDS; EXTREMITY/TRUNK: RATIO OF EXTREMITY SKINFOLDS DIVIDED BY TRUNK SKINFOLDS.

These results indicate that the trunk subcutaneous fat of males could be more sensitive to be reduced in response to training. This adaptation agrees with the fact that males are less prone to increase their food intake following exercise in comparison to females. However, since these data were only collected in non obese individuals, they would need to be reproduced in a sample of obese subjects. Finally, these results raise the pertinence to conduct further experiments dealing with the association between alterations in fat distribution and the regulation of food intake.

IMPLICATIONS OF TRAINING-INDUCED CHANGES IN FAT AND FAT DISTRIBUTION ON PLASMA GLUCOSE AND INSULIN

It is well established that the hypertrophy of fat cells is related to insulin resistance (Salans and Dougherty, 1971) and that obese individuals are more predisposed to develop type II diabetes. In addition, results presented in this symposium as well as data of other published studies indicate that central fat deposition is an independent risk factor of insulin resistance and type II diabetes (Kissebah et al., 1982; Krotkiewski et al., 1983b). On the other hand, exercise-training is known to produce a substantial improvement in insulin sensitivity. This concept has been introduced by Björntorp et al. (1970) who reported that a training program induces a decrease in insulinaemia without any detrimental effect on glucose tolerance. These investigators also demonstrated that athletes display much lower levels of insulin than non-trained individuals (Björntorp et al. 1972). Numerous studies which compared trained to non-trained subjects have subsequently reproduced this concept (Lohmann et al., 1978; LeBlanc et al., 1979; Tremblay et al., 1983, 1985b). This improved insulin sensitivity in trained individuals has also been confirmed by the euglycemic clamp technique to assess insulin stimulated glucose disporal (Rosenthal et al., 1983; Yki-Järvinen and Koivisto, 1983). Since the athletes are generally characterized by low levels of adiposity and fat cell size (Després et al., 1983, 1984b), it is tempting to associate their high level of insulin sensitivity to their reduced adiposity.

In response to a 16 week training program, Leon et al. (1979) observed a reduction of 43% in the insulin response to glucose. Interestingly, a reduction in fat mass of 5.9 kg was also induced by this program, which is concordant with the hypothesis relating training-induced changes in insulin and those in fatness.

In the present chapter, this hypothesis is discussed in making reference to the three following methodological approaches: 1) acute effect of exercise; 2) comparison of trained to non-trained subjects; 3) relationship between training-induced changes in plasma insulin and glucose and those in fat and fat distribution.

Acute effect of exercise

The impact of one bout of prolonged vigorous exercise is not sufficient to alter significantly body fat and fat distribution. On the other hand, significant reductions in insulinaemia have been found following one bout of prolonged exercise in obese (Fahlen et al., 1972; Holm et al., 1978; Koivisto et al., 1980) and lean individuals (LeBlanc et al, 1981), indicating that exercise can influence plasma insulin without morphological changes.

Comparison of trained to non-trained individuals

As indicated above, individuals practicing prolonged aerobic exercise on a regular basis display lower insulin levels than non-trained persons without any deterioration in glucose tolerance. In an attempt to explain such an adaptation, LeBlanc et al. (1979) analyzed the relationship between fitness indicators and the response of plasma insulin to an intravenous glucose injection using partial correlation analysis. Their results showed that plasma insulin levels were more closely related to the adiposity than to the $\dot{V}O_2$ max of subjects. More recently, we investigated this relationship in 9 trained and 23 non-trained individuals who were subjected to an oral glucose tolerance test (Perron et al., 1986). Correlation analyses revealed no significant association between plasma insulin and body fat mass or various subcutaneous fat indicators. Furthermore, we also compared insulinaemia of the two groups in eliminating the intergroup difference in percent body fat. This was achieved first by covariance analysis and second by comparing subsamples of five trained and non-trained subjects paired with respect to percent body fat. These two comparisons showed that even when adiposity is equal between the groups, a much higher insulin sensitivity was observed in the trained subjects.

Relationship between training-induced changes in plasma insulin and changes in fat and fat distribution

The association between training-induced changes in body fat and those in insulinaemia has been frequently investigated in obese individuals and no evidence of a link between changes in these two variables has been reported (Björntorp et al., 1970; Krotkiewski et al., 1979, 1984). This is concordant with recent data obtained in our laboratory in 6 pairs of monozygotic twins following a 22 day training protocol. Indeed, no association was found between changes in plasma insulin and those in body fat (Després et al., submitted). However, it is interesting to note that a significant positive correlation was observed between changes in the trunk/extremity skinfolds ratio and changes in plasma insulin. This latter observation suggests that changes in central body fat could partly explain the beneficial effect of exercise-training on insulin sensitivity.

In the latter study, we also obtained data suggesting that the response in insulinaemia to training could be partly genetically determined (Tremblay et al., 1987). With respect to this concept, further studies are needed to determine whether the influence of heredity on the adaptation in insulinaemia to exercise-training is mediated by changes in fat distribution.

CONCLUSIONS

Studies reviewed in this chapter indicate that exercise-training can induce moderate to high fat losses provided that a large quantity of aerobic exercise is performed over a long period of time. This can be accompanied by substantial changes in central subcutaneous fat. However, further studies are needed to establish whether such an effect reflects a preferential depletion in comparison to changes in central deep fat and extremity subcutaneous fat. Males are more sensitive to lose body fat and central subcutaneous fat than females, in response to training, probably due to a lower postexercise compensation in energy intake. Training-induced changes in body fat do not seem to be an important determinant of the high insulin sensitivity characterizing trained individuals. The latter adaptation could however be explained by changes in fat distribution.

REFERENCES

Applegate, E.A., Upton, D.E., Stern, J.S. (1982). Food intake, body composition and blood lipids following treadmill exercise in males and females rats. Physiol. Behav. 28: 917-920.

Bahr, R., Ingnes, I., Vaage, O., Sejersted, O.M., Newsholme, E.A. (1987). Effect of duration of exercise on excess postexercise O_2 consumption. J. Appl. Physiol., 62: 485-490.

Björntorp, P., De Jounge, K., Sjöstrom, L., Sullivan, L. (1970). The effect of physical training on insulin production in obesity. Metabolism, 19: 631-638.

Björntorp, P., Fahlen, M., Grimby, G., Gustafson, A., Holm, J., Renström, P., Schersten, T. (1972). Carbohydrate and lipid metabolism in middle-aged, physically well-trained men. Metabolism, 21: 1037-1044.

Després, J.P., Savard, R., Tremblay, A., Bouchard, C. (1983). Adipocyte diameter and lipolytic activity in marathon runners: Relationship with body fatness. Eur. J. Appl. Physiol. 51: 223-230.

Després, J.P., Bouchard, C., Savard, R., Tremblay, A., Marcotte, M., Thériault, G. (1984a). The effect of a 20-week endurance training program on adipose tissue morphology and lipolysis in men and women. Metabolism, 33: 235-239.

Després, J.P., Bouchard, C., Savard, R., Tremblay, A., Marcotte, M., Thériault, G. (1984b). Level of physical fitness and adipocyte lipolysis in humans. J. Appl. Physiol., 56: 1157-1161.

Desprês, J.P., Bouchard, C., Tremblay, A., Savard, R., Marcotte, M. (1985). Effects of aerobic training on fat distribution in male subjects. Med. Sci. Sports Exerc., 17(1): 113-118.

Desprês, J.P., Moorjani, S., Tremblay, A., Poehlman, E.T., Lupien, P.J., Nadeau, A., Bouchard, C. (submitted). Heredity and changes in plasma lipids and lipoproteins following short-term exercise-training in man: association with changes in adipose tissue distribution and plasma insulin.

Fahlen, M., Stenberg, J., Björntorp, P. (1972). Insulin secretion in obesity after exercise. Diabetologia, 8: 141-144.

Gwinup, G. (1975). Effect of exercise alone on the weight of obese women. Arch. Int. Med ., 135: 676-680.

Holm, G., Björntorp, P., Jagenberg, R. (1978). Carbohydrate, lipid and amino acid metabolism following physical exercise in man. J. Appl. Physiol., 45: 128-131.

Kissebah, A.H., Vydelingum, N., Murray,R., Evans, D.J., Hontz, A.J., Kalkhoff, R.K., Adams, P.W. (1982). Relation of body fat distribution to metabolic complications of obesity. J. Clin. Endocrinol. Metab. 54: 254-260.

Koivisto, V.A., Soman, V.R., Felig, P. (1980). Effects of acute exercise on insulin binding to monocytes in obesity. Metabolism, 29: 168-172.

Krotkiewski, M., Mandroukas, K., Sjöström, L., Sullivan, L., Wetterqvist, H. Björntorp, P. (1979). Effects of long-term physical training on body fat, metabolism, and blood pressure in obesity. Metabolism, 28: 650-658.

Krotkiewski, M., Bylund-Fallenius, A.C., Holm, J., Björntorp, P., Grimby, G., Mandroukas, K. (1983a). Relationship between muscle morphology and metabolism in obese women. The effects of long-term physical training. Eur. J. Clin. Invest., 13: 5-12.

Krotkiewski, M., Björntorp, P., Sjöström, L., Smith, J. (1983b). Impact of obesity on metabolism in men and women: Importance of regional adipose tissue distribution. J. Clin. Invest. 72: 1150-1162.

Krotkiewski, M., Björntorp, P., Holm, G., Marks, V., Morgan, L., Smith, U., Feurle, G.E. (1984). Effect of physical training on insulin, connecting peptide (C-peptide), gastric inhibitory polypeptide (GIP) and pancreatic polypeptide (PP) level in obese subjects. Int., J. Obesity, 8: 193-199.

Leblanc, J., Nadeau, A., Boulay, M., Rousseau-Migneron, S., (1979). Effects of physical training and adiposity on glucose metabolism and 125 I-insulin binding. J. Appl. Physiol., 46: 235-239.

Leblanc, J., Nadeau, A., Richard, D., Tremblay, A. (1981). Studies on the sparing effect of exercise on insulin requirements in human subjects. Metabolism, 30: 1119-1124.

Leon, A.S., Conrad, J., Hunninghake, D.M., Serfass, R. (1979). Effects of a vigorous walking program on body composition, and carbohydrate and lipid metabolism of obese young men. Am. J. Clin. Nutr., 32: 1776-1787.

Lohmann, D., Liebold, F., Heilmann, W., Senger, H., Pohl, A. (1978). Diminished insulin response in highly trained athletes. Metabolism, 27: 521-524.

Mackeen, P.C., Franklin, B.A., Nicholas, W.C., Buskirk, E.R. (1983). Body composition, physical work capacity and physical activity habits at 18-month follow-up of middle-aged women participating in an exercise intervention program. Int. J., Obesity, 7: 61-71.

Maxfield, M.E. (1971). The indirect measurement of energy expenditure in industrial situations. Am. J. Clin. Nutr., 24: 1126-1138.

Moody, D.L., Wilmore, J.H., Girandola, R.N., Royce, J.P. (1972). The effects of a jogging program on the body composition of normal and obese high school girls. Med. Sci. Sports, 4: 210-213.

Nance, D.M., Bromley, B., Barnard, R.J., Gorski, R.A. (1977). Sexually dimorphic effects of forced exercise on food intake and body weight in the rat. Physiol. Behav., 19: 155-158.

Oscai, L.B., Molé, P.A., Krusak, L.M., Holloszy, J.O. (1973). Detailed body composition analysis of female rats subjected to a program to swimming. J. Nutr., 103: 412-418.

Perron, L., Mitchell, D., Tremblay, A., Després, J.P., Nadeau, A., Bouchard, C. (1986). The role of body fat in insulin sensitivity of endurance athletes. Diabète & Métabolisme, 12: 233-238.

Rosenthal, M., Haskell, W.L., Solomon, R., Widstrom, A., Reaven, G.M. (1983). Demonstration of a relationship between level of physical training and insulin-stimulated glucose utilization in normal humans. Diabetes, 32: 408-411.

Salans, L., B., Dougherty, J.W. (1971). The effect of insulin upon glucose metabolism by adipose cells of different size. J. Clin. Invest., 50: 1399-1410.

Tremblay, A., Nadeau, A., Leblanc, J. (1983). The influence of high carbohydrate diet on plasma glucose and insulin of trained subjects. Eur. J. Appl. Physiol., 50: 155-160.

Tremblay, A., Després, J.P., Leblanc, C., Bouchard, C. (1984a). Sex dimorphism in fat loss in response to exercise-training. J. Obes. weight Reg., 3: 193-203.

Tremblay, A., Després, J.P., Bouchard, C. (1984b). Adipose tissue characteristics of ex-obese long distance runners. Int. J. Obes., 8: 641-648.

Tremblay, A., Fontaine, E., Nadeau, A, (1985a). Contribution of the post exercise increment in glucose storage to variations in glucose-induced thermogenesis in endurance athletes. Can. J. Physiol. Pharmacol., 63: 1165-1169.

Tremblay, A., Fontaine, E., Nadeau, A. (1985b). Contribution of the exercise-induced increment in glucose storage to the increased insulin sensitivity of endurance athletes. Eur. J. Appl. Physiol., 54: 231-236.

Tremblay, A., Fontaine, E., Poehlman, E.T., Mitchell, D., Perron, L., Bouchard, C. (1986). The effect of exercise-training on resting metabolic rate in lean and moderately obese individuals. Int. J. Obes., 10: 511-517.

Tremblay, A., Poehlman, E.T., Nadeau, A., Pérusse, L., Bouchard, C. (1987). Is the response of plasma glucose and insulin to short-term exercise-training genetically determined? Horm. Metab. Res., 19: 65-67.

Vague, J. (1947). La différenciation sexuelle: Facteur déterminant des formes de l'obésité. La Presse Médicale, 30: 339-340.

Vague, J. (1956). The degree of masculine differentiation of obesities. Am. J. Clin. Nutr., 4(1): 20-34.

Woo, R., Garrow, J.S., Pi-Sunyer, F.X. (1982). Voluntary food intake during prolonged exercise in obese women. Am. J. Clin. Nutr., 36: 478-484.
Yki-Jävinen, H., Koivisto, V.A. (1983). Effects of body composition on insulin sensitivity. Diabetes, 32: 965-969.

Fat Distribution During Growth and Later Health Outcomes
pages 313–332 © 1988 Alan R. Liss, Inc.

ALTERATION IN DISTRIBUTION OF ADIPOSE TISSUE IN RESPONSE TO
NUTRITIONAL INTERVENTION

John H. Himes

Department of Health and Nutrition Sciences,
Brooklyn College, City University of New York,
Brooklyn, NY 11210

INTRODUCTION

Adipocytes from different body sites may differ
considerably in metabolic activity related to lipogenesis
and lipolysis (Smith et al., 1975; Rebuffe-Scrive et al.,
1985). On a gross morphological level, this intersite
variation in cellular activity probably contributes to
variability in the anatomical distribution of adipose
tissue depots. Significantly, variation in the distribution of adipose tissue, and patterns of distribution, may
be associated with metabolic and cardiovascular disease and
related risk factors (see other contributors to the symposium).

Positive energy balance favors lipid storage in
adipose tissue and negative energy balance favors lipid
mobilization from adipose tissue. Because dietary intervention often changes energy balance, it is of interest to
inquire if adipose tissue depots respond differently to
dietary manipulation. Moreover, particularly in adults,
where disease risks have been documented for distributional
patterns of adipose tissue, it is of interest to determine
whether diet-induced changes in fat distribution suggest
altered disease risk with nutritional intervention.

Most of the available data pertaining to alterations
in adipose tissue distribution with nutritional intervention concern changes in subcutaneous fat thicknesses, and
to a lesser extent, body circumferences. It is unfortunate
for the present concern that much of the literature on

nutritional interventions has focused on changes in total body composition. Accordingly, when measurements of subcutaneous fat thicknesses are included, often only sums of skinfold thicknesses are reported as indicators of total body fat, making it impossible to evaluate differential site responses. Also, there are few data differentiating between responses of internal depots and subcutaneous adipose depots to nutritional intervention.

The notions of nutritional intervention and alteration in the distribution of adipose tissue imply change: change in nutritional intake and energy balance in the former, and differential responses, or changes, in amount of adipose tissue among various fat depots in the latter. Meaningful evaluation of change requires at least short-term longitudinal data; these data require more complex analyses than do evaluations of status from cross-sectional data. Further, relative to cross-sectional analyses, change analyses demand greater reliability of measurement, and they usually require larger sample sizes (Himes, 1987). Clues for possible intervention effects may be drawn from cross-sectional samples, but verification of these effects require preintervention-postintervention designs.

For this report, the main focus is studies of nutritional intervention, where the primary intervention affecting energy balance was dietary intake. For example, interventions including a large exercise component are not included. Often, specific associations with energy intakes are not reported so intervention effects must be inferred from associations with changes in body weight. Associations with body weight per se, rather than body fat are appropriate here because there are usually significant changes in lean tissue in response to nutritional intervention (Forbes, 1987). Nutritional interventions for pregnant women are not considered. Finally, studies of developmental changes in fat distribution in children without nutritional intervention are not considered to avoid possible confounding of nutritional factors by endocrine-mediated changes and other normal developmental phenomena.

NUTRITIONAL INTERVENTIONS

Studies of nutritional interventions affecting energy

balance have been conducted in a variety of circumstances
that may be important for interpreting results. Therapeu-
tically, nutritional interventions may increase energy
intakes in undernourished individuals, or decrease intakes
in overnourished or obese individuals. These treatments may
be given to individuals across a wide age range.
Experimental nutritional interventions may increase or
decrease energy intakes of adequately nourished individuals. Because of ethical constraints, these experimental
interventions have been carried out almost exclusively on
young adults. Effects of nutritional intervention on
adipose tissue distribution, then, may vary according to
the nutritional status and age of individuals, as well as
the direction of the intervention's contributions to energy
imbalance. Clearly, within such broad categories of
nutritional status and nutritional intervention there is
considerable variation in the exact statuses, the nature of
treatments, and the responses measured.

In addition to these chief general descriptors of
studies of dietary energy intervention, other factors that
may modify treatments or outcomes include: genetic factors
(including sex), activity, physiological state, disease,
medication, and health- and nutrition-related behaviors.
In most cases, there is insufficient data to evaluate
systematically the roles that each of these interacting
factors play in the response of adipose tissue distribution
to nutritional intervention. Nevertheless, these factors
have compelling biological reasons for being considered
when interpreting results from past studies and in the
planning of future studies.

Cross-Sectional Findings

Variability in subcutaneous fat thickness is significantly associated with body weight in well-nourished
adults. Table 1 presents previously unpublished partial
regression coefficients of six skinfold thicknesses and
weight, while controlling age, for a sample of French
Canadian adults (Bouchard et al., 1985; Himes and Bouchard,
1985). These partial regression coefficients (slopes)
describe the rates of increase in skinfold thickness (mm)
per kg of body weight across the observed variability in
these measures. Importantly, these estimates have been
corrected for attenuation due to random measurement error

TABLE 1. Relationships between skinfold thicknesses and weight (mm/kg) in French Canadians from partial regression coefficients (b) of skinfolds on weight, controlling for age, and adjusted for measurement reliability (Rel. $\underline{r}$)

Skinfold	Rel. r	Men (n=400) Mean (mm)	b (mm/kg)	SE_b	Women (n=414) Mean	b (mm/kg)	SE_b
Triceps	0.96	9.8	0.21	0.01	18.5	0.41	0.02
Biceps	0.92	5.1	0.12	0.01	9.5	0.32	0.02
Subscapular	0.96	15.5	0.42	0.02	16.3	0.57	0.03
Suprailiac	0.93	13.0	0.43	0.03	14.9	0.65	0.03
Abdominal	0.96	19.9	0.58	0.03	21.1	0.63	0.04
Medial Calf	0.88	7.3	0.18	0.01	17.3	0.43	0.03

(McNemar, 1969). To the degree that measures of fatness vary among sites in measurement reliability, the relative magnitudes of uncorrected coefficients of regression and correlation using these measures cannot be interpreted with confidence.

In the men (Table 1), the skinfold-weight coefficient is largest for the abdominal skinfold and smallest for the biceps skinfold. For women, suprailiac and abdominal skinfolds have the largest coefficients with weight and biceps skinfold has the smallest. Within men, variability among skinfolds in weight relationships is very close to the ordinal magnitude of mean skinfold thickness, although this pattern is less clear in women. When men and women are compared, women, who have greater mean skinfolds at corresponding sites, also have greater skinfold-weight coefficients. In each sex, skinfolds at trunk sites have greater slopes of skinfold thickness per unit of weight than do skinfolds measured on the extremities. These six skinfold sites are not sufficient for meaningful comparisons between upper-body sites and lower-body sites.

Garn (1957) has reported fat thickness-weight correlations, uncorrected for measurement reliability, for 100 well-nourished young white men. These correlations were based on measurements of subcutaneous fat from radiographs taken at twelve sites. There was considerable variability among sites in weight correlations (range 0.35-0.62), with fat thicknesses measured at the iliac-spine and mid-trochanteric sites most highly correlated (0.58, 0.62), and fat thicknesses at the lateral leg, medial arm, and posterior leg least correlated with weight (0.35-0.38). If the twelve sites are regrouped according to body location, average $\underline{r}$'s for trunk and extremity sites are 0.53 and 0.44, respectively (difference significant, p less than 0.05). Based on these data, the average correlation with weight for upper-body sites is 0.49, and for lower-body sites 0.45 (difference not significant). Findings from other cross-sectional studies support a trunk/extremity difference in correlations of subcutaneous fat thicknesses and weight, as well as a smaller upper-body/lower-body difference in weight correlations (Borkan and Norris, 1977; Lewis et al., 1960), although these findings are not universal (Badora, 1975).

Review of cross-sectional data on associations of subcutaneous fat thicknesses and weight in well-nourished children provide little evidence of systematic patterns of correlations according to specific site, or according to trunk/extremity or upper-body/lower-body dichotomies (Reynolds, 1951; Malina, 1972). Cross-sectional samples of healthy children have been compared and differences in fatness have been attributed to socioeconomic factors, including nutrition. Nevertheless, findings from these studies have been equivocal in demonstrating consistent site-specific sensitivities of various skinfolds (McKay et al., 1971; Bogin and MacVean, 1981; Mueller, 1986).

Multiple fat thicknesses have not been included in most studies comparing clinically malnourished children with better-nourished controls. Available data indicate generally reduced subcutaneous fat thicknesses compared with controls, but no obvious patterns of differential responsiveness of particular fat thicknesses (Pharaon et al., 1965; Keet et al., 1970).

Nonintervention Studies Of Weight Change

If changes in weight observed over time for groups of adults are assumed to be of primarily nutritional origin, associations between changes in weight and changes in subcutaneous fat thicknesses may suggest differential responses of adipose tissue depots. These kinds of studies are less well controlled than intervention studies and one cannot separate nutritional effects from those resulting from other factors that may affect body weight and subcutaneous fatness, e.g., normal development, disease, activity, aging, medication, smoking, etc.

Regression coefficients for five-year changes in four skinfold thicknesses relative to changes in weight have been reported by Garn et al. (in press) for 620 healthy men and women 20-49 years of age. Sex-specific rates of change in skinfold thickness (mm) per kg of weight were greatest for abdominal and iliac skinfolds (1.03-1.36 mm/kg), and least for triceps skinfold (0.64, 0.66 mm/kg); rates for subscapular skinfold were intermediate (0.77, 0.87 mm/kg). Regression coefficients did not differ significantly between those losing weight over the period and for those gaining weight, when these groups were compared. In other studies, increments in subcutaneous fat thicknesses on trunk sites have been shown to be more highly correlated with weight increments than fat thicknesses measured on the extremities (Comstock and Stone, 1972; Borkan and Norris, 1977).

A trunk vs. extremity difference in associations between nonintervention changes in fat thicknesses and weight gains probably exists in adults. Nevertheless, the exact magnitudes of these relationships among changes are difficult to estimate in some cases because the analytic approaches used have not accounted for effects of regression to the mean and for measurement reliabilities; these factors would be expected to have appreciable effects in this kind of analysis of change (Lord, 1963).

Nutritional Rehabilitation Of The Undernourished

Generally, interventions for the undernourished include studies of nutritional rehabilitation of clinically malnourished children and adults, and studies of nutritional supplementation of chronically, but less severely malnourished children.

Subcutaneous fat thicknesses of clincially malnourished children generally increase rapidly with nutritional

TABLE 2. Changes in mean measurements of 25 clinically malnourished children before and after seven weeks of high-energy feeding (calculated from Brooke and Wheeler, 1976)

Measure	Admission	Treated	Change	% Change
Weight (kg)	5.8	8.4	2.6	45
Biceps Skf. (mm)	4.1	6.5	2.4	58
Biceps Skf. Area (mm^2)*	218	461	243	111
Triceps Skf. (mm)	5.5	10.2	4.7	85
Triceps Skf. Area (mm^2)*	295	721	426	144
Subscapular Skf. (mm)	3.4	7.5	4.1	121
Suprailiac Skf. (mm)	3.8	9.8	6.0	158
Arm Circ. (cm)	10.8	14.3	3.5	32

* calculated according to Himes et al. (1980).

rehabilitation (Himes, 1980). Brooke and Wheeler (1976) fed 25 seriously malnourished Jamaican children a high-fat, high energy (199 kcal/kg/day) diet for seven weeks. Mean age on admission was 1.17 years, and diagnoses were marasmus, kwashiorkor, or marasmic-kwashiorkor. Based on mean values at admission and after treatment, absolute and relative changes in weight, arm circumference, four skinfolds, and estimated fat areas have been calculated (Table 2).

While there was no control group for comparisons, the treatment period was short and the median expected increments during treatment are very small, e.g. weight, 0.35 kg (Baumgartner et al., 1986). On an absolute basis, suprailiac skinfold thickness showed the largest gains, followed by triceps, subscapular, and biceps skinfolds. On a percentage basis, trunk skinfolds (suprailiac and subscapular), had larger gains than the arm skinfolds.

Expressing intervention-related changes in fat thicknesses as percentages standardizes the changes relative to initial fat thicknesses. Nevertheless, an initially larger fat thickness that gains an equivalent percentage as does a smaller thickness, has actually gained more fat in absolute terms. So, for example, the 4.7 mm gain in the compressed double fold of skin and subcutaneous tissues over the triceps (Table 2), represents a greater absolute increase in subcutaneous adipose tissue than the corresponding 4.1 mm at the subscapular site, even though the percentage changes indicate greater proportional change for the subscapular thickness. The absolute gains are more desirable than relative gains, if the intent is to reflect the site-specific differentials in adipocyte hypertrophy and hyperplasia in response to nutritional rehabilitation. Direct comparison of sites assumes identical skinfold compression among sites, which may not be so (Himes et al., 1979).

Unfortunately, straightforward interpretations of changes in the distribution of subcutaneous adipose tissue, resulting from the skinfold thickness data (Table 2) are hampered by large differences in shape and size of the trunk and extremities underlying the subcutaneous tissues. Theoretical cross-sectional areas of the annuli of fat have been estimated from limb circumferences and corresponding fat thickness to help reduce the effects of underlying shape differences, but these area estimates are not without problems of interpretation (Himes et al., 1980). For the data in Table 2, triceps fat area showed a greater gain than the corresponding fat area calculated from the biceps skinfold, and relative gain in triceps fat area was second only to that of suprailiac skinfold thickness.

Nutritional rehabilitation of severely undernourished adults is accompanied by rapid increases in subcutaneous fat thickness. Russell and Mezey (1962) reported increments in skinfolds, measured at five sites, accompanying weight gains in three young women treated dietarily for anorexia nervosa for 32 to 41 days. The most rapid mean increases per kg of body weight were observed for the abdominal skinfold (0.44 mm/kg) and for the thigh skinfold (0.39 mm/kg). In descending order, the mean rates of other skinfold increases relative to weight gain were 0.28 mm/kg (axillary), 0.07 mm/kg (lateral arm), and 0.05 mm/kg (subscapular). The observed rates of skinfold increases in these anorexic women are considerably less than estimates from cross-sectional data (Table 1) and from nonintervention weight-change studies (Garn et al., in press). Clearly, in these women much of the dietary energy contributed to replenishment of protein stores, glycogen, and internal lipids; weight gains were estimated to contain an average of 16% water.

Subscapular skinfold thickness increased at a slightly greater rate relative to weight gain than did triceps thickness when undernourished men were given high-protein (100g/day) diets that were isocaloric (2240 kcal/day) with previous low-protein (27 g/day) basal diets (Barac-Nieto et al., 1979). Presumably, these increases in subcutaneous fat thickness resulted from the residual energy obtained from sparing gluconeogenic protein losses.

Men nutritionally rehabilitated as part of the Minnesota Starvation Experiment (Keys et al., 1950) regained in body circumferences to approximate or exceed prestarvation basal values. At the end of a 20-week rehabilitation period, abdominal circumference had the greatest rate of increase (0.69 cm/week) followed by circumferences of the thigh (0.24 cm/week), arm (0.33 cm/week), and calf (0.24 cm/week). Rates of gain in circumferences with nutritional rehabilitation in these men showed positive dose response relationships with categories of caloric intakes.

Dietary rehabilitation of 13 men restricted previously to 1000 kcal/day for 24 days was accompanied by rapid increases in body circumferences and subcutaneous fat thicknesses (Brozek et al., 1957). In absolute terms, trunk circumferences increased more than limb circumferences, with abdominal circumference having the largest mean gain. Skinfolds measured at the waist and juxtanavel sites showed the greatest increments with recovery (0.86, 0.70 mm/kg), although increments in a mid-abdominal skinfold were no greater than those observed for triceps skinfold thickness (0.25 mm/kg).

Findings regarding responses of subcutaneous fat thicknesses to nutritional supplementation in mildly or moderately malnourished children are difficult to interpret. Protein-supplemented New Guinean school children had significantly smaller increments in triceps skinfold than unsupplemented controls, and supplemented children had significant decrements in subscapular skinfolds compared with corresponding increments in control children (Lampl et al., 1978). In these same children there was a significant positive supplementation effect on stature and weight. Correlations between lifetime high-protein supplement intake and three skinfold thicknesses (triceps, subscapular, medial calf) were negative for three-year-old Guatemalan children (Martorell et al., 1982). Corresponding supplementation correlations with weight and length were significantly positive. Thus, the supplementation effected taller and heavier, but leaner children.

Compared with control school children in Kenya who were losing subcutaneous fat at the triceps and subscapular sites, children participating in a school feeding program had significantly smaller annual losses in fat thicknesses (Pieters et al., 1977). The feeding effects, i.e., decreases in rates of normal developmental fat loss, were more pronounced in subscapular skinfold thickness than in triceps skinfold thickness.

Interpretations of the supplementation effects on subcutaneous fat distribution are complicated because children have been studied during periods of normal developmental decreases in fat thicknesses. Even so, if supplementation favors more positive energy balance, one would not anticipate total cumulative intakes of supplement to be negatively associated with subcutaneous fat thicknesses, as observed in the Guatemala study. Significant positive associations between nutritional supplementation and increases in skinfold thickness over a 13-week period have been reported (Malcolm, 1970).

Overfeeding Experiments In The Adequately Nourished

Six pairs of male monozygotic twins were overfed by Poehlman et al. (1986). Subjects ate an additional 1000 kcal/day above measured energy expenditures. Means of fat-related variables before and after the period of overfeeding show considerable variation among skinfold sites in response to the additional calories (Table 3). In absolute terms, the trunk skinfold thicknesses tended to increase more with the overfeeding than the extremity skinfolds; although, while suprailiac increased most, chest skinfold increased the least.

Sims et al. (1968) overfed nine men for 200 days. Based on measurements from standardized photographs, the authors reported changes in radii for selected body regions, relative to changes in densitometrically-determined percentage body fat. Greatest changes in body breadths were reported for the abdomen (3.01 mm/%), chest (1.94 mm/%) and at the trochanters (1.76 mm/%). Smallest

TABLE 3. Changes in mean fat-related variables in six pairs of twins after 22 days of overfeeding (Poehlman et al., 1986)

Variable	Before	After	Diff	% Diff	Change/ kg wt
Weight (kg)	65.1	67.3	2.2	3.4	—
Fat Mass (kg)	11.8	13.1	1.3	11.0	0.59
Triceps Skf. (mm)	6.9	7.9	1.0	14.5	0.45
Biceps Skf. (mm)	4.0	4.4	0.4	10.0	0.18
Subscapular Skf. (mm)	9.5	10.3	0.8	8.4	0.36
Abdominal Skf. (mm)	11.6	13.0	1.4	12.1	0.64
Suprailiac Skf. (mm)	11.5	13.2	1.7	14.8	0.77
Calf Skf. (mm)	5.6	5.9	0.3	5.3	0.14
Thigh Skf. (mm)	8.0	8.7	0.7	8.8	0.32
Axillary Skf. (mm)	6.7	7.2	0.5	7.5	0.23
Chest Skf. (mm)	5.4	5.6	0.2	3.7	0.09
Ave Trunk Skf. (mm)	8.9	9.9	1.0	11.2	0.45
Ave Extremity Skf. (mm)	6.1	6.7	0.7	11.5	0.32

changes were observed for the calf (0.43 mm/%), forearm (0.46 mm/%), and neck (0.48 mm/%). Available overfeeding experiments then, show measures of trunk fatness to respond more to imposed excess calories than measures of extremity fatness.

Experimental Weight Loss In The Adequately Nourished

Lehman et al. (1893) reported differential losses among three skinfolds for two subjects undergoing experimental fasts of 6 and 10 days each. For one subject, greatest losses were at chest and abdominal sites and least at the lateral thigh, while the other subject experienced greatest skinfold loss at the lateral thigh. The authors state the fast-associated subcutaneous fat losses were larger at the sites with greater subcutaneous thicknesses initially. Changes in body circumferences of a subject undergoing a voluntary 31-day fast have been reported by Benedict (1915). Girth of the abdomen decreased most in absolute and relative terms, and girths of calf and biceps decreased least.

Short-term rapid weight losses of wrestlers attempting

to make lower weight categories for competition are associated with significant changes in body circumferences and skinfold thicknesses. In a five-day experiment, 10 collegiate wrestlers were measured daily (Singer and Weiss, 1968). The dimension to show a significant decrease earliest in the experimental period was waist girth (2nd day), followed by abdominal and subscapular skinfolds (3rd day), and thigh girth, triceps skinfold, cheek skinfold, anterior thigh skinfold and suprailiac skinfold (4th day).

After 24-weeks of semistarvation, men participating in the Minnesota Starvation Experiment experienced greatest absolute reduction in circumference of the abdomen, followed by circumferences of thigh, arm and calf (Keys et al., 1950). Similar ordinal relationships for reductions in body circumferences have been reported for other semistarvation experiments (Benedict et al., 1919; Brozek et al., 1957).

Thirteen young men maintained on 1000 kcal/day for 24 days had differential responses among nine sites in radiographic fat thickness (Garn and Brozek, 1956; Brozek et al., 1957). Largest median rates of loss in subcutaneous fat per kg of weight were observed for centrally located sites, i.e., ilium, trochanter, deltoid (0.5-0.7 mm/kg). Particularly on the distal extremities, the median rates of loss of subcutaneous fat associated with caloric restriction were small (0.1-0.3 mm/kg). On the leg, a given site of measurement differed by as much as three-fold in rate of fat loss.

While subcutaneous tissues responded differentially in absolute terms to the period of negative energy balance, amount of fat lost was positively correlated with fat thicknesses before weight reduction (Garn and Brozek, 1956). This association between fat loss and initial status was such that the relative distribution of subcutaneous fat among sites was unchanged after the dietary restriction, and general patterns of subcutaneous fat distribution persisted (Garn, 1955).

It is important to note, however, that if relative distributions of subcutaneous fat are stable with energy restriction, perforce there must be significant absolute differences among depots in rates of fat mobilization, proportional to the variance in initial subcutaneous fat thicknesses. In other words, if responses of adipose tissue are proportional to initial stores, sites with larger stores must mobilize fat proportionally faster than sites with smaller stores; a ten percent decrease in a thick depot constitutes absolutely more fat loss than a ten percent decrease in a thin depot.

Weight Reduction In The Obese

Bray et al. (1978) reported correlation coefficients for associations between weight loss and changes in selected body circumferences and skinfold thickness for a series of 23 obese adults, treated with behavior therapy and anorectic drugs. Highest correlations with weight loss were observed for biceps circumference (0.83) and subscapular skinfold thickness (0.74), and iliac circumference had the lowest correlation with weight loss (0.40). Weight-loss correlations with circumferences of thigh, waist, and chest were intermediate (0.59-0.67). Because of the small sample size, the 95% confidence intervals about the correlation coefficients are approximately ± 0.23, so only the extreme correlations probably reflect real differences in associations with weight loss.

Correlation coefficients relating loss of total body fat in 76 obese women to concomitant changes in body circumferences and skinfold thicknesses have been reported by Wadden et al.(in press). Circumferences and skinfolds were measured at similar locations. Changes in triceps and 10th rib circumferences were more highly correlated with fat loss than skinfold thicknesses measured at the same sites; although, this pattern did not hold for chest circumference and subscapular skinfold thickness. How much of the circumference-skinfold difference in fat-loss correlations is due to relatively more reliable measurements of the circumferences is not known. For these women, there was no obvious trunk/extremity difference in magnitude of correlations with fat loss.

The ratio of waist circumference to hip circumference in these women (Wadden et al., in press) did significantly decrease with weight reduction, indicating waist circumference changed relatively more than did hip circumference. The waist-hip ratio was not related to weight loss for a separate sample of hospitalized obese women (Lanska et al.,

1985). A fat distribution score based on the ratio of photogrametrically-determined waist diameter to thigh diameter decreased significantly with a 9 kg weight loss in obese women (Ashwell et al., 1978); but there was no significant correlation between change in this score and changes in actual or relative weight.

DISCUSSION

Table 4 summarizes the major patterns of findings from the reviewed literature, according to the types of studies and nutritional interventions. For studies demonstrating considerable differences among sites in responses to nutritional intervention, there is a general pattern of centrally located sites showing greater responses than extremity sites. Often, thigh sites respond to a degree similar to trunk sites, and usually thigh sites respond to a greater extent than arm sites or distal leg sites.

The cross-sectional data do not suggest systematic differential sensitivity to nutritional intervention among sites for healthy children, nor do available data regarding supplementation of mildly malnourished children. Studies of weight reduction in obese adults do not support the notion of consistent differential responses to dietary treatment among adipose depots. Overall, because of the selection of sites, the data are insufficient to document consistent patterns of upper body/lower body depot differences in response to nutritional intervention.

Besides the relative paucity of data from which to draw firm conclusions, the available studies are frought with methodological and analytical problems that make interpretations difficult. That body circumferences and subcutaneous fat thicknesses, especially skinfolds, are measured with appreciable error is well known (Mueller and Malina, 1987). Further, it is likely that these errors are exaggerated in the obese (Bray et al., 1978). To the degree that measures indicating adipose tissue distribution vary in the degree of reliability with which they are measured, statistical analyses of these variables, without accounting for measurement error, may be misleading (Fleiss and Shrout, 1977). Seldom have reported analyses of alteration of fat distribution in response to nutritional

TABLE 4. Summary of findings from the literature regarding alteration of adipose distribution in response to nutritional intervention.

Type	Different Responses	Most Effect	Least Effect	Trunk/ Extremity
Cross-Sectional				
adult	yes	abd s* iliac s	biceps s calf s	++
child	no			
Nonintervention Weight Change				
adult	yes	abd s iliac s	triceps s calf s	++
Rehabilitation of Undernourished				
adult	yes	abd s,c** thigh s	calf c	++
child	yes	iliac s	biceps s	+
Supplementation				
child	no			
Overfeeding				
adult	yes	abd s,c	calf s,c	++
Experimental Weight Loss				
adult	yes	abd c iliac s	calf s,c	++
Obesity Weight Loss				
adult	no			

* s = skinfold or radiographic fat thickness
** c = circumference

intervention considered errors of measurement. Further, nutritional intervention studies are at particular risk in this regard because of their emphasis on evaluation of change and the sensitivity of these analyses to measurement error (Himes, 1987).

Many of the studies reviewed based conclusions of effects or associations on product-moment correlation coefficients. Correlation coefficients are inappropriate for this purpose because they confound the actual relationship between the two variables of interest with the standard deviations of the variables (Greenland et al., 1986). A better measure of the relationship is the unstandardized regression coefficient or partial regression coefficient, corrected for measurement reliabilities.

A final common problem in evaluating change is failure to account for regression to the mean (Lord, 1963). Because nutritional intervention deals with extreme groups, e.g., undernourished and obese, change in measures of adipose tissue distribution in response to the intervention are particularly prone to suffer from regression effects. Statistical approaches such as gain scores or value-added scores can obviate problems with regression to the mean and provide more reliable estimates of true change (Healy and Goldstein, 1978).

The data reviewed here were seldom derived from studies designed to answer the particular question of whether adipose tissue distribution is altered in response to nutritional intervention. It should be clear that the data are fragmentary and conclusions must be considered provisional, pending more focused studies that consider or control for possible interacting factors, and that are analyzed in a manner to minimize known deficiencies in existing studies. Nevertheless, the total weight of the available data support the notion of considerable variability among adipose tissue depots in response to selected nutritional interventions. On the average, central trunk sites appear to respond more rapidly to imposed caloric imbalance than do sites on the extremities.

Casting these general conclusions in terms of altering disease risks associated with central obesity must be done with caution. Increasing adipose tissue deposition at centrally located sites with nutritional intervention in acutely malnourished individuals cannot be logically associated with increased disease risk. Clearly, at some point, one must be concerned with the levels of total fat associated with disease risk, as well as patterns of fat distribution. To the extent that central fatness is a risk factor for disease in non obese individuals, the available data suggest that caloric restriction may improve the fat pattern associated with risk. The available data do not show convincingly that this pattern of preferential central-fat loss systematically occurs in the obese when treated with dietary restriction.

Certainly, the gross morphological changes in adipose tissue distribution in response to nutritional intervention are incompletely known. More complete understanding of site-specific responses of adipose depots to nutritional intervention require more comprehensive studies that include concomitant measures of lipogenesis and lipolysis on the cellular level.

REFERENCES

Ashwell M, Chinn S, Stalley S, Garrow JS (1978). Female fat distribution - a photographic and cellularity study. Int J Obesity 2:289-302.

Badora G (1975). The distribution of subcutaneous fat tissue in young women and men. Stud Phys Anthrop 1:91-108.

Barac-Nieto M, Spurr GB, Lotero H, Maksud MG, Sahners HW (1979). Body composition during nutritional repletion of severely malnourished men. Am J Clin Nutr 32:981-991.

Baumgartner RN, Roche AF, Himes JH (1986). Incremental growth tables: supplementary to previously published charts. Am J Clin Nutr 43:711-722.

Benedict FG (1915). "A Study of Prolonged Fasting." Washington DC: Carnegie Institute Pub No 203.

Benedict FG, Miles WR, Roth P, Smith HM (1919). "Human Vitality and Efficiency Under Prolonged Restricted Diet." Washington DC: Carnegie Institute Pub No 280.

Bogin B, Mac Vean RB (1981). Nutritional and Biological determinants of body fat patterning in urban Guatemalan children. Hum Biol 53:259-268.

Borkan GA, Norris AH (1977). Fat redistribution and the changing body dimensions of the adult male. Hum Biol 49:495-514.

Bouchard C, Savard R, Despres J-P, Tremblay A, LeBlanc C (1985). Body composition in adopted and biological siblings. Hum Biol 57:61-75.

Bray GA, Greenway FL, Molitch ME, Dahms WT, Atkinson RL, Hamilton K (1978). Use of anthropometric measures to assess weight loss. Am J Clin Nutr 31:769-773.

Brooke OG, Wheeler EF (1976). High energy feeding in protein-energy malnutrition. Arch Dis Childh 51:968-971.

Brozek J, Grande F, Taylor HL, Anderson JT, Buskirk ER, Keys A (1957). Changes in body weight and body dimensions in men performing work on a low calorie carbohydrate diet. J Appl Physiol 10:412-420.

Comstock GW, Stone RW (1972). Changes in body weight and
  subcutaneous fatness related to smoking habits. Arch
  Envion Health 24:329-334.
Fleiss JL, Shrout PE (1977). The effects of measurement
  errors on some multivariate procedures. AM J Pub Hlth
  67:1188-1191.
Forbes GB (1987). "Human Body Composition. Growth, Aging,
  Nutrition, and Activity." New York: Springer-Verlag.
Garn SM (1955). Relative fat patterning: An individual
  characteristic. Hum Biol 27:75-89.
Garn SM (1957). Selection of body sites for fat
  measurement. Science 125:550-551.
Garn SM, Brozek J (1956). Fat changes during weight loss.
  Science 124:682.
Garn SM, Sullivan TV, Hawthorne VM (in press).
  Differential rates of fat change relative to weight
  change at different body sites. Int J Obesity.
Greenland S, Schlesselman JJ, Criqui MH (1986). The
  fallacy of employing standardized regression coefficients
  and correlations as measures of effect. Am J Epidemiol
  123:203-208.
Healy MJR, Goldstein H (1978). Regression to the mean.
  Ann Hum Biol 5:277-280.
Himes JH (1980). Subcutaneous fat thickness as an
  indicator of nutritional status. In Greene LS, Johnston
  FE (eds): "Social and Biological Predictors of
  Nutritional Status, Physical Growth, and Neurological
  Development, "New York: Academic Press, pp 9-32.
Himes JH (1987). Purposeful assessment of nutritional
  status. In Johnston FE (ed): "Nutritional Anthropology,"
  New York: Alan R. Liss, pp 1-15.
Himes JH, Bouchard C (1985). Do the new Metropolitan Life
  Insurance weight-height tables correctly assess body
  frame and body fat relationships? Am J Pub Hlth
  75:1076-1079.
Himes JH, Roche AF, Siervogel RM (1979). Compressibility
  of skinfolds and the measurement of subcutaneous fatness.
  Am J Clin Nutr 32:1734-1740.
Himes JH, Roche AF, Webb P (1980). Fat areas as estimates
  of total body fat. Am J Clin Nutr 33:2093-2100.
Keet MP, Hansen JDL, Truswell AS (1970). Are skinfold
  measurements of value in the assessment of suboptimal
  nutrition in young children? Pediat 45:965-972.
Keys A, Brozek J, Henschel A, Michelsen F, Taylor HL
  (1950). "The Biology of Human Starvation." Minneapolis:
  Univ Minnesota Press.

Lampl M, Johnston FE, Malcolm LA (1978). The effects of
  protein supplementation on growth and skeletal maturation
  of New Guinean school children. Ann Hum Biol 5:219–227.
Lanska DJ, Lanska MJ, Hartz AJ, Kalkhoff RE, Rupley D,
  Rimm AA (1985). A prospective study of body fat
  distribution and weight loss. Int J Obesity 9:241–246.
Lehmann C, Mueller F, Munk I, Senator H, Zuntz N (1893).
  Untersuchungen an zwei hungerden Menchen. Arch path
  Anat Physiol 131:1–228.
Lewis HE, Masterson JP, Rosenbaum S (1960). Body weight
  and skinfold thickness of men on a polar expedition.
  Clin Sci 19:551–561.
Lord FM (1963). Elementary models for measuring change.
  In Harris CW (ed): "Problems in Measuring Change,"
  Madison Wisconsin: Univ Wisconsin Press, pp 21–38.
Malcolm LA (1970). "Growth and Development in New Guinea.
  A study of the Bundi People of the Madang District."
  Madang: Institute of Human Biology.
Malina RM (1972). Skinfold-body weight correlations in
  Negro and White children of elementary school age.
  Am J Clin Nutr 25:861–863.
Martorell R, Habicht J-P, Klein RE (1982). Anthropometric
  indicators of change in nutritional status in
  malnourished populations. In Underwood BA (ed):
  "Methodologies for Human Population Studies in Nutrition
  Related to Health," Washington DC: US GPO, pp 96–110.
McKay DA, Lim RKH, Notaney KH, Dugdale AE (1971).
  Nutritional assessment by comparative growth achievement
  in Malay children below school age. Bull Wld Hlth Org
  45:233–242.
McNemar Q (1969). "Psychological Statistics." Fourth ed,
  New York: John Wiley and Sons.
Mueller WH (1986). Environmental sensitivity of different
  skinfold sites. Hum Biol 58:499–506.
Mueller WH, Malina RM (1987). Relative reliability of
  circumferences and skinfolds as measures of body fat
  distribution. Am J Phys Anthrop 72:437–439.
Pharaon HM, Darby WJ, Shammout HA, Bridgforth EB, Wilson CS
  (1965). A year-long study of the nutriture of infants
  and pre-school children in Jordan. J Trop Pediat 2:1–39.
Poehlman ET, Tremblay A, Despres J-P, Fontaine E, Perusse
  L, Theriault G, Bouchard C (1986). Genotype-controlled
  changes in body composition and fat morphology following
  overfeeding in twins. Am J Clin Nutr 43:723–731.
Pieters JJL, de Moel JPC, van Steenbergan WM, van der
  Hoeven WJM (1977). Effect of school feeding on growth of

children in Kirinyaga District, Kenya. E Afr Med J
54:621-630.

Rebuffe-Scrive M, Enk L, Crona N (1985). Fat cell
metabolism in different regions in women. Effect of
menstrual cycle, pregnancy, and lactation. J Clin Invest
75:1973-1976.

Reynolds EL (1951). The distribution of subcutaneous fat
in childhood and adolescence. Monog Soc Res Child
Develop 14, No 2 (serial No 52).

Russell GFM, Mezey AG (1962). An analysis of weight gain
in patients with anorexia nervosa treated with high
calorie diets. Clin Sci 23:449-461.

Sims EA, Goldman RF, Gluck CM, Horton ES, Kelleher PC,
Rowe DW (1968). Experimental obesity in man. Trans
Assoc Am Physicians 81:153-169.

Singer RN, Weiss SA (1968). Effects of weight reduction on
selected anthropometric, physical, and performance
measures of wrestlers. Res Quart 39:361-369.

Smith U, Hammerston J, Bjorntorp P, Kral JG (1979).
Regional differences and effect of weight reduction on
human fat cell metabolism. Europ J Clin Inves 9:327-332.

Wadden TA, Stunkard AJ, Johnston FE, Wang J, Pierson RN,
Van Itallie TB, Costello E, Rena M (in press). Body fat
deposition in adult obese women. Part II: Changes in fat
distribution accompanying weight reduction. Am J Clin
Nutr.

Fat Distribution During Growth and Later Health Outcomes
pages 333–350 © 1988 Alan R. Liss, Inc.

OBESITY: FUTURE DIRECTIONS FOR RESEARCH

George A. Bray and Frank L. Greenway

Department of Medicine, University of Southern California, Los Angeles, California 90033 and the Department of Medicine, University of California at Los Angeles, Los Angeles, California 90291

INTRODUCTION

My assignment has been to review possible future directions for research to solve important problems relating to obesity and its health implications. To accomplish this task, I will first review the information available in 1977 and the progress we have made in the past ten years in four major areas. These will be: 1) Improvements in our techniques for estimating body composition; 2) The epidemiologic base on which health risks associated with obesity can be estimated; 3) Improved understanding of the mechanisms which control food intake, metabolism of fat cells and energy expenditure; and 4) Treatments for obesity. In each of these four areas, the status in 1977 will be briefly summarized and the additional information developed over the next ten years presented in outline form. This will be followed by some recent studies from our laboratory on the modification of regional fat distribution. We will ask the question, "Can regional fat distribution be modulated?" and will summarize three recent studies from our laboratory on this question. Finally, a summary of future directions will be proposed based on recent developments.

1.   Improved techniques for measuring body composition

In 1977 a variety of techniques were available for estimating body dimensions and the body composition.

Table 1

OBESITY-BODY COMPOSITION

1977	1987
Anthropometry	Bioelectric Impedance
Density	Computed Tomography
Isotope Dilution	Magnetic Resonance Images
Ultrasound	Neutron Activation

The most widely used of these techniques are still of great use and are based on anthropometry, including measurements of height and weight, skinfold thickness, body circumferences and body breadths. Beginning with the work of Behnke (Behnke and Wilmore, 1974), the technique of density measurement for estimating body fat came into wide use and was the 'gold standard' for measuring body composition in the past 40 years (Lohman, 1981). Various chemical, radioactive and non-radioactive isotopes have also been used for estimating various body compartments for more than 10 years (Bray, 1976; Garrow, 1978; Moore et al., 1963). Total body water can be estimated from the dilution of antipyrine as well as from tritiated water (^3H_2O) or deuterium oxide (D_2O). Body fat can be directly estimated from dilution xenon or cyclopropane. The final major technique available for measuring body composition in 1977 was the use of the naturally occurring isotope of potassium (^{40}K).

During the last ten years a number of new and sophisticated techniques have been added to the armamentarium which allow not only quantitation of fat and non-fat components in the body but also accurate estimate of their regional distribution. The first of these is the measurement of impedance or body conductivity (Segal et al., 1985). The total body electrical conductivity system has been developed for grading meat in terms of fat content and has been recently applied to the measurement of body fat in human beings. The expense of this instrument, however, will limit its current usefulness. A simple technique for estimating body impedance, however, may see more widespread use if formulas can be developed for reliably estimating fat from this technique which involves attaching electrodes to an arm and leg and measuring the intermediate impedance. The computed tomography can be used to give estimates of subcutaneous and intra-abdominal fat and has been applied for this purpose by several laboratories (Sjostrom et al., 1981). Even more elegant pictures contrasting subcutaneous and intra-abdominal fat can be obtained by magnetic resonance imaging (MRI). In these pictures the fat depots stand out as white compared to the tissues which contain water and other components (Cohn et al., 1980). Finally, a total body neutron activation allows estimates not only of total composition of water and fat but also of calcium, protein and other components. Utilizing these techniques our ability to quantitate total fat and estimate its regional distribution has been markedly improved during the past decade.

2.   The epidemiologic base for estimating the risks of obesity

In contrast with the elegant laboratory techniques which have become available for estimating body fatness and its distribution, the application of these techniques to population studies lags far behind. In 1977 there were several important studies available from which concerns about obesity and health were estimated.

Table 2

ESTIMATING RISKS FOR OBESITY

1977	1987
Build and Blood Pressure 1959	Build Study 1980
Health Examination Survey 1961-3	National Health Examination Surveys, 1971-74; 1976-80
Framingham Study 18 years	Framingham Study - 30 years
Ten State Nutrition Survey	American Cancer Society Study
Cross-Town Manhattan Study	Scandanavian Studies

These included several life insurance studies (Society of Actuaries, 1959), the 18-year follow-up of the Framingham Study (Kannel and Gordon, 1979), the seven country study of Keys and his collaborators (Keys et al., 1984) and the Pooling project (Pooling Project, 1978). The life insurance studies have consistently suggested that increased body weight was associated with higher mortality and that the major causes of this excess risk were heart disease, digestive diseases and diabetes.

Several prospective studies, however, suggested that obesity was not an independent risk factor for mortality but rather that obesity might have its effects through its association with hypertension or with diabetes. Data from long term follow-up studies from Canadian Air Force pilots in the Manitoba project

(Rabkin et al., 1977) and for younger individuals in the Los Angeles civil servants study suggested that a different picture might emerge with newer data.

Over the past ten years several new studies have appeared which have solidified our understanding of the relationships of weight and obesity to health. The Build Study of 1979 (Society of Actuaries, 1979) from the life insurance industry confirmed their earlier findings. The Framingham data at 26 and 30 years (Feinlieb, 1985; Hubert et al., 1983) indicated a similar relationship between weight and mortality as estimated in the life insurance studies, with a minimum mortality rate associated with an entry body mass index of 22 for all age groups. In addition, the 26-year follow-up indicated that obesity was an important predictor of risk of heart attacks, particularly among women. The American Cancer study with its 750,000 people also demonstrated the important relationship between increasing body mass and the risks for heart disease, diabetes mellitus and digestive diseases (Lew and Garfinkel, 1979). This study also made clear that certain forms of cancer, particularly those of the uterus, ovary and breast in women and prostate and colon in men also showed a small but significant increase, particularly in the very heavy groups. Finally, two Scandanavian studies have added to our knowledge base. The large population base study in Norway showed the similarity of mortality for under and overweight individuals of both sexes at all ages confirming the relationship in previous studies (Waaler, 1983). Finally, the studies in Gothenberg (Lapidus et al., 1984; Larsson et al., 1984) and in Milwaukee (Kissebah et al., 1982) demonstrated the important relationship between abdominal fat and risk for diabetes, hypertension, stroke, cardiovascular disease and overall mortality. Indeed, recognition of the importance of increased abdominal fat for all of the risks associated with obesity provides one of the important advances of the past decade and focuses on key questions which need answering in the years ahead.

3. Mechanisms for positive fat balance

Development of obesity implies deposition of increased amounts of fat or alternatively a positive fat balance. Understanding the processes by which this occurs has been steady, but less dramatic than our understanding of the relative risks described above.

Table 3

MECHANISMS FOR OBESITY

Food Intake - 1977	Food Intake - 1987
Calories Do Count	Hyperphagia NOT essential
Dual Center Hypothesis	Autonomic Hypothesis
Monoamine neurotransmitters	Peptide Neurotransmitters

Fat Cells - 1977	Fat Cells - 1987
Hyperplastic Obesity	Hyperplasia After Puberty
Fat Cells Fixed at Puberty	Alpha-2 inhibitory and
	Beta-stimulatory receptors
Beta-Receptor and Lipolysis	
	Lipoprotein Lipase as
	Gatekeeper
	Adipsin

Thermogenesis - 1977	Thermogenesis - 1987
Basal RMR related to	RMR is familial
surface area	
	Sympathetic component in TEF
TEF NOT Different in Obese	
	Sodium Pump, Brown Fat
Luxusconsumption present	and futile Cycles
	implicated in Obesity

In 1977 the statement "calories do count" would have been widely accepted. The anatomic basis for considering the problem of obesity focused on the dual center hypothesis with the ventromedial satiety and lateral feeding centers (Bray and York, 1972). The principal neurotransmitters were considered to be monoaminergic and to involve norepinephrine and dopamine.

In the past decade our focus has shifted from the dual center hypothesis with two anatomic nuclei to a dual control mechanism involving in important ways, the control of the autonomic nervous system (Bray and York, 1979). Thus those conditions associated with reduced body fat (lateral hypothalamic lesions) appear to have increased sympathetic activity and those with increased body fat (ventromedial hypothalamic lesions);

genetic obesity to have reduced activity of the sympathetic nervous system (Bray, 1987).

The role of calories has also changed. It is now apparent that most experimental types of obesity can develop in the absence of increased quantity of food intake (Bray, 1987). The most striking and complex development in the area of food intake has come from the recognition that numerous peptides found in the gastrointestinal tract are also found in the brain and that many of these have important effects on food intake. Three groups of endogenous opioid peptides have been identified and characterized during the past decade, and two of them can stimulate feeding. Similarly two peptides from the family of pancreatic polypeptides are also known to stimulate food intake when injected to the paraventricular nucleus (Leibowitz, 1986).

On the other hand, several peptides have been identified which have potent inhibitory effects on food intake. These include cholecystokinin, calcitonin and corticotrophin releasing factor (Morley, 1985). Corticotriphin releasing factor (CRF) is of particular interest because adrenalectomy has been demonstrated to reverse weight gain or its progression in essentially all forms of experimental obesity (Bray, 1987). Since corticotrophin releasing factor increases in the brain and presumably in the cerebral spinal fluid of animals following adrenalectomy, this peptide may play an important role in this process.

Finally, in addition to the ventromedial and lateral hypothalamic areas, it has become clear that the paraventricular nucleus with its rich supply of peptides is also important in the regulation of food intake. Modulating this system are not only the monoamines norepinephrine and epinephrine, but also clearly serotonin. As will be noted below, drugs related to the metabolism of serotonin have become agents in the treatment of obesity because any agent which enhances serotonin or serotonin-like effects is associated with a reduction in body weight.

In 1977 Hirsch and his colleagues (Hirsch and Batchelor, 1976) along with Bjorntorp and his associates (Bjorntorp, 1974) had clearly identified the hyperplastic and hypertrophic types of obesity. Moreover, it was dogma at that time that the hyperplastic type of obesity developed in childhood and that by the end of puberty, the number of fat cells was fixed.

It had also become clear by 1977 that in human beings, adipose tissue triglyceride stores arose primarily from fatty acids obtained from circulating lipoproteins and that lipoprotein lipase thus played a crucial role in the entry of fatty acids from circulating triglycerides into the adipose tissue pool of fatty acids (Greenwood, 1985).

Over the past decade our views about the time in which multiplication of new fat cells ends has changed. In experimental animals it is now clear that the number of cells of animals in some fat deposits can increase after the end of the pubertal growth spurt (Faust et al., 1978). There is also data in human beings suggesting that increasing fat stores in adult life may also be associated with an increase in the number of fat cells (Sjostrom and William-Olsson, 1981). Knowledge about the mechanisms controlling lipolysis have increased substantially. The beta receptor mediated activation of adenylate cyclase with the formulation of cyclic AMP were already known in 1977 (Burns et al., 1981). However, it has become clear that there is an important alpha-2 adrenergic inhibitory system operative in human fat cells and that this alpha-2 adrenergic inhibitory system varies from one fat deposit to another (Lafontan et al., 1979). It now appears that the major differences associated with regional fat deposits relate to the density of the alpha-2 adrenergic receptors on human fat cells.

It has also been demonstrated that lipoprotein lipase, the so-called gatekeeper for fat storage by fat cells, remains high following weight loss (Schwartz and Brunzell, 1981) whereas most other abnormal parameters of obesity tend to return to normal. Some have suggested that this high activity of LPL may play an important role in the tendency to regain weight after weight loss.

In 1977 the relationship of energy expenditure to body surface area, body weight and fat free mass had been clearly demonstrated (Bray, 1976; Garrow, 1978). Based on the work of Sims and his colleagues (Sims et al., 1986) as well as that of Miller and associates in London (Miller and Mumford, 1967a; Miller et at., 1967b), the concept of individual differences in response to excess energy intake, categorized as those who gain weight easily and those who gain weight with difficulty (luxusconsumption), has reemerged from a period where this concept was thought to have succumbed (Newburgh, 1944). Mechanisms for this effect were poorly understood and it provided one of the fascinating developments of the past decade (Rothwell and Stock, 1981).

Studies on weight gain during overfeeding have demonstrated important genetic components in this process

(Bouchard, 1985). Not only are genetic components demonstrated in the process of ease or difficulty of weight gain, but also in the familial association of resting energy expenditure within families (Bogardus et al., 1986). Studies on the mechanisms for differences have suggested a role for the sympathetic nervous system, which is activated during intravenous infusion of glucose and insulin (Ravussin et al., 1983). It has been shown that part of the increased oxygen consumption produced by infusing glucose and insulin can be blocked by administration of a beta adrenergic blocking drug (Acheson et al., 1983). This suggests that there are beta receptors which mediate energy expenditure related to glucose disposal. Changes in energy efficiency during weight gain and weight loss have sparked renewed interest in the question of whether weight cycling, that is, gaining and losing and regaining weight, may be more hazardous than maintaining a stable weight (Brownell, 1982).

4.   Treatment of obesity

In 1977 a number of treatments were used for obese patients.

Table 4

1977	1987
Diet and Exercise	Diet and Exercise
Behavior Modification	Behavior Modification
Starvation	Very Low Calorie Diets
Appetite Suppressants	Appetite Suppressants
Thyroid Hormone	Serotonin-like Drugs
Jejunoileal Bypass	Thermogenic Drugs
	Jaw-Wiring
	Vagotomy
	Gastric Restriction

Diet and exercise were the standard recommendations, with new varieties of dietary advice being being published each year to captivate the gullible. Behavior modification was already in wide use. Pioneering studies with this approach were first published in 1967 and the ensuing ten years had seen the practical application of these ideas become widely disseminated. It was clear even then that programs which incorporated behavior modification techniques had improved short and long term results.

Starvation or the zero calorie diet was waning in popularity. Introduced in 1959, it had spread widely as a way of getting weight off quickly in the hospital. Problems such as hypotension, kidney stones, loss of protein and poor long term results lead to the introduction of diets with only small amounts of protein. Gradually these evolved into the very low calorie diets, sometimes mistakenly called protein-sparing modified fasts. The past 10 years has seen an explosion in the use of these diets, both under medical supervision and without. It would appear desirable to have very low calorie diets under medical supervision.

The early 1970's saw the release by the Food and Drug Administration of three new appetite suppressants which were derivatives of amphetamine. Due to abuse and addiction to amphetamine, all drugs in this group received a bad name with a resultant decrease in their usage. Although there are many trials with these drugs, the use of a good behavioral Craighead program can do as well as in many instances (Stunkard et al., 1980, Dahms et al., 1978). With the recognition that serotonin played an important role in reducing food intake (Blundell, 1984) and that thermogenic mechanisms were important in regulating body weight (Rothwell and Stock, 1981), new approaches to drug therapy were developed. Trial drugs for both of these mechanisms are now being tested.

The surgical approaches to obesity have evolved rapidly. Jejuno-ileal bypass, an operation which connected the first 35 cm or so of jejunum to the terminal 10 cm of ileum, was in wide use in 1977. By the end of the decade, however, it had been largely replaced by gastric restrictive operations. The metabolic and inflammatory consequences of J-I bypass were unacceptable. In contrast the number of complications associated with gastric restriction has been less. Weight loss, however, may not be as good. Jaw-wiring is less invasive than gastric surgery but less effective in the long run. One major use of jaw-wiring has been as a technique of rapid weight loss prior to a gastric operation. Vagotomy has been given a trial in treatment of obesity but has not received wide use. Surgical treatment is palliative. For massively obese individuals, it may be the best we currently have to offer, but it is still only palliative.

4.   Treatment of regional deposits

Nearly ten years ago Dr. Greenway and I became aware of studies by Smith et al. (1979) and by Kral et al. (1977) demonstrating that during weight loss after jejuno-ilieal bypass, fat was absorbed more slowly from the femoral region in women than from the abdominal region. The demonstration that there were differences in the dose response characteristics to norepinephrine between femoral and abdominal regions and in the presence of norepinephrine but not in the presence of isoproterenol suggested that a major difference between the thigh and abdomen might be the alpha adrenergic inhibitory system. This suggested that direct application of isoproterenol or adrenergic blockade might enhance fat loss in the femoral region. We have tested these ideas in three separate studies, utilizing the symmetrical nature of the legs to measure changes in circumference of the placebo treated thigh with that of the thigh treated with active agent.

Study 1.

In the first study 0.2 ul of isoproteronol (10^{-5}M) was injected at 4 cm intervals to encircle one thigh and compared to saline injections on the other. Five women were treated three times weekly for four weeks. The data from this study are summarized in figure 1. All patients were put on a diet of 20 kcal/kg ideal

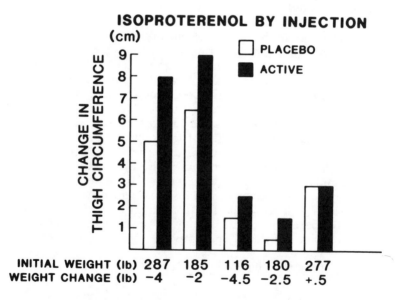

Figure 1. Isoproterenol by injection.

body weight. The weight loss and change in thigh circumference can be seen in this table. In all five women there was a decrease in circumference on the treated side compared to the untreated side. This preliminary study indicated that over a four-week treatment period a small but significant differential change in circumference of one thigh could be produced. When we calculated the amount of triglyceride which would come from a reduction of the circumference size as estimated in relation to the total energy deficit predicted from the weight loss, assuming that two-thirds of it was triglyceride, we estimated that somewhere between 10 and 50% of the total triglyceride consumed during treatment came from the treated thigh.

Study 2.

Since the isoproteronol study had demonstrated that differential fat absorption was possible, a second study was designed to evaluate several active agents in a single cream. For this purpose the cream, aquafor, was prepared in a placebo form containing small concentrations of yohimbine (2.5×10^{-4}M), aminophylline (1.3×10^{-2}M), or forskolin, a beta adrenergic

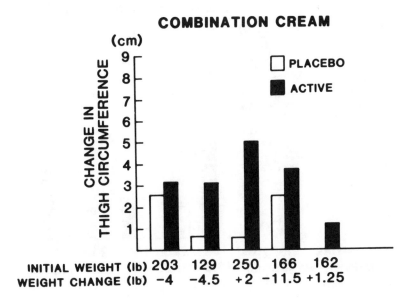

Figure 2. Combination cream.

adenylate cyclase activator ($1.2 \times 10^{-5}M$). For this study the two thighs were initially soaked with $MgSO_4$ 600-900 mOsm for 30 minutes prior to rubbing on the cream. Cream applications were done in a blind fashion by a laboratory technician on a daily basis five days a week for four weeks. The results are shown in figure 2. Subjects were on a weight loss diet. The circumference of the treated thigh decreased more than the placebo treated thigh. Again, our calculations of the quantity of fat which would be required assuming the entire thigh was a cyclinder composed of triglyceride provided an estimate of between 10 and 50% of fat from the treated thigh.

Study 3

This study was a follow-up to Study 2 using each of the three components in the combination cream as separate treatments. These data summarized in figure 3a-c. Again, the same effects are observed. The yohimbine effect was suggestive but not statistically significant in the four women but the other two treatments were statistically significant. From all of the

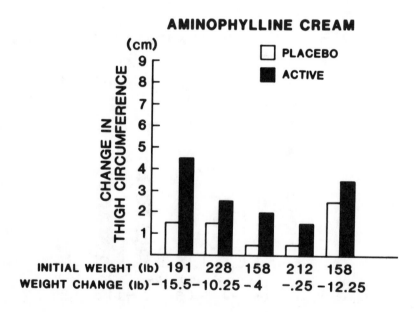

Figure 3a. Aminophylline cream.

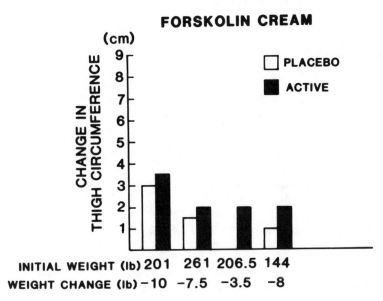

Figure 3b. Forskolin cream.

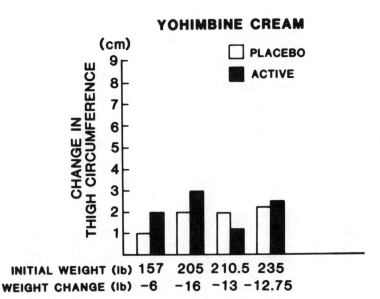

Figure 3c. Yohimbine cream.

data, we would tentatively suggest it is possible by topical application to modify fat storage by utilizing selective adrenergic agents.

SUMMARY AND RECOMMENDATIONS

From this review of advances in our knowledge over the past ten years, several conclusions and recommendations are possible.

Table 5

RECOMMENDATIONS FOR NEXT DECADE

1. Study mechanisms for local fat deposition and for this effect on health.

2. Examine basis for interaction of peptides and monoamines in control of single meals versus long term regulation of fat.

3. Identify genetic markers for obesity, and the environmental system with which they act.

4. Develop improved methods of treatment.

First, regional fat distribution, particularly the deposition of fat in the abdominal and probably the intra-abdominal region, is a far more important health hazard than a comparable increase in fat in other regions. The important questions remaining to be answered are whether intra or extra abdominal subcutaneous fat are equally important and why fat accumulates in one region as opposed to another. One possible clue to this mechanism is the data of Evans and Kissebah (1983), who have shown a correlation between free testosterone and upper body or abdominal fat. The mechanisms by which testosterone is increased in some women and the differential effects in men are questions of utmost importance.

A second area of considerable importance is our understanding of food intake. In clinical treatment protocols there appears to be a maximal weight loss of about 10 kg, even with prolonged treatment. This suggests that there must be redundancy in the control mechanisms for fat stores and raises the possibility that effective treatment of obesity may require more than a single approach. Additional information about the regulation of food intake and its role in the development of obesity, will certainly come from enhanced understanding of the mechanisms by which adrenalectomy reverses or prevents the development of experimental types of obesity. Clarifying the role of the centrally acting peptides in feeding may also have important clinical dividends. A third area of considerable importance is the role of genetic and environmental interaction in individuals who gain weight easily. Understanding of the mechanisms for familial aggregation of energy expenditure may provide important clues to the cellular mechanisms by which these genetic factors are manifested and thus to the potential differences in risk for developing obesity. Finally, treatments for obesity are woefully inadequate. Recent data suggests that weight cycling, the so-called rhythm method of girth control or the yo-yo syndrome may be hazardous to one's health. This needs to be clearly documented. Newer approaches to the therapy of obesity, particularly the abdominal type of obesity, are of importance because of the risks which individuals with this type of fat distribution have for the development of diabetes, hypertension, stroke and heart attack. In conclusion, I would suggest that the past decade has seen great strides and that we are standing on the threshold of an exciting era in the understanding of obesity and the approaches for its effective treatment of disorders of positive fat balance.

REFERENCES

Acheson K, Jequier E, Wahren J (1983). Influence of B-Adrenergic blockade on glucose-induced thermogenesis in man. J Clin Invest 72:981-986

Behnke AR, Wilmore JH (1974). Evaluation of body build and composition. Englewood Cliffs, NJ: Prentice-Hall.

Bjorntorp P (1974). Effects of age, sex, and clinical conditions on adipose tissue cellularity in man. Metab 11:1091-1102.

Blundell JE (1984). Serotonin and appetite. Neuropharmacol 23:1537-1552.

Bogardus C, Lillioja S, Ravussin E, Abbott W, Zawadzki JK, Young A, Knowler WC, Jacobowitz R, Moll PP (1986). Familial dependence on the resting metabolic rate. N Engl J Med 315:96-100.

Bouchard C (1985). Body composition in adopted and biological siblings. Hum Biol 57:61-75.

Bray GA (1987). Obesity--A disease of nutrient or energy balance? Nutr Rev 45(2):33-43.

Bray GA (1979). Obesity in America. Washington, DC DHEW Publ No (NIH) 79-359.

Bray GA, York DA (1979). Hypothalamic and genetic obesity in experimental animals: An autonomic and endocrine hypothesis. Physiol Rev 59:719-809.

Bray GA (1976). The obese patient: Major problems in internal medicine. Philadelphia: Saunders, pp 1-450.

Bray GA, York DA (1971). Genetically transmitted obesity in rodents. Physiol Rev 51:598-646.

Brownell KD (1982). Obesity: Understanding and treating a serious, prevalent, and refractory disorder. J Consult Clin Psychol 50:820-840.

Burns TW, Langley PE, Terry BE, Bylund DB, Hoffman BB, Tharp MD, Lefkowitz RJ, Garcia-Saintz JA, Fain JN (1981). Pharmacological Characterizations of Adrenergic Receptors in Human Adipocytes. J Clin Invest 67:467-475.

Chapman JM, Coulson AH, Clark VA, Borun ER (1971). The differential effect of serum cholesterol, blood pressure and weight on the incidence of myocardial infarction and angina pectoris. J Chronic Dis 23:631-647.

Cohn SH, Vartsky D, Yasumura S, Sawitsky A, Zanzi I, Vaswani A, Ellis KJ (1980). Compartmental body composition based on total-body nitrogen, potassium, and calcium. Endocrinol Metab 2:E524-E530.

Dahms WT, Molitch ME, Bray GA, Greenway FL, Atkinson RL, Hamilton K (1978). Treatment of obesity: Cost-benefit assessment of behavioral therapy, placebo, and two anorectic drugs. Am J Clin Nut 31:774-778.

Faust IM, Johnson PR, Stern JS, Hirsch J (1978). Diet-induced adipocyte number increase in adult rats: A new model of obesity. Am J Physiol 235:E279-E286.

Feinleib M (1985). Epidemiology of obesity in relation to health hazards. Ann Int Med 106:1019-1024.

Garrow JS (1982). New approaches to body composition. Am J Clin Nutr 35:1152-1158.

Garrow JS (1978). Energy balance and obesity in man. New York: Elsevier, 2nd Ed.

Greenwood MRC (1985). Adipose tissue: Cellular morphology and development. Ann Int Med 103:996-999.

Hirsch J, Batchelor B (1976). Adipose tissue cellularity in human obesity. Clin Endocrinol Metab 5:299-311.

Hubert HB, Feinleib N, McNamara PM, Castelli WP (1983). Obesity as an independent risk factor for cardiovascular disease: A 26-year follow-up of participants in the Framingham Heart Study. Circ 67(5):968-977.

Kannel WB, Gordon T (1979). Physiological and medical concomittants of obesity: The Framingham study. In Bray GA (ed): Obesity in America. DHEW Publication No (NIH) 79-359, Washington, DC: U.S. Government Printing Office, pp 125-153.

Keys A, Menotti A, Aravanis C, Blackburn H, djordevic BS, Buzina R, Dontas AS, Fidanza F, Karvonen MJ, Kimura N, Mohacek I, Nedeljkovic S, Puddu V, Punsar S, Taylor HL, Conti S, Kromhout D, Toshima H (1984). The seven countries study: 2,289 deaths in 15 years. Prev Med 13:141-154.

Kissebah AH, Vydelingum N, Murray N, Evans DJ, Hartz DJ, Kalkoff RK, Adams PW (1982). Relation of body fat distribution to metabolic consequences of obesity. J Clin Endocrinol Metab 54:254-260.

Kral JG, Bjorntorp P, Schersten T, Sjostrom L (1977). Body composition and adipose tissue cellularity before and after jejuno-ileostomy in severely obese subjects. Europ J Clin Invest 7:413-419.

Lafontan M, Dang-Tran L, Berlan M (1979). Alpha adrenergic antilipolytic effect of adrenaline in human fat cells of the thigh. Comparison with adrenaline responsiveness of different fat deposits. Europ J Clin Invest 9:261-266.

Lapidus T, Bengtsson LC, Larsson B, Pennert K, Rybo E, Sjostrom L (1984). Distribution of adipose tissue and risk of cardiovascular disease and death: A 12 year follow-up of participants in the population study of women in Gothenburg, Sweden. Br Med J 289:1257-1261.

Larsson B, Svardsudd K, Welin L, Wilhelmsen L, Bjorntorp P, Tibblin G (1984). Abdominal adipose tissue distribution, obesity, and risk of cardiovascular disease and death: 13 year follow-up of participants in the study of men born in 1913. Brit Med J 288:1401-1404.

Leibowitz S (1986). Brain monamines and peptides: Role in the control of eating behavior. Fed Proc 45:1396-1403.

Lew EA, Garfinkel L (1979). Variations in mortality by weight among 750,000 men and women. J Chron Dis 32:563-576.

Lohman TG (1981). Skinfolds and body density and their relation to body fatness: A review. Hum Biol 53:181-225.

Miller DS, Mumford P (1967a). Gluttony. I. An experimental study of overeating low- or high-protein diets. Am J Clin Nutr 20:1212-1222.

Miller DS, Mumford P, Stock NJ (1967b). Gluttony. II. Thermogenesis in overeating man. Am J Clin Nutr 20:1223-1229.

Moore FD, Olesen KH, McMurrey JD, Parker HV, Ball MR, Boyden CM (1963). The body cell mass and its supporting environment in body composition in health and disease. Philadelphia, PA: Saunders, p. 23.

Morley JE, Levine AS (1985). The pharmacology of eating behavior. Ann Rev Pharmacol Toxicol 25:127-146.

Newburgh LH (1944). Obesity: 1. Energy metabolism. Physiol Rev 24:18-31.

The Pooling Project Research Group (1978). Relationship of blood pressure, serum cholesterol, smoking habit, relative weight and ECG abnormalities to incidences of major coronary events: Final report of the Pooling Project. J Chron Dis 31:201-306.

Rabkin SW, Mathewson FAL, Hsu PH (1977). Relation of body weight to development of ischemic heart disease in a cohort of young North American men after a 26-year observation period: The Manitoba Study. Am J Cardiol 39:452-458.

Ravussin E, Bogardus C, Schwartz RS, Robbins DC, Wolfe RR, Horton ES, Danforth E Jr., Sims EH (1983). Thermic effect of infused glucose and insulin in man. Decreased response with increased insulin resistance in obesity and noninsulin-dependent diabetes mellitus. J Clin Invest 72:893-902.

Rothwell NJ, Stock MJ (1981). Regulation of energy balance. Ann Rev 1:235-56.

Schwartz RS, Brunzell JD (1981). Increase of adipose tissue lipoprotein lipase activity with weight loss. J Clin Invest 67:1425-1430.

Segal KR, Gutin B, Presta E, Wang J, Van Itallie TB (1985). Estimation of human body composition by electrical impedance methods: A comparative study. J Appl Physiol 58(5):1565-1571.

Sims EAH (1986). Energy balance in human beings: The problems of plenitude. Vit Horm 43:1-43.

Sjostrom L (1986). Determination of total adipose tissue and body fat in women by computed tomography, K 40, and tritium. Am J Physiol 250(6):E736-E745.

Sjostrom L, William-Olsson T (1981). Prospective studies on adipose tissue development in man. Int J Obes 5:597-604.

Smith O, Hammersten J, Bjorntorp P, Kral JG (1979). Regional differences and effect of weight reduction on human fat cell metabolism. Europ J Clin Invest 9:327-332.

Society of Actuaries (1979). Build study of 1979. Society of Actuaries and Association of Life Insurance Medical Directors of America.

Society of Actuaries (1959) Build and blood pressure study. Society of Actuaries, Chicago, IL.

Stunkard AJ, Wilcox ON, Craighead L, O'Brien R (1980). Controlled trial of behaviour therapy, pharmacotherapy, and their combination in the treatment of obesity. Lancet II:1045-1047.

Waaler HT (1983). Height, weight and mortality: The Norwegian experience. Acta Medica Scan 679:1-55.

Index

Abdominal fat
  and blood pressures, 244–255
    and measurement of fat distribution,
      245–247
  and Cushing's disease, 169
  early detection, 31
  exercise-training and alterations in, 300
  and glucose tolerance in diabetic Wistar
    fatty rat, 290–292
  measurement of, 263
  and morbidity and mortality, 4, 31, 119,
    122
    and exercise-training studies, 299
  and plasma lipids and lipoproteins, 247
    sex differences in, 222–236
  as predictor of angina pectoris and myo-
    cardial infarction, 247–248
  sex differences in children and youth, 97
  see also Abdominal obesity; Metabolic
    differences in fat depots; Waist/hip
    circumference ratio
Abdominal obesity
  and metabolic disturbances, 6, 244–245
    phenomena involved in, 5
  and risk
    compared with obesity, 6
    compared with other risk factors, 6
  see also Abdominal fat; Waist/hip cir-
    cumference ratio
Abdominal skinfold measurements, without
    adjustment for heaviness or fatness, in
    study of inherited fat distribution, 116;
    see also Abdominal fat; Abdominal
    obesity
Additive genetic effect
  for abdominal skinfold measurements
    without adjustment for heaviness
    or fatness, 116
  and inheritance of total body fat, 103–107
  see also Heredity
Adipocytes

high-density lipoprotein metabolism, and
    association between abdominal fat
    and plasma high-density lipopro-
    tein-cholesterol, 232–235
hypertrophy, insulin resistance and, 305
intersite variation in metabolic activity,
    313
and obesity, research findings on,
    337–339
subcutaneous abdominal, high density
    binding sites of, 232
in women
  enlargment and increased number of,
    165
  in femoral compared to abdominal re-
    gion, 164
Adipocytometry, and hypertrophic and hy-
    perplastic obesities, 15
Adipose tissue
  computed tomography measurements of,
    45–58
    accuracy and reproducibility of,
      46–49
    and anthropometric predictions of vis-
      ceral adipose tissue volume,
      54–55
    and determination of adipose tissue
      areas, 46–48
    in fat distribution studies, 15–16, 63
    and intra-portal-drained and extra per-
      itoneal cava-drained fat, 51–53
    mathematical algorithms for, 48–49
    and measurement of body composi-
      tion, 334
    and prediction of visceral adipose tis-
      sue volume, 55–56
    ratios between total and subcutaneous,
      metabolic disturbances and,
      56–57
    regional determinations, 50–53
  sexual differences in

351